Understanding Kidney Diseases

Understanding Kidney Disease

Hugh C. Rayner • Mark E. Thomas
David V. Milford

Understanding Kidney Diseases

Second edition

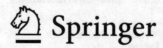

Hugh C. Rayner
Birmingham Heartlands Hospital
Birmingham
UK

Mark E. Thomas
Birmingham Heartlands Hospital
Birmingham
UK

David V. Milford
Birmingham Children's Hospital
Birmingham
UK

ISBN 978-3-030-43029-0   ISBN 978-3-030-43027-6   (eBook)
https://doi.org/10.1007/978-3-030-43027-6

This Springer imprint is published by the registered company Springer Nature Switzerland AG
The registered company address is: Gewerbestrasse 11, 6330 Cham, Switzerland

Foreword to the First Edition

Great teachers make their subjects appealing. Doctors Rayner, Thomas and Milford have certainly done that for renal science and kidney medicine. They have taken up-to-date molecular biology, physiology made complicated at medical school, innovative therapeutics and an intimate understanding of twenty-first century holistic healthcare, and moulded a superb monograph accessible to students, vital for doctors in training and definitely of value for all practitioners of kidney care.

Kidney disease is common, harmful and treatable. Early detection, accurate diagnosis, systematic monitoring and evidence-based interventions are the key to improving outcomes. Doctor Rayner and colleagues bring their experience as front-line clinicians, researchers and educators to explain kidney problems clearly and concisely, simplifying where possible and highlighting areas of controversy or ambiguity where necessary.

Given the central role of the kidneys in maintaining the *milieu intérieur,* it is not surprising that kidney diseases provide a route to understanding a range of other metabolic, immunological and genetic conditions. This book balances clarity in describing these classic disorders with insights into the interaction between diseases in multimorbid patients. The compassion of the authors as practicing physicians is revealed in the excellent chapter on planning for transplantation or dialysis.

Those who have the pleasure of reading this book will gain a deep understanding of kidney diseases, knowledge of contemporary treatments and familiarity with systems to manage populations and personalise care. They will be better doctors and able to apply the lessons learned in whichever branch of medicine they practice.

Reviews of the First Edition

An Excellent Nephrology Textbook for Medical Students and Junior Doctors

Renal medicine is often deemed to be a complex subject for many medical students and junior doctors. There is currently a paucity of resources which helps them understand and appreciate this fascinating speciality. This book is thus a valuable tool for both students and doctors in training as the book teaches the subject of renal medicine in a very practical and enjoyable manner.

I really like the format of each chapter in this book. Each chapter begins with an outline of the key points to help focus the reader's mind. In addition, there are also several case studies and beautiful illustrations which help to explain the fundamental aspects of each chapter.

The authors have successfully covered a wide breadth of topics within the speciality without overwhelming the reader with too much factual knowledge. This concise and well-written book will not only enhance the reader's understanding of renal medicine but also increase the confidence of both students and junior doctors when they assess a patient with kidney disease.

I thoroughly recommend this book to all medical students and junior doctors.

Weng Chin Oh
UK and Ireland Renal SpR Club

This book goes a long way to remediating the deficiencies [of other books] and is a must-have for any medical student or junior doctor struggling with the subject, as well as for doctors in training considering a career in renal medicine.

In this book the authors do not just manage to impart knowledge and information, but a career's worth of experience. This book can be used well as a reference tool.

Matthew Graham-Brown
Renalmed.co.uk

Customer Reviews

A Brilliant Guide for Medical Students, and Beyond!

Having just started specialty medical rotations as part of my fourth year clinical studies, this book has proved invaluable for my learning and understanding of kidney disease and renal medicine. I really like the structure of the book and the contextualised case examples per chapter. A definite must-have book for students and doctors alike!

Great for Students

I have just started the clinical part of medical school and this textbook has been great—it has pretty much everything you need to know about the kidneys in it, set out clearly and well explained.

Book Well Worth Reading

Beautifully written, clear and to the point. Reads like a storybook. I would highly recommend to anyone who feels nephrology is too complex and complicated to understand.

Great Book!

Easily laid out, great for quickly brushing up nephrology skills.

Donal O'Donoghue OBE
First NHS National Clinical Director for Kidney Care
London, UK

Foreword to the Second Edition

Understanding Kidney Diseases is already in its second edition after only 4 years. This is a remarkable achievement for any new clinical textbook. What makes this book so special and so successful?

Reading the various chapters makes it obvious that it is written by experienced clinicians for clinicians, as well as for others dealing with kidney disease. Each chapter provides descriptions with detailed data on actual patients. You feel like you are attending teaching rounds, where full histories, physical findings and laboratory data are presented and then discussed. The authors actually invoke Dr. Osler, the father of clinical medicine. They succeed in following his style of clinical case discussions that include pathophysiology and treatment options.

As the title of this book says, its goal is to teach "understanding". In clinical medicine it is the understanding of interrelated pathophysiology that allows clinicians to keep the wealth of individual facts together in their minds. There is a huge amount of factual knowledge transmitted in this book even though it is remarkably easy reading. This combination is a rare and amazing achievement of Dr. Hugh Rayner and his two co-authors.

The headings of chapters are refreshingly original; they entice you to continue by suggesting that the text will be fun to read. This second edition has an expanded section on Acid-Base and a new chapter on Stone Disease. The new Frequently Asked Questions chapter gives answers uniquely in plain English, thus teaching understandable communication with kidney patients. The focus on quality-of-life and end-of-life issues is welcome for dealing with advanced kidney disease. It is great that these topics were integrated with straight science, a rarity in textbooks. A large appendix of multiple-choice questions gives readers the opportunity to help their retention of factual knowledge. Furthermore, each chapter provides highly relevant and recently updated references to allow readers the opportunity for more in-depth reading on particular issues and gain further understanding of the factual statements in the text.

This book on the understanding of the many complex topics and pathophysiologies in kidney disease will be invaluable for practicing clinicians in general medicine and in nephrology. I congratulate Drs. Rayner, Thomas and Milford for making teaching so exemplary, learning so enjoyable and the clinical facts so easy to understand and remember.

Vivant sequentes

Prof Friedrich K. Port MD, MS, FACP
University of Michigan
Ann Arbor, MI, USA

Words with Pictures: The Gift of Graphical Data Presentation

This book can be seen as a successful product of the experience of information technology in renal clinical practice over four decades. It builds on the 1980s exploration of renal clinical IT, skilfully distilled using clinical and educational principles. It presents a general incorporation of those piecemeal insights, especially the gift of graphical data presentation. This was one of the earliest applications of computers in the clinic, and it turbo-charged the early enthusiasts in their unconstrained delving into the possibilities of digital renal clinical support (https://renal.org/history/history-of-renal-it/).

We are addressing fundamentals here. Clinical events in renal disease, and the laboratory data that calibrate them, come from an antecedent past and are destined to resolve in a conceivable future. These trajectories offer time-series that can be better understood through some form of notation. Our most familiar time-series is a written musical score—a completed trajectory, the repeated patterns of which bring deep satisfaction.

Before digitisation, published diagrams of illness trajectories were likewise drawings of completed clinical features and measurements. In real time, an incomplete, unfolding picture of a disorder is the inestimable value of graphical data presentation. Such pictorial integration of events and findings is a core guide to effective clinical practice for all but the "graphically tone-deaf". This second edition exposes and transfers clinical experience by emphasising and rehearsing those pictures.

The discrimination of a diagnostic signal from noise is a quintessential skill of the clinician. The camouflage of appearances must be penetrated to reveal the patterns of disease. An unstructured clinical situation appears chaotic (a cacophony) until some virtual order is introduced, either by the evolution of serial evidence or by revelation, in the recognition of a pattern in events. Such patterns come in various forms but a graphical message is the easiest to read and troubleshoot.

A verified pattern of disorder allows the relaxation of anxious diagnostic effort, a considered prediction of outcome and balanced treatment decisions. These are the basis of convincing reassurance of the patient and the best-founded route to their taking back some control of their well-being.

Renal Medicine was an ideal specialty in which to develop clinical IT and continues to supply model scenarios for exploring new digital techniques. This volume from experienced polymaths is a secure guide as the digital revolution rages on. The graphical portraits of renal disorders bring them comprehensively within the grasp of aspiring clinicians and serve to promote career-long habits of clinical engagement.

Es Will FRCP, FBRS
Chairman of the British Renal Computing Group 1982-8,
Secretary of the UK Renal Registry 1997-2007

Preface

Kidney diseases are common: in 2017 an estimated 850 million adults had kidney disease worldwide [1]. In 2013, reduced GFR was associated with 4% of deaths [2]. So, being proficient in assessing and managing someone with a kidney disease is an essential skill for all doctors.

This book provides you with the information and explanations you need to understand kidney diseases. The chapters follow the sequence taken during a consultation in a clinic or when clerking a patient on the ward. At each stage we explain the principles and concepts underlying the things that may make kidney medicine seem difficult.

Time is an important factor in kidney diseases. The same diagnosis can cause different symptoms and signs as the disease progresses over days, months, years and decades. It can be hard to make sense of one disease that presents in many different ways. To overcome this problem, we have included over 200 figures, including lots of graphs and charts. As Arthur Brisbane, the American newspaper editor said: "Use a picture. It's worth a thousand words".

The commonest chart is the graph of the eGFR (estimated glomerular filtration rate). This shows you how kidney function changes over time and helps you to make a diagnosis, decide when to do tests, monitor response to treatment, and plan dialysis and transplantation. Crucially, it also shows patients how they are getting on.

We have illustrated the book with case examples based upon patients we have cared for. Details have been altered to protect confidentiality and the patients have given written consent for information about them to be used. We hope their stories make the diseases more understandable and memorable. Throughout the book, we have included references to detailed reviews and original research studies if you wish to explore items in greater depth.

The first edition of this book discussed the value of writing outpatient letters directly to patients. The Academy of Medical Royal Colleges in the UK has since endorsed this as best practice and published guidance about how to do it [3]. An educational article in the *British Medical Journal* builds upon that guidance [4]. Clinic letters written to patients help them understand their condition and its treatment. In this edition we have included some frequently asked questions. We suggest you use these as an exercise in communicating effectively with patients. We have provided answers written in plain English for you to compare.

We dedicate this book to people who live with kidney disease and the clinicians who care for them.

Birmingham, UK   Hugh C. Rayner
Birmingham, UK   Mark E. Thomas
Birmingham, UK   David V. Milford

References

1. Jager KJ, Kovesdy C, Langham R, Rosenberg M, Jha V, Zoccali C. A single number for advocacy and communication—worldwide more than 850 million individuals have kidney diseases. Nephrol Dialysis Transplant. 2019;34(11):1803–5. https://doi.org/10.1093/ndt/gfz174.
2. Global Burden of Disease 2013 GFR Collaborators; CKD Prognosis Consortium; Global Burden of Disease Genitourinary Expert Group. Global cardiovascular and renal outcomes of reduced GFR. J Am Soc Nephrol. 2017;28(7):2167–79. https://doi.org/10.1681/ASN.2016050562. https://jasn.asnjournals.org/content/jnephrol/28/7/2167.full.pdf.
3. The Academy of Medical Royal Colleges. Please write to me—writing outpatient clinic letters to patients. Guidance. 2018. http://www.aomrc.org.uk/wp-content/uploads/2018/09/Please_write_to_me_Guidance_010918.pdf.
4. Rayner H, Hickey M, Logan I, Mathers N, Rees P, Shah R. Writing outpatient letters to patients. BMJ 2020;368. https://www.bmj.com/content/368/bmj.m24.

Acknowledgements

We are indebted to the following for their contributions:

Roger Adkins, Colin Aldridge, Lise Bankir, Morgan Cleasby, Indy Dasgupta, Simon Dodds, Jo Ewing, John Evans, Agnes Fogo, Jonathan Freedman, Matthew Graham-Brown, Aarn Huissoon, Thirumala Krishna, Chris Lote, Donal O'Donoghue, Fritz Port, Michael Riste, Steve Smith, David Tudway, Es Will, Teun Wilmink, Chris Winearls.

Clinical images by *mediahub.agency*.

Additional artwork by Anthony Williams and Andrea Tibbitts.

Disclaimer

Although every effort is made to ensure that the information in this book is accurate, the ultimate responsibility for assessment and treatment of a patient rests with the practicing physician. Neither the publishers nor the authors can be held responsible for errors or for any consequences arising from the use of information contained herein.

Contents

About the Authors

Hugh C. Rayner gained a first-class degree in physiology at Cambridge University before qualifying with honours at the London Hospital Medical College in 1981. He was awarded an MD from the University of Leicester for studies on experimental models of kidney disease. After a number of training posts, including a year as clinical fellow in Melbourne, Australia, he was appointed as a consultant in renal and general medicine in Birmingham in 1993, teaching renal medicine to undergraduates and trainee doctors.

As part of his studies for the Diploma in Medical Education from Dundee University in 1996, he presented a dissertation on the interpretation of serum creatinine and published a consensus curriculum for undergraduate renal medicine [1]. He retired from clinical nephrology practice in December 2019.

Mark E. Thomas studied Biological Sciences and Medicine as an undergraduate at King's College London and Westminster Medical School. After postgraduate training, he was a Research Fellow at Washington University Medical School in St Louis, USA, for three years, studying models of proteinuric renal disease. This interest continued during Senior Registrar training in Leicester. He has been a Consultant Nephrologist and Physician in Birmingham since 1998.

He has had a clinical research interest in acute kidney injury (AKI) for some years, including earlier detection and intervention in AKI. He is chief investigator for the Acute Kidney Outreach to Reduce Deterioration and Death (AKORDD) study, a large pilot study of AKI outreach. He has chaired clinical guideline development groups for AKI, anaemia management in CKD and end of life care for the UK National Institute for Health and Care Excellence (NICE).

David V. Milford commenced basic paediatric training in 1983 and higher paediatric training at Sheffield Children's Hospital in 1986. He undertook research in the Department of Nephrology, Birmingham Children's Hospital, into the epidemiology of diarrhoea-associated haemolytic uraemic syndrome resulting in several major publications and a thesis for Doctor of Medicine. He was appointed consultant nephrologist at Birmingham Children's Hospital in 1992. His interests include hypertension, acute kidney injury and renal transplantation.

Reference

1. Rayner HC. A model undergraduate core curriculum in adult renal medicine. Med Teacher. 1995;17:409–12.

The Anatomy of the Kidney

The kidneys are complex and beautiful organs. Anatomical studies using light and electron microscopy reveal their complex internal structure (Figs. 1.1, 1.2, 1.3, 1.4 and 1.5).

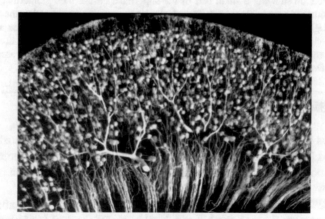

Fig. 1.1 Longitudinal section through the cortex and outer medulla of a rabbit kidney in which the artery has been injected with white Microfil. Microfil has filled the arteries, arterioles, glomerular tufts and the early part of the post-glomerular capillaries in the cortex and outer medulla. (Courtesy of Dr. Lise Bankir, Centre de Recherche des Cordeliers, Paris, France)

© Springer Nature Switzerland AG 2020
H. C. Rayner et al., *Understanding Kidney Diseases*,
https://doi.org/10.1007/978-3-030-43027-6_1

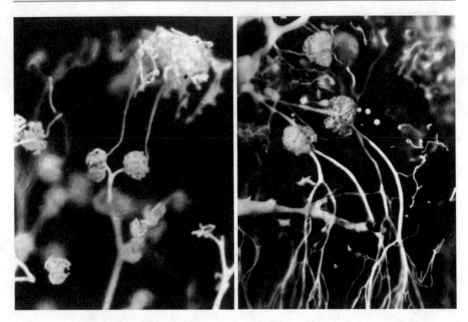

Fig. 1.2 Rabbit kidney injected with white Microfil through the renal artery. **Left:** detail of a longitudinal section showing a small part of the superficial cortex. The glomerular tufts of two superficial glomeruli are visible with their post-glomerular capillaries located in the very superficial cortex. **Right:** detail of a longitudinal section showing part of the deep cortex and the outer stripe of the outer medulla. The glomerular tufts of two juxtamedullary glomeruli are visible with their efferent arterioles that run towards the outer medulla where they give rise to vascular bundles. (Courtesy of Dr. Lise Bankir, Centre de Recherche des Cordeliers, Paris, France)

Turning Blood into Urine

The kidneys play a central role in homeostasis [2]. They use exquisite sensory mechanisms [3] to regulate blood pressure, water [4], sodium [5], potassium [6], acidity [7], bone minerals [8], and haemoglobin. But their core function is the excretion of the waste products of metabolism in urine.

About 22% of the cardiac output of blood goes to the kidneys and about 20% of the plasma passing through the kidneys is filtered. Of the 170 L of glomerular filtrate produced per day, 99% is reabsorbed as it flows along the nephrons, leaving only about 1.5 L to emerge as urine.

Filtration occurs through the glomerular filtration barrier [9]. This is made up of five layers [10] (Fig. 1.6):

- the glycocalyx covering the surface of the endothelial cells
- holes (fenestrations) in the glomerular endothelial cells
- the glomerular basement membrane
- the slit diaphragm between the foot-processes of the podocytes
- the sub-podocyte space between the slit diaphragm and the podocyte cell bodies

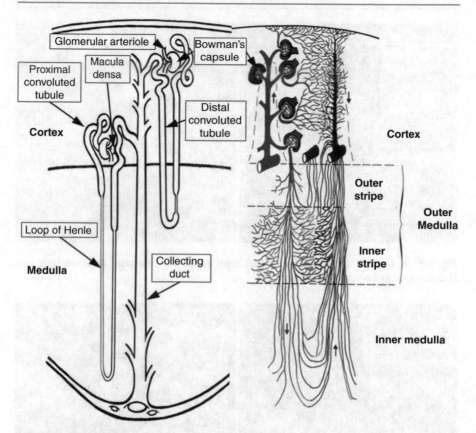

Fig. 1.3 Nephrons and their blood supply. **Left**: a short looped- and a long looped-nephron. **Right**: the different vascular territories and their location in the four renal zones. For clarity, the cortex has been widened and the inner medulla compressed

The structure, arrangement and electrical charge of the collagen protein molecules that form the filtration barrier determine the composition of glomerular filtrate. So, glomerular filtration is both size-selective and charge-selective; molecules that are too large or too highly charged cannot get through.

A substantial amount of albumin does get through the barrier—between 3.3 and 5.7 g per day. Some of this passes through the podocytes by transcytosis [11]. Angiotensin II increases the amount of albumin passing through the barrier. Almost all the filtered albumin is reabsorbed into the proximal tubular cells [12].

The 80% of plasma that is not filtered flows through the peritubular capillaries. Here, active transporters on the surface of the proximal tubules next to the capillaries pump large and protein-bound molecules into the tubular cell and then out into the lumen. This is important for the excretion of many endogenous toxins and drugs [13].

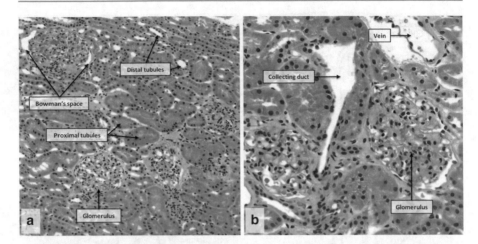

Fig. 1.4 (**a**, **b**) Light micrographs of normal renal cortex with the main structures indicated. Haematoxylin and eosin; (**a**) ×100, (**b**) ×200

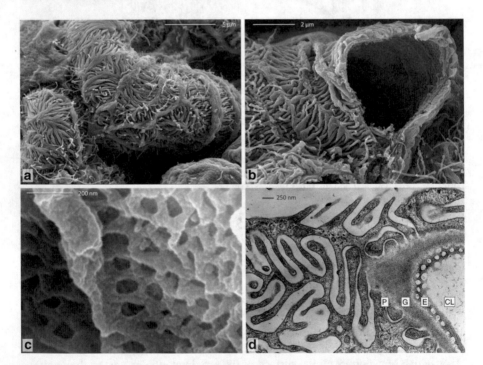

Fig. 1.5 Scanning electron micrographs of a mouse glomerular capillary. (**a**) The surface of a capillary showing podocyte (5000× by SecretDisc). (**b**) A cut open capillary revealing the endothelial lining (10,000× by SecretDisc). (**c**) The inner surface showing fenestrations in the endothelial cells (100,000× by SecretDisc). (**d**) Transmission electron micrograph of a section of glomerular capillary wall showing the layers that form the glomerular filtration barrier. *CL* Capillary Lumen, *E* Endothelial cell fenestrations, *G* Glomerular basement membrane, *P* Podocyte slit diaphragm. (Image **d** made available by James D. Jamieson and the Department of Cell Biology, Yale University School of Medicine. Original 3.25 in. × 4 in. lantern slides were scanned at 600 dpi. Original magnification ×16,000. The original work has been cropped and modified with labels) [1]

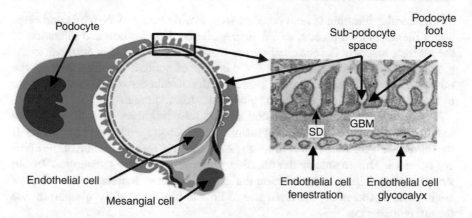

Fig. 1.6 The cells and five structural components that form the glomerular filtration barrier. *SD* slit diaphragm, *GBM* glomerular basement membrane

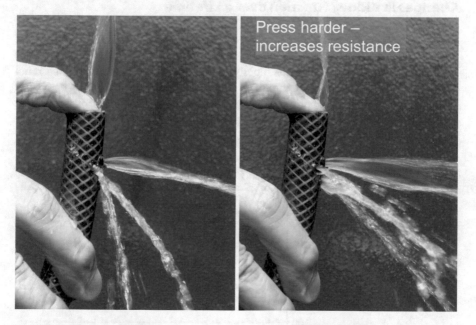

Fig. 1.7 The hose from the tap represents the afferent arteriole. Holes have been made near the end of the hose to represent fenestrations in the glomerular capillary wall. Pressing the finger on the end of the hose simulates increased resistance in the efferent arteriole. This increases glomerular filtration pressure and flow rate

A simple model of the haemodynamics of glomerular filtration can be made from a garden hose (Fig. 1.7).

Glomerular filtration is held constant over a wide range of systemic and renal artery pressures by a process called autoregulation. Constriction and dilatation of the afferent arteriole is controlled by the macula densa, which is adjacent to the glomerulus. The macula densa senses the flow of sodium chloride through the tubule next to it. When this flow is increased, the macula densa causes constriction of the afferent arteriole to reduce the glomerular filtration rate.

Conversely, if the pressure of blood flowing into the kidney falls, the resistance in the afferent arteriole is reduced to maintain the pressure within the glomerulus. If the inflow pressure continues to drop, angiotensin II causes constriction of the efferent arteriole. This maintains the filtration pressure within the glomerulus. In our simple model (Fig. 1.7) pressing on the end of the hose represents the effect of angiotensin II, increasing the resistance to flow of blood out of the glomerulus via the efferent arteriole.

Changes in Kidney Function over a Lifetime

In the uterus, only about 2% of cardiac output goes to the kidneys. Excretion of waste products produced by the foetus is via the placenta. In the first week after birth, kidney blood flow increases rapidly as flow in the aorta increases and renal vascular resistance falls. By 1 month of age it has doubled and by 1 year it has reached adult levels in proportion to body size. Similarly, glomerular filtration rate (GFR) is about 10% of the adult value at birth, rises rapidly in the first month, and reaches adult levels by 1 year of age (Fig. 1.8).

Fig. 1.8 Glomerular filtration rate (GFR) measured by a single injection technique in infants aged up to 13 months. (Redrawn using data from [14])

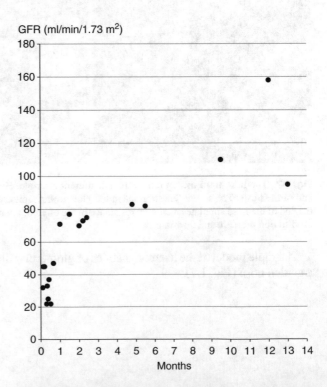

There is huge variation between people in the number of glomeruli per kidney. The average is approximately 800,000 but numbers can vary ninefold from approximately 200,000 to 1,800,000 [15].

There is less variation between people in GFR because the size and filtration rate per glomerulus increases as the number of glomeruli decreases. On average, glomeruli are twice as big in people with the fewest glomeruli compared to those with the most. Enlarged glomeruli are found in people who are born prematurely, have a low birth weight, massive obesity, hypertension and cardiovascular disease, and are associated with an increased risk of chronic kidney disease [16, 17].

After the age of about 45 years there is a steady decline in the number of functioning nephrons as glomeruli undergo sclerosis. This is reflected in a decline in kidney blood flow and GFR (Fig. 1.9). In males at age 40 years the mean kidney blood flow is 600 mL/min/1.73 m² and GFR is 120 mL/min/1.73 m². By age 80 years these have reduced to 300 and 70 mL/min/1.73 m² respectively [18]. Values for females are similar. Urine albumin excretion does not change with age [19].

Fig. 1.9 Changes in glomerular filtration rate (GFR) with age. GFR was measured using the 'gold standard' inulin clearance method in 75 healthy males. Error bars indicate standard deviation of the mean. Outer lines indicate standard deviation of the distribution. (Redrawn from [17])

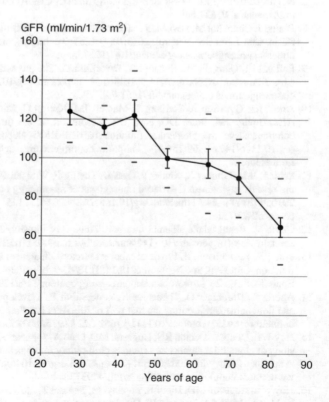

References

1. Farquhar MG, Wissig SL, Palade GE. Glomerular permeability. J Exp Med. 1961;113:47–66. http://www.cellimagelibrary.org/images/37178.
2. Hoenig MP, Zeidel ML. Homeostasis, the Milieu Intérieur, and the wisdom of the nephron. Clin J Am Soc Nephrol. 2014;9(7):1272–81. https://doi.org/10.2215/CJN.08860813. http://cjasn.asnjournals.org/content/9/7/1272.full.
3. Pluznick JL, Caplan MJ. Chemical and physical sensors in the regulation of renal function. Clin J Am Soc Nephrol. 2015;10(9):1626–35. https://doi.org/10.2215/CJN.00730114. https://cjasn.asnjournals.org/content/10/9/1626.long.
4. Danziger J, Zeidel ML. Osmotic homeostasis. Clin J Am Soc Nephrol. 2015;10(5):852–62. https://doi.org/10.2215/CJN.10741013. http://cjasn.asnjournals.org/cgi/pmidlookup?view=long&pmid=25078421.
5. Palmer LG, Schnermann J. Integrated control of Na transport along the nephron. Clin J Am Soc Nephrol. 2015;10(4):676–87. https://doi.org/10.2215/CJN.12391213. https://cjasn.asnjournals.org/content/10/4/676.long.
6. Subramanya AR, Ellison DH. Distal convoluted tubule. Clin J Am Soc Nephrol. 2014;9(12):2147–63. https://doi.org/10.2215/CJN.05920613. http://cjasn.asnjournals.org/content/9/12/2147.full.
7. Curthoys NP, Moe OW. Proximal tubule function and response to acidosis. Clin J Am Soc Nephrol. 2014;9(9):1627–38. https://doi.org/10.2215/CJN.10391012. http://cjasn.asnjournals.org/content/9/9/1627.full.
8. Blaine J, Chonchol M, Levi M. Renal control of calcium, phosphate, and magnesium homeostasis. Clin J Am Soc Nephrol. 2015;10(7):1257–72. https://doi.org/10.2215/CJN.09750913. https://cjasn.asnjournals.org/content/10/7/1257.long.
9. Pollak MR, Quaggin SE, Hoenig MP, Dworkin LD. The glomerulus: the sphere of influence. Clin J Am Soc Nephrol. 2014;9(8):1461–9. https://doi.org/10.2215/CJN.09400913. http://cjasn.asnjournals.org/content/9/8/1461.full.
10. Arkill KP, Qvortrup K, Starborg T, Mantell JM, Knupp C, Michel CC, Harper SJ, Salmon AHJ, Squire JM, Bates DO, Neal CR. Resolution of the three dimensional structure of components of the glomerular filtration barrier. BMC Nephrol. 2014;15:24. https://doi.org/10.1186/1471-2369-15-24. http://link.springer.com/article/10.1186/1471-2369-15-24/fulltext.html.
11. Schießl IM, Hammer A, Kattler V, Gess B, Theilig F, Witzgall R, Castrop H. Intravital imaging reveals angiotensin II–induced transcytosis of albumin by podocytes. J Am Soc Nephrol. 2016;27(3):731–44. https://doi.org/10.1681/ASN.2014111125. https://jasn.asnjournals.org/content/27/3/731.
12. Gekle M. Renal tubule albumin transport. Annu Rev Physiol. 2005;67:573–94. http://www.annualreviews.org/doi/abs/10.1146/annurev.physiol.67.031103.154845.
13. Wang K, Kestenbaum B. Proximal tubular secretory clearance: a neglected partner of kidney function. Clin J Am Soc Nephrol. 2018;13(8):1291–6. https://doi.org/10.2215/CJN.12001017. Epub 2018 Feb 28. https://cjasn.asnjournals.org/content/13/8/1291.long.
14. Aperia A, Broberger O, Thodenius K, Zetterström R. Development of renal control of salt and fluid homeostasis during the first year of life. Acta Paediatr Scand. 1975;64:393–8. http://onlinelibrary.wiley.com/doi/10.1111/j.1651-2227.1975.tb03853.x/abstract.
15. Hoy WE, Douglas-Denton RN, Hughson MD, Cass A, Johnson K, Bertram JF. A stereological study of glomerular number and volume: preliminary findings in a multiracial study of kidneys at autopsy. Kidney Int. 2003;63:S31–7. https://doi.org/10.1046/j.1523-1755.63.s83.8.x. http://www.nature.com/ki/journal/v63/n83s/full/4493733a.html.
16. Hoy WE, Hughson MD, Diouf B, Zimanyi M, Samuel T, McNamara BJ, Douglas-Denton RN, Holden L, Mott SA, Bertram JF. Distribution of volumes of individual glomeruli in kidneys at autopsy: association with physical and clinical characteristics and with ethnic group. Am

J Nephrol. 2011;33(Suppl 1):15–20. https://doi.org/10.1159/000327044. http://www.karger.com/Article/FullText/327044.

17. Davies DF, Shock NW. Age changes in glomerular filtration rate, effective renal plasma flow, and tubular excretory capacity in adult males. J Clin Invest. 1950;29(5):496–507. https://doi.org/10.1172/JCI102286. PMCID: PMC436086. http://www.jci.org/articles/view/102286.

18. Crump C, Sundquist J, Winkleby MA, Sundquist K. Preterm birth and risk of chronic kidney disease from childhood into mid-adulthood: national cohort study. BMJ. 2019;365:l1346. https://doi.org/10.1136/bmj.l1346. https://www.bmj.com/content/365/bmj.l1346.long.

19. Hommos MS, Glassock RJ, Rule AD. Structural and functional changes in human kidneys with healthy aging. J Am Soc Nephrol. 2017;28(10):2838–44. https://doi.org/10.1681/ASN.2017040421. https://www.ncbi.nlm.nih.gov/pmc/articles/PMC5619977.

Measuring Kidney Function: How to Use Laboratory Tests to Measure Glomerular Filtration Rate

2

How Can Kidney Function Be Measured?

To assess someone's kidney function, we would ideally measure their glomerular filtration rate (GFR). This can be done using a radioisotope tracer that is cleared from the blood solely by glomerular filtration, such as Cr-51 EDTA or Tc-99m DTPA. This technique is useful for research and when precise measurements of GFR are required but it is impractical for routine repeated measurements.

Routine assessment of kidney function uses the concentration of a substance produced by the body: creatinine, urea or cystatin C. The concentration of these substances is determined by the balance between the rates of their production and excretion. When the rates of production and excretion remain stable, equilibrium is reached.

The rate of excretion of a substance by filtration depends upon the volume filtered per unit of time and the concentration of the substance in the filtrate. If the volume filtered per unit of time—the glomerular filtration rate—is kept constant, the concentration in the blood depends upon the production rate. If the production rate is kept constant, the concentration in the blood depends upon the excretion rate.

When production and excretion are stable and in equilibrium, the volume of water in which a substance is dissolved does not affect its concentration. For example, patients who are chronically fluid overloaded do not have a lower concentration of urea due to dilution. Conversely, the higher concentration of urea found in patients who are dehydrated is due to the reduced excretion of urea, not haemoconcentration.

The ideal substance to be used to measure glomerular filtration would be produced at a constant rate, freely filtered by glomeruli, and neither reabsorbed nor secreted by the tubules. Creatinine fulfils some but not all of these criteria. It is released into the bloodstream at a fairly constant rate from the breakdown of creatine in healthy skeletal muscles and is freely filtered by the glomeruli. However, 10 to 20% of total creatinine excretion is by secretion into the tubules. As GFR declines,

© Springer Nature Switzerland AG 2020

H. C. Rayner et al., *Understanding Kidney Diseases*,

https://doi.org/10.1007/978-3-030-43027-6_2

Fig. 2.1 Simultaneous measurements of serum creatinine and GFR (by inulin clearance) in over 100 individuals. The continuous line represents the relationship between serum creatinine and GFR that would be found if creatinine was only filtered by glomeruli and not secreted by the tubules. (Redrawn from [1])

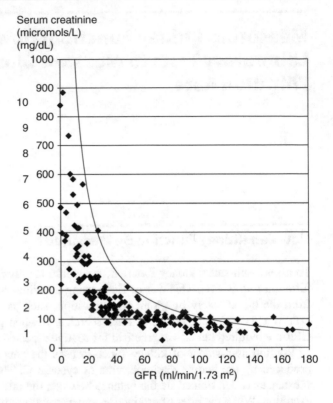

tubular secretion keeps the creatinine concentration lower than would otherwise be the case. This is shown by comparing measurements of serum creatinine and GFR (Fig. 2.1).

The curved relationship between creatinine and GFR makes changes in serum creatinine hard to interpret. Figure 2.2 shows a graph of serum creatinine against time in a man with declining kidney function. The shape of the line suggests that the rate of loss of kidney function accelerates over the years.

If we now add in GFR values, it is clear that kidney function has actually declined at a constant rate over the whole period (Fig. 2.3).

Because of the inverse curved relationship between GFR and creatinine, the drop in eGFR from 116 to 60 during the first 5 years causes a smaller increase in serum creatinine than the decline from 60 to 30 over the next 3 years.

How Can GFR Be Estimated from Serum Creatinine?

To make serum creatinine results easy to interpret we need to convert them into estimates of the GFR (eGFR). Equations to do the conversion have been derived from databases containing simultaneous measurements of GFR, by a radioisotope clearance technique, and serum creatinine concentration. The four-variable

MDRD equation was derived from measurements performed on adult patients with chronic kidney disease in the Modification of Diet in Renal Disease (MDRD) study [2].

eGFR values are standardised to a body surface area of 1.73 m² and so their calculation does not require the patient's body weight. This makes it possible for the laboratory to provide eGFR values automatically from the patient's age and sex. As the laboratory does not usually have reliable information about ethnicity, the adjustment for Afro-Caribbean race is done manually.

The MDRD Equation [2]

For serum creatinine values in µmol/L, the equation is:

GFR (mL/min/1.73 m²) = 175 × (Creat/88.4)$^{-1.154}$ × (Age)$^{-0.203}$ × (0.742 if female) × (1.212 if black race)

For serum creatinine values in mg/dL, the equation is:

GFR (mL/min/1.73 m²) = 175 × (Creat)$^{-1.154}$ × (Age)$^{-0.203}$ × (0.742 if female) × (1.212 if black race)

This equation uses serum creatinine values calibrated against isotope dilution mass spectrometry (IDMS).

For children, different equations are available [3]. The commonest used is the Schwarz equation [4].

The Schwarz Equation [4]

GFR (mL/min/1.73 m²) = (0.413 × Height in cm × 88.4)/Creatinine in µmol/L

GFR (mL/min/1.73 m²) = (0.413 × Height in cm)/Creatinine in mg/dL

For adolescents, an average of the child and adult eGFR estimates should be used [5].

Are eGFR Estimates Accurate and Reliable?

The 90% confidence intervals of the estimates are wide. Using the MDRD equation, 90% of estimates are within 30% of the directly measured GFR and 98% within 50%. In children using the Schwarz equation, 80% of estimates are within 30% of the measured GFR. The estimates are less accurate in people with very abnormal body composition, such as amputees and malnourished patients.

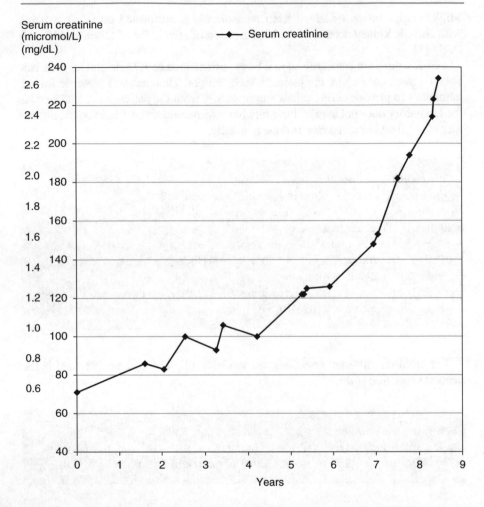

Fig. 2.2 A graph of serum creatinine against time in a man with declining kidney function

The MDRD equation was derived from patients known to have kidney disease and a raised serum creatinine. It is inaccurate for estimating GFR from serum creatinine values in the normal range, i.e. outside the dataset used to derive the formula, for example in pregnancy [6]. The eGFR is not appropriate for situations in which a more accurate measurement of GFR is required, such as in the assessment of a potential kidney transplant donor.

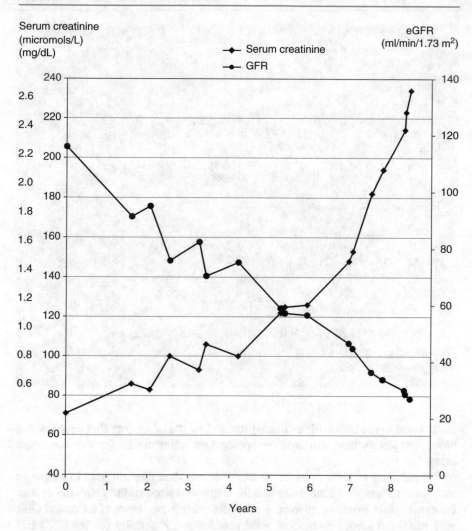

Fig. 2.3 A graph of serum creatinine and GFR against time in a man with declining kidney function

Because the MDRD equation underestimates the true GFR when serum creatinine values are in the normal range, people are at risk of being labelled as having kidney disease based upon these estimates. To reduce this, guidelines recommend that laboratories use the CKD-EPI equations [7]. CKD-EPI gives estimates that are closer to the measured GFR at lower levels of serum creatinine, applying a different equation when creatinine is in the normal range [8, 9].

The CKD-EPI Equations [8]

Black

Female
- Serum creatinine
- ≤62 μmol/L (≤0.7 mg/dL) $GFR = 166 \times (Scr/0.7)^{-0.329} \times (0.993)^{Age}$
- >62 μmol/L (>0.7 mg/dL) $GFR = 166 \times (Scr/0.7)^{-1.209} \times (0.993)^{Age}$

Male
- ≤80 (≤0.9) $GFR = 163 \times (Scr/0.9)^{-0.411} \times (0.993)^{Age}$
- >80 (>0.9) $GFR = 163 \times (Scr/0.9)^{-1.209} \times (0.993)^{Age}$

White or other ethnicity

Female
- ≤62 (≤0.7) $GFR = 144 \times (Scr/0.7)^{-0.329} \times (0.993)^{Age}$
- >62 (>0.7) $GFR = 144 \times (Scr/0.7)^{-1.209} \times (0.993)^{Age}$

Male
- ≤80 (≤0.9) $GFR = 141 \times (Scr/0.9)^{-0.411} \times (0.993)^{Age}$
- >80 (>0.9) $GFR = 141 \times (Scr/0.9)^{-1.209} \times (0.993)^{Age}$

CKD-EPI = Chronic Kidney Disease Epidemiology Collaboration

Scr = serum creatinine in mg/dL (μmol/L/88.4)

Age in years for ≥18

It is best to use the eGFR estimate provided by the laboratory that analysed the blood sample as that will include appropriate adjustments for the creatinine assay.

The accuracy of GFR estimates is less relevant when they are used to follow an individual patient over time. Here it is the shape and slope of the graph rather than the exact values that is of interest. Studies comparing the slopes of estimated GFR with measured GFR values show good correlations, especially for the CKD-EPI equation [10, 11]. Patient-related factors affect the measured and estimated GFR slopes in a similar way.

One way to validate the use of eGFR graphs is to compare them with graphs of measured GFR in patients with similar pathological processes. Figure 2.4 shows sequential measurements of GFR from five patients with autosomal dominant polycystic kidney disease (ADPKD). The trajectory of GFR is linear, although the gradient varies between patients. Graphs of estimated GFR from ADPKD patients with declining kidney function also follow a linear trajectory [13] (Fig 2.5).

Fig. 2.4 Measurements of
GFR using inulin or
Cr-EDTA clearance from
five patients with
autosomal dominant
polycystic kidney disease
(ADPKD). The rate of
decline is more rapid than
found in most patients with
ADPKD [12]

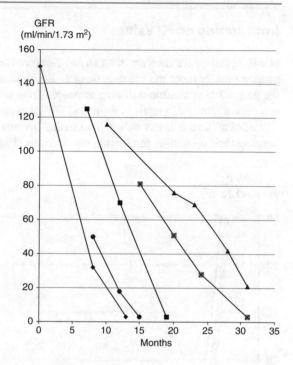

Fig. 2.5 eGFR graphs
from three patients with
ADPKD, chosen to show
the wide variation in the
eGFR gradient between
patients

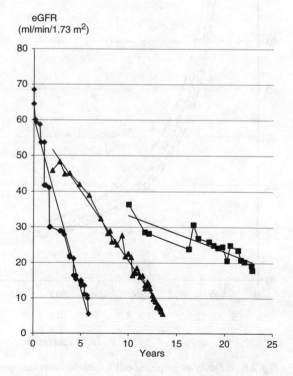

Interpreting eGFR Values

eGFR equations for men and women are different because, on average, men contain proportionately more muscle than women. Body composition also changes with age, the proportion of muscle declining as people grow older. Including these factors, we can draw a family of graphs of estimated GFR versus serum creatinine (Fig. 2.6).

Females have a lower eGFR than males for any given serum creatinine value because their creatinine production rate is lower (Fig. 2.7).

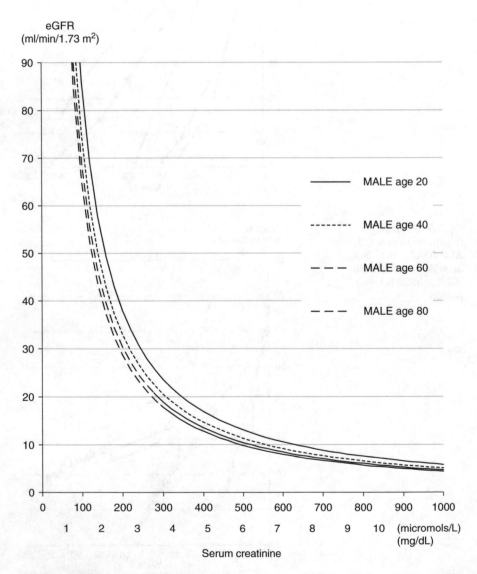

Fig. 2.6 A family of graphs of eGFR against serum creatinine, showing how the estimated GFR falls with age (MDRD equation)

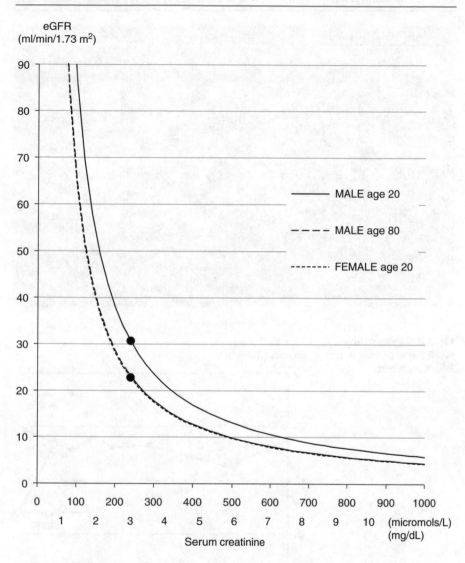

Fig. 2.7 eGFR calculated for a female aged 20 and males aged 20 and 80 years (MDRD equation). For a male with a serum creatinine = 240 µmol/L (2.7 mg/dL) altering the sex to female, or the age from 20 to 80 years, reduces the eGFR from 31 to 23 mL/min/1.73 m². The line for a male aged 80 is almost identical to that for a female aged 20 years

To derive the correct eGFR, the laboratory must be provided with the correct sex and date of birth. Using an incorrect adjustment causes a significant error in the estimate, giving either false alarm or false reassurance, as shown by the following cases (Patients 2.1 and 2.2).

Patient 2.1 Biochemical 'Sex Change'
Mr Edwards was shocked to be told by his GP that he needed to go back to the kidney clinic and talk about possible dialysis because his kidney function had suddenly dropped from 25 to 18 (Fig. 2.8).

Careful study of the laboratory report revealed the mistake:

```
Patient: 123456         John Edwards
Date of Birth   14/08/1948
Sex Female
Sample B,13.0763622 (BLOOD) Collected 16 Jun 2013
08:00 Received 16 Jun 2013 12:00
Urea & Electrolytes
Sodium            141    mmol/L         (133 - 146)
Potassium         5.0    mmol/L         (3.5 - 5.3)
Urea              19.6   mmol/L         (2.5 - 7.8)
Creatinine        235    μmol/L         (50 - 98)
Estimated GFR     18     ml/min/1.73m²
```

Fig. 2.8 Apparent drop in eGFR due to an error in the laboratory report

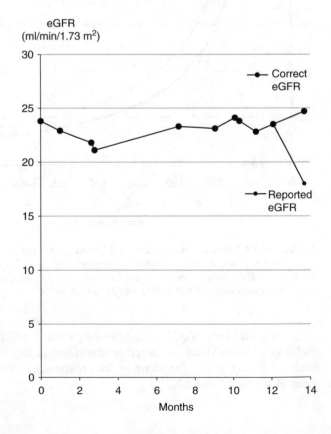

Patients with family names that are also used as first names are at particular risk of being labelled with the wrong sex (Patient 2.2).

Patient 2.2 Biochemical 'Sex-Change'

Mrs Tracey Paul was delighted to be told at her routine diabetes clinic review that her kidney function had improved (Fig. 2.9).

Unfortunately, the good news was an error; her kidney was declining after all. The error was picked up when a doctor questioned how serum creatinine and eGFR had both increased. Here is her laboratory report:

```
Patient: 234567          Tracey Paul
Date of Birth    02/07/1937
Sex Male
Sample B, 13.0343712 (BLOOD) Collected 15 Apr 2014
Received 15 Apr 2014 15:38
Urea & Electrolytes
Sodium           139    mmol/L        (133 - 146)
Potassium        4.9    mmol/L        (3.5 - 5.3)
Urea             16.7   mmol/L        (2.5 - 7.8)
Creatinine       144    µmol/L        (50 - 98)
Estimated GFR    41     ml/min/1.73m²
Previous results:
```

Date	Sodium	Potassium	Urea	Creatinine	eGFR
15.01.2014	141	5.0	14.8	126	37

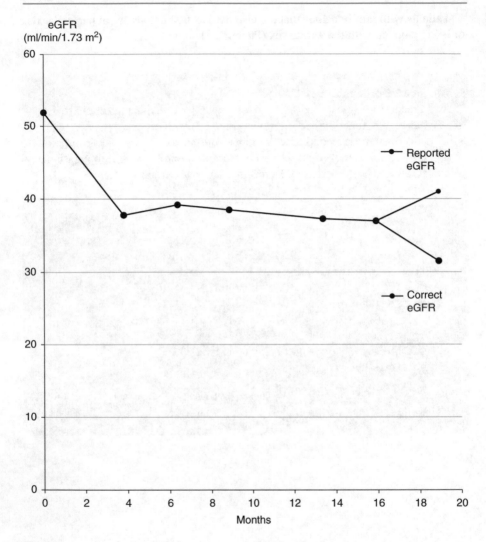

Fig. 2.9 Apparent rise in eGFR due to an error in the laboratory report

The estimated GFR needs to be adjusted for Afro-Caribbean race but not for other ethnicities (Fig. 2.10). This is because of genetically determined differences in skeletal muscle between racial groups. Compared to white Caucasians, black African people have 30–40% higher activities of a number of enzymes involved in phosphagenic metabolic pathways, including creatine kinase [14].

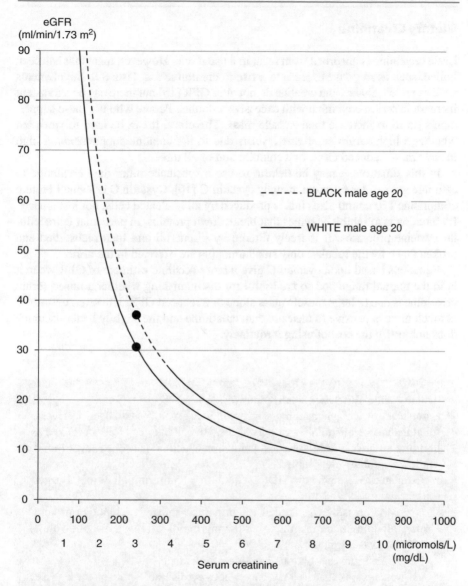

Fig. 2.10 eGFR calculated for white and black males aged 20 years (MDRD equation). For a man with a serum creatinine = 240 μmol/L (2.7 mg/dL), altering the race from white to black increases the eGFR by 21%, from 31 to 37 mL/min/1.73 m²

Not All Changes in Serum Creatinine Are Caused by Changes in GFR

Changes in serum creatinine do not necessarily indicate that the glomerular filtration rate has changed. Three factors other than GFR affect the serum creatinine concentration: dietary creatinine, muscle mass and secretion of creatinine by the tubules.

Dietary Creatinine

Little creatinine is absorbed from meat in a usual diet. However, meat that has been boiled, such as in goulash, leads to a rise in creatinine that lasts 8 h. Supplements such as protein shakes and creatine do not alter GFR [15] but there can be a transient increase in serum creatinine with excessive amounts. People who use these supplements do so to increase their muscle mass. Therefore, it can be hard to work out whether a high serum creatinine level is due to the creatine supplements, a high muscle mass, reduced GFR, or a combination of all three.

In this situation, it may be helpful to use a substance other than creatinine to estimate glomerular filtration, namely cystatin C [16]. Cystatin C is a small protein comprising 120 amino acids that is produced by all nucleated cells, not just muscle. Its function is to inhibit enzymes that break down proteins, in particular extracellular cysteine proteases. It is freely filtered by glomeruli and then reabsorbed and broken down by the tubules; only small amounts are excreted in the urine.

Equations based upon cystatin C give a more accurate estimate of GFR when it is in the normal range and so are useful for distinguishing whether a raised serum creatinine is due to large muscle mass alone or a reduced GFR. However, cystatin C is much more expensive to measure than creatinine and the slightly better accuracy does not justify the cost of using it routinely.

Patient 2.3 Big Muscles or Small Kidneys?
Emershan was a fit and healthy 33-year old black man. He had been a successful athlete, specialising in sprint distances. He had had his U&E's checked as part of a number of tests for chest pains, for which no cause was ever found. These were the results (Table 2.1).

Estimated GFR using the MDRD equation = 55 mL/min/1.73 m² (adjusted for black race)

His blood pressure was normal and urinalysis showed no blood or protein. Urinary albumin:creatinine ratio was 0.2 mg/mmol (2 mg/g). A kidney ultrasound scan was normal.

He ate a normal diet with no creatine supplements.

He was anxious that he may have a kidney disease. To resolve the issue, serum cystatin C was measured. The result, 0.93 mg/L, gave an eGFR using the CKD-EPI Cystatin C (2012) equation of 95 mL/min/1.73 m². He was reassured.

He was reassured that there was no evidence of kidney disease.

Table 2.1 Emershan's blood results

Sodium	139 mmol/L	(133–146)		
Potassium	4.4 mmol/L	(3.5–5.3)		
Urea	4.3 mmol/L	(2.5–7.8)	BUN	12.0 mg/dL
Creatinine	130 μmol/L	(64–111)	Creatinine	1.47 mg/dL

Changes in Muscle Mass

Creatinine production is proportional to a patient's skeletal muscle mass. If a patient loses or gains a lot of muscle, the serum creatinine concentration will change independently of GFR. For example, patients who are seriously ill requiring care in an intensive therapy unit (ITU) can lose a substantial amount of body weight. As a result, their serum creatinine can be up to one-third lower after the illness. This can lead to an underestimate of the number of patients left with kidney damage on discharge from the ITU [17].

Tubular Secretion of Creatinine

The equations used to estimate GFR take the tubular secretion of creatinine into account. However, problems arise when a patient is given a drug that blocks secretion of creatinine by the tubules. The most commonly used drug that does this is the antibiotic trimethoprim [18]. The anti-arrhythmic dronedarone has the same effect in some patients [19].

Treatment with these drugs will cause the eGFR to drop, even though the true GFR has not changed (Patient 2.4).

Patient 2.4 The Trimethoprim Effect

Rick, a longstanding kidney transplant patient, was troubled by recurrent *Escherichia coli* urinary infections. These responded well to long-term treatment with alternating courses of trimethoprim and cephalexin. Each time Rick took trimethoprim the eGFR dropped and he was worried that his transplant was being damaged (Table 2.2).

The serum urea was the clue that the tubular effect of trimethoprim was causing a rise in creatinine. It did not change with the serum creatinine, suggesting that the true GFR was unchanged.

Table 2.2 Sequential biochemical results in a kidney transplant patient receiving prophylactic antibiotics

Date	Urea (mmol/l)	Creatinine (μmol/L)	BUN (mg/dL)	Creatinine (mg/dL)	eGFR (mL/min/1.73 m²)	Antibiotic
22 Oct 2017	13.3	168	37.3	1.90	40.2	TMP
05 Nov 2017	13.0	166	36.4	1.88	40.8	TMP
21 Jan 2018	12.6	136	35.3	1.54	51.5	Ceph
27 May 2018	11.7	167	32.8	1.89	40.4	TMP
26 Aug 2018	12.5	147	35.0	1.66	46.9	Ceph

TMP trimethoprim, *Ceph* cephalexin

Serum Urea and Creatinine: Different Measures of Kidney Function

Changes in serum urea can give useful additional information about what is happening to kidney function. Urea and creatinine are both filtered by the glomeruli but only urea can diffuse across cell membranes and be reabsorbed from the tubules.

The amount of urea reabsorbed is determined by the rate of flow of filtrate along the nephron. When the rate slows, more urea is reabsorbed and the rate of excretion falls (Fig. 2.11).

How does this difference affect a patient's results? Consider two people: one with polycystic kidneys (ADPKD), the other with normal kidneys but low blood pressure due to prolonged diarrhoea. In the man with ADPKD, half of the nephrons have been affected by cysts and do not function; his total GFR is half-normal. However, the GFR in the nephrons that are functioning is normal and he produces a normal volume of urine per day.

In the man with diarrhoea and low blood pressure, the nephrons are filtering at half the normal rate so his GFR is also half-normal. To compensate for the hypovolaemia, salt and water are reabsorbed from the tubules into the blood and the flow of filtrate along the nephrons is slow. Urine volume is reduced.

Fig. 2.11 Effect of urine volume on the rate of excretion of urea, calculated as the urea clearance. (Redrawn from clearance values reported in [20]. Data are from samples taken from Harold Austin, published in 1921 [21])

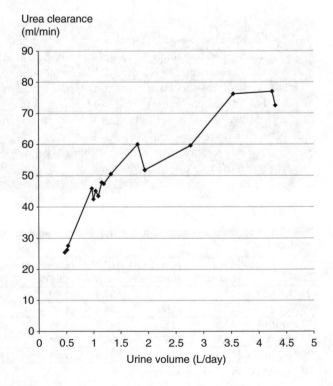

Table 2.3 Calculation of the urea-to-creatinine ratio

	ADPKD	Low blood pressure
Urea (mmol/L)	10.2	33.5
BUN (mg/dL)	28.6	93.8
Creatinine (μmol/L)	160	160
Creatinine (mg/dL)	1.8	1.8
eGFR (mL/min/1.73 m²)	38.9	38.9
Urea-to-creatinine ratio	10,200 ÷ 160 = **63.8**	33,500 ÷ 160 = **209.4**
BUN-to-creatinine ratio	28.6 ÷ 1.8 = **15.9**	93.5 ÷ 1.8 = **51.9**

Because the total glomerular filtration rate is halved, the concentration of creatinine is doubled in both patients. However, in the second patient, the slower flow of filtrate along the nephrons allows more urea to diffuse out of the tubules into the blood. As a result, the serum urea concentration is higher in the second patient than in the first.

Calculating the ratio of serum urea to serum creatinine shows this effect (Table 2.3).

A urea-to-creatinine ratio >100 (BUN-to-creatinine ratio >20) is often said to indicate dehydration but it can occur in any situation in which the flow of filtrate along the nephrons is slowed. It is a marker of a pre-renal or, more precisely, pre-glomerular cause of kidney impairment.

References

1. Shemesh O, Golbetz H, Kriss JP, Myers BD. Limitations of creatinine as a filtration marker in glomerulopathic patients. Kidney Int. 1985;28(5):830–8. http://www.nature.com/ki/journal/v28/n5/pdf/ki1985205a.pdf.
2. Levey AS, Bosch JP, Lewis JB, Greene T, Rogers N, Roth D. A more accurate method to estimate glomerular filtration rate from serum creatinine: a new prediction equation. Modification of Diet in Renal Disease Study Group. Ann Intern Med. 1999;130(6):461–70. PubMed: 10075613. http://annals.org/article.aspx?articleid=712617.
3. Schwartz GJ, Work DF. Measurement and estimation of GFR in children and adolescents. Clin J Am Soc Nephrol. 2009;4(11):1832–43. https://doi.org/10.2215/CJN.01640309. http://cjasn.asnjournals.org/content/4/11/1832.full.
4. Schwartz GJ, Muñoz A, Schneider MF, Mak RH, Kaskel F, Warady BA, Furth SL. New equations to estimate GFR in children with CKD. J Am Soc Nephrol. 2009;20:629–37. https://doi.org/10.1681/ASN.2008030287. http://jasn.asnjournals.org/content/20/3/629.full.
5. Ng DK, Schwartz GJ, Schneider MF, Furth SL, Warady BA. Combination of pediatric and adult formulas yield valid glomerular filtration rate estimates in young adults with a history of pediatric chronic kidney disease. Kidney Int. 2018;94(1):170–7. https://doi.org/10.1016/j.kint.2018.01.034. https://www.kidney-international.org/article/S0085-2538(18)30184-4/fulltext.
6. Smith M, Moran P, Ward M, Davison J. Assessment of glomerular filtration rate during pregnancy using the MDRD formula. BJOG. 2008;115:109–12. http://onlinelibrary.wiley.com/doi/10.1111/j.1471-0528.2007.01529.x/full.
7. KDIGO. Clinical practice guideline for the evaluation and management of chronic kidney disease. 2012. www.kdigo.org/clinical_practice_guidelines/pdf/CKD/KDIGO_2012_CKD_GL.pdf.

8. Levey AS, Stevens LA, Schmid CH, Zhang YL, Castro AF 3rd, Feldman HI, Kusek JW, Eggers P, Van Lente F, Greene T, Coresh J, CKD-EPI (Chronic Kidney Disease Epidemiology Collaboration). A new equation to estimate glomerular filtration rate. Ann Intern Med. 2009;150(9):604–12. http://www.ncbi.nlm.nih.gov/pmc/articles/PMC2763564/.
9. Kilbride HS, Stevens PE, Eaglestone G, Knight S, Carter JL, Delaney MP, Farmer CK, Irving J, O'Riordan SE, Dalton RN, Lamb EJ. Accuracy of the MDRD (Modification of Diet in Renal Disease) study and CKD-EPI (CKD Epidemiology Collaboration) equations for estimation of GFR in the elderly. Am J Kidney Dis. 2013;61(1):57–66. https://doi.org/10.1053/j.ajkd.2012.06.016. Epub 2012 Aug 11. http://www.ajkd.org/article/S0272-6386(12)00941-9/abstract.
10. Xie D, Joffe MM, Brunelli SM, Beck G, Chertow GM, Fink JC, Greene T, Hsu C-y, Kusek JW, Landis R, Lash J, Levey AS, O'Conner A, Ojo A, Rahman M, Townsend RR, Wang H, Feldman HI. A comparison of change in measured and estimated glomerular filtration rate in patients with nondiabetic kidney disease. Clin J Am Soc Nephrol. 2008;3(5):1332–8. http://www.ncbi.nlm.nih.gov/pmc/articles/PMC2518808/.
11. Padala S, Tighiouart H, Inker LA, Contreras G, Beck GJ, Lewis J, Steffes M, Rodby RA, Schmid CH, Levey AS. Accuracy of a GFR estimating equation over time in people with a wide range of kidney function. Am J Kidney Dis. 2012;60(2):217–24. http://www.ncbi.nlm.nih.gov/pmc/articles/PMC3399947/.
12. Franz KA, Reubl FC. Rate of functional deterioration in polycystic kidney disease. Kidney Int. 1983;23:526–9. http://www.nature.com/ki/journal/v23/n3/pdf/ki198351a.pdf.
13. Yu ASL, Shen C, Landsittel DP, Grantham JJ, Cook LT, Torres VE, Chapman AB, Bae KT, Mrug M, Harris PC, Rahbari-Oskoui FF, Shi T, Bennett WM, Consortium for Radiologic Imaging Studies of Polycystic Kidney Disease (CRISP). Long-term trajectory of kidney function in autosomal-dominant polycystic kidney disease. Kidney Int. 2019;95(5):1253–61. https://doi.org/10.1016/j.kint.2018.12.023. Epub 2019 Mar 4. https://www.kidney-international.org/article/S0085-2538%2819%2930104-8/fulltext.
14. Ama PF, Simoneau JA, Boulay MR, Serresse O, Thériault G, Bouchard C. Skeletal muscle characteristics in sedentary black and Caucasian males. J Appl Physiol (1985). 1986;61(5):1758–61. http://jap.physiology.org/content/61/5/1758.
15. Lugaresi R, Leme M, de Salles Painelli V, Murai IH, Roschel H, Sapienza MT, Herbert Lancha AH, Gualano B. Does long-term creatine supplementation impair kidney function in resistance-trained individuals consuming a high-protein diet? J Int Soc Sports Nutr. 2013;10:26. https://doi.org/10.1186/1550-2783-10-26. http://www.jissn.com/content/10/1/26.
16. Stevens LA, Coresh J, Schmid CH, Feldman HI, Froissart M, Kusek J, Rossert J, Van Lente F, Bruce RD, Zhang YL, Greene T, Levey AS. Estimating GFR using serum Cystatin C alone and in combination with serum creatinine: a pooled analysis of 3418 individuals with CKD. Am J Kidney Dis. 2008;51(3):395–406. https://doi.org/10.1053/j.ajkd.2007.11.018. http://www.ncbi.nlm.nih.gov/pmc/articles/PMC2390827/.
17. Prowle JR, Kolic I, Purdell-Lewis J, Taylor R, Pearse RM, Kirwan CJ. Serum creatinine changes associated with critical illness and detection of persistent renal dysfunction after AKI. Clin J Am Soc Nephrol. 2014;9(6):1015–23. https://doi.org/10.2215/CJN.11141113. http://cjasn.asnjournals.org/content/9/6/1015.abstract.
18. Berg KJ, Gjellestad A, Nordby G, Rootwelt K, Djøseland O, Fauchald P, Mehl A, Narverud J, Talseth T. Renal effects of trimethoprim in ciclosporin- and azathioprine-treated kidney-allografted patients. Nephron. 1989;53(3):218–22. http://www.karger.com/Article/Abstract/185747.
19. Duncker D, Oswald H, Gardiwal A, Lüsebrink U, König T, Schreyer H, Klein G. Stable cystatin C serum levels confirm normal renal function in patients with dronedarone-associated increase in serum creatinine. J Cardiovasc Pharmacol Ther. 2013;18(2):109. http://cpt.sagepub.com/content/18/2/109.abstract.
20. Van Slyke DD. The effect of urine volume on urea excretion. J Clin Invest. 1947;26:1159–67. http://www.ncbi.nlm.nih.gov/pmc/articles/PMC439461/pdf/jcinvest00386-0111.pdf.
21. Austin JH, Stillman E, Van Slyke DD. Factors governing the excretion rate of urea. J Biol Chem. 1921;46:91–112. http://www.jbc.org/content/46/1/91.full.pdf.

Plot All the Dots: How Graphs Reveal the History of Someone's Kidney Disease

Good doctors are skilled at taking a patient's history. As Sir William Osler[1] famously said: "Listen to your patient; he is telling you the diagnosis".

Patients with kidney disease often have no symptoms, but we can modify Osler's advice to: "Look at your patient's eGFR graph; it is telling you the kidney history".

In other words:

Plot all

the dots!

Viewing eGFR values as a column of figures is not enough; your brain cannot adjust for the different time intervals between the results to see the trends. Also, there may be so many results that you cannot view them all at once. Drawing a graph overcomes all of these problems [1].

The eGFR graph helps both clinicians and patients make sense of what is happening. And with this greater understanding, patients are more likely to successfully modify their lifestyle or adhere to treatment.

The more complete the dataset you use to draw the graph the better. It may require detective work and telephone calls to different pathology laboratories to track down all the old results (Patient 3.1). You may need to convert previous serum creatinine results into estimated GFR values, as explained in Chap. 2. These GFR estimates may be slightly less accurate than those provided by the laboratory as they may use uncorrected serum creatinine values. However, they give valuable information about long-term trends in kidney function.

---

[1]William Osler (1849–1919), a Canadian physician, was one of the four founding professors of Johns Hopkins Hospital in Baltimore, Maryland, United States. Osler created the first speciality training program for physicians and was the first to provide bedside clinical training. He has been described as the "Father of Modern Medicine".

© Springer Nature Switzerland AG 2020
H. C. Rayner et al., *Understanding Kidney Diseases*,
https://doi.org/10.1007/978-3-030-43027-6_3

Patient 3.1 Hunting Out the History

Arthur, a 70 year old man with diabetes, was referred by his GP for advice about how to improve the control of his blood pressure and glucose. This is a table of his eGFR results for the previous two and a half years (Table 3.1).

The variation in the time intervals between the results makes it hard to interpret the table of numbers. A graph of the results resolves this problem (Fig. 3.1).

The variation in these results makes it difficult to estimate the rate of decline in GFR. Further searching of the laboratory database uncovered some older results that had been stored using a different patient identification number. The pathology database had not automatically merged these with the more recent records. When this was done manually, the trend over 10 years was revealed (Fig. 3.2).

Table 3.1 Sequential eGFR results over two and a half years

	eGFR
18/04/2016	51.3
07/11/2016	47.8
10/02/2017	52.0
23/07/2017	37.9
20/08/2017	51.5
10/10/2017	56.4
29/07/2018	44.5
30/10/2018	46.1

Fig. 3.1 Trend in eGFR over two and a half years

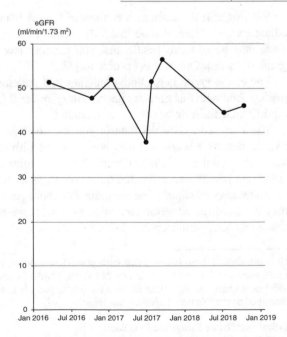

Fig. 3.2 Trend in eGFR
over 10 years

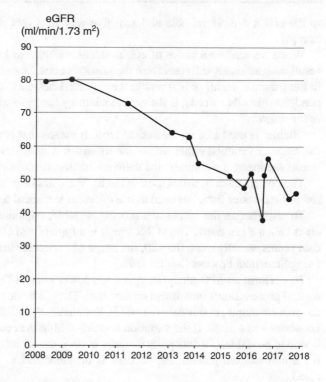

eGFR
(ml/min/1.73 m²)

Once you have tracked down all the eGFR results and plotted a complete graph, the next step is to interpret it correctly.

Variation in eGFR

If you took blood from the same person every day for 1 week, the seven serum creatinine results would not all be the same. They would vary above and below an average value. This is caused by biological variation in the person's true GFR from day to day combined with measurement variation in the laboratory assay.

The minimum difference between two measurements that is statistically significant is called the Reference Change Value (RCV). The RCV is calculated by combining the biological and analytical variation of the substance being analysed. The RCV for eGFR at an eGFR of 60 is about 10 mL/min/1.73 m². At an eGFR of 30 it is about 6 mL/min/1.73 m² [2]. These values are smaller than the RCV for GFR measured directly, showing how reliable the eGFR estimates are for monitoring kidney function [3].

These figures suggest that eGFR is an insensitive way of measuring changes in kidney function. However, the RCV is a statistical comparison of only two values. Patients with kidney disease usually have many more than two readings to compare. Comparing multiple values averages out the analytical variation, making the trend in the eGFR a more reliable and sensitive way to detect change in kidney function [4].

When we analyse a series of eGFR values we want to know whether the latest result is significantly different from the previous ones. Does it indicate a real change in the patient's health or is it within the expected range of variation of their known condition? In other words, is the patient's kidney function stable or is there a signal in the noise?

'Stable' is used as a mathematical term. It means that both the mean eGFR and the range of variation either side of the mean are constant over time. If the eGFR is stable, the mean is stationary and there are no non-random signals.

The comparative statistics used in the RCV are not helpful for analyzing sequential or time-series data. We need to use different statistical tests.

To test whether the output of a process is stable, sequential data are plotted on a chart called a run chart. The eGFR graph is a type of run chart. If we have enough data points, usually more than 20, the range of expected variation can be estimated using Statistical Process Control (SPC).

To perform an SPC analysis, upper and lower control limits (sometimes called natural process limits) are drawn on the chart. They indicate the range beyond which the process output, in this case the eGFR, is statistically unlikely to occur by chance, i.e. about 3 in a 1000. If the variation remains within the control limits, the process is said to be stable. If a data point deviates outside the limits or meets statistical tests for a non-random pattern, the process is unstable and a 'special cause' is indicated [5].

An SPC chart can sometimes be helpful for analysing a series of eGFR results.

Patient 3.2 Using an SPC Chart to Analyse Variation in eGFR
Marjorie was aged 82 and had CKD stage 4 due to diabetes and hypertension. Her eGFR was stable over 5 years. She then presented to hospital with cellulitis of her leg and hypotension. She was treated with antibiotics and allowed home.

Reviewing her eGFR results, the value on presentation was below the lower control limit (LCL) on a SPC chart drawn using all her previous results (BaseLine©, www.SAASoft.com) (Fig. 3.3). This was a warning that the sepsis was affecting her kidneys.

Six weeks later she returned to hospital more unwell. Her eGFR had dropped to 5. The clinical significance of the value taken previously was now clear (Fig. 3.4).

With intensive treatment over the following month her eGFR returned to its previous mean baseline.

Fig. 3.3 Statistical Process Control chart of eGFR values over 5 years. When the patient presented to hospital with cellulitis, the eGFR was below the lower control limit. This indicates that the deviation was significantly greater than expected from the previous normal variation for the patient. *UCL* upper control limit, *LCL* lower control limit

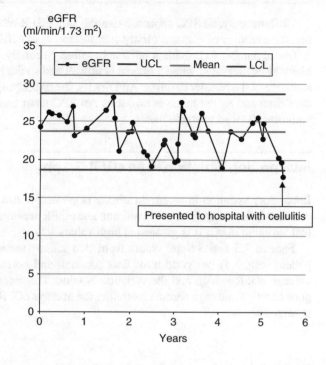

Fig. 3.4 Statistical Process Control chart showing acute kidney injury with recovery to previous baseline. *UCL* upper control limit, *LCL* lower control limit

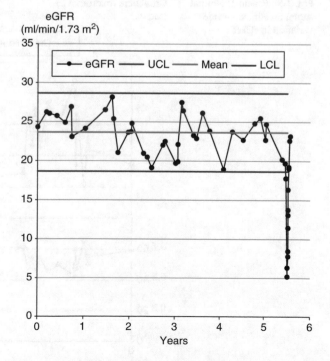

Unfortunately, an SPC approach to analysing eGFR results is usually not possible, for a number of reasons. Firstly, measurements of eGFR may be too infrequent or few in number to provide a reliable baseline. Secondly, kidney function is more likely to be measured when a patient is unwell and so the results may not be representative of the healthy baseline. And finally, the underlying GFR is often declining over time and so the mean is unstable. An SPC chart cannot be used to interpret variation about an unstable mean.

Interpreting Variation in an eGFR Graph

Laboratory variation in serum creatinine is greatest at low values because of inaccuracies in the assay. Because creatinine and eGFR are inversely related, this means that variation in eGFR is greatest at high values.

Figures 3.5 and 3.6 are charts from two kidney transplant patients. The first patient (Fig. 3.5) has good transplant function and normal serum creatinine; the average eGFR is high and the variation is wide. The second patient (Fig. 3.6) has poor function and high serum creatinine; the average eGFR is low and the variation is narrower.

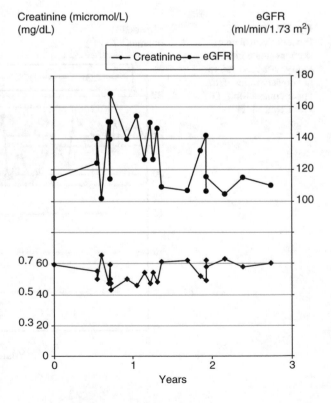

Fig. 3.5 Patient 1: Normal serum creatinine —wide variation in eGFR

Fig. 3.6 Patient 2: High serum creatinine—narrow variation in eGFR

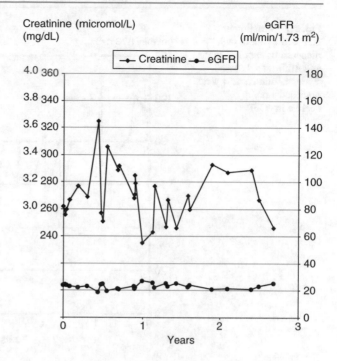

The range of variation in eGFR also depends upon the underlying kidney disease. Patients with wide variation in GFR may be having multiple episodes of 'micro' acute kidney injury. This pattern is associated with a greater risk of decline in eGFR over the long term and an increased risk of mortality [6].

Patient 3.3 Wide Variation in eGFR Predicts a Poor Outcome
Natasha had type 1 diabetes. Her blood glucose control had been very poor despite a multiple daily dose regimen, so she used an insulin pump. To make matters worse, she had Addison's disease and suffered from recurrent urinary infections. Infections caused her to have Addisonian crises with hypotension and acute kidney injury. Her eGFR varied widely for a number of years and then showed a declining trend (Fig. 3.7). As the eGFR fell, the variation around the trendline narrowed.

Fig. 3.7 Variation in
eGFR in a patient with
diabetes, urinary infections
and Addison's disease.
Wide variation over 4 years
preceded a rapid
decline in eGFR

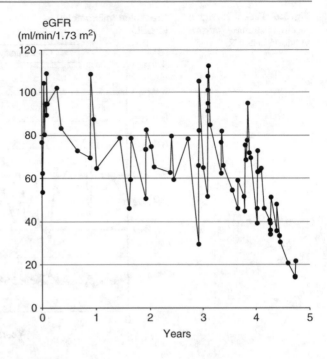

Linking an eGFR Graph to Clinical Events over Time

Clinical judgement and experience are needed to interpret eGFR graphs; it is a skill that requires practice. The more you use graphs of eGFR and other clinical measurements, the more skilled you will be at seeing links—sometimes surprising ones—between changes in data and clinical events. You can become familiar with common patterns in eGFR graphs by studying the examples throughout this book, such as Patients 3.4 and 3.5.

Patient 3.4 The Effect of Intravenous Fluids

Mrs. Ivy Flewyd was referred to the kidney clinic because of concern about a decline in her eGFR, from 45 mL/min/1.73 m^2 in March 2015 to 25 in September 2015.

Plotting the full eGFR graph showed that before March 2015 her eGFR had varied between 28 and 35 (Fig. 3.8). In March 2015 she had been admitted to hospital and had received intravenous fluids for a number of days. This had temporarily improved her kidney function, lowering the serum urea and creatinine and increasing the eGFR.

An ultrasound scan showed that both kidneys were small with reduced cortical thickness, changes that had been present on a scan 5 years previously. The most recent urea and eGFR values had merely returned to her usual range and were no cause for concern.

Fig. 3.8 Changes in serum urea and eGFR due to intravenous fluids

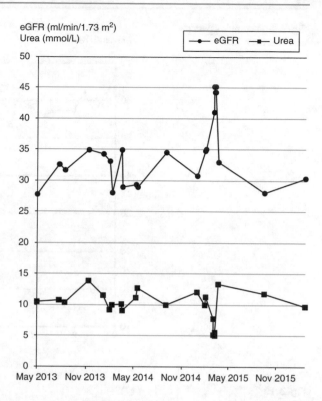

eGFR (ml/min/1.73 m²)
Urea (mmol/L)

● eGFR ■ Urea

May 2013 Nov 2013 May 2014 Nov 2014 May 2015 Nov 2015

Patient 3.5 Interpreting a More Complex eGFR Graph

Mr. Fish was 76 years old. He had diabetes and so had regular checks of his kidney function. Here is his eGFR graph (Fig. 3.9).

The graph can be divided into four periods (Fig. 3.10).

In the first period, the eGFR values are between 70 and 50 and the trend is slowly downwards due to his advancing age and diabetic nephrosclerosis.

In the second period, the trend turns abruptly downwards. Mr. Fish was unaware that his poor urinary stream and occasional incontinence were due to chronic urinary retention. It was only after a number of eGFR measurements showing worsening function that he was referred to a nephrologist, who palpated his grossly distended bladder.

At the start of the third period, a urinary catheter was inserted. This led to a rapid initial improvement in eGFR followed by a slower increase.

In the fourth period, the eGFR varies above and below a stable mean eGFR of 35, indicating residual non-progressive kidney damage.

This example comes from a time when eGFR was not routinely reported. One wonders how much of Mr. Fish's kidney function could have been saved if the decline in his eGFR during period 2 had been noticed and acted upon sooner.

Fig. 3.9 A complex pattern
of eGFR over time

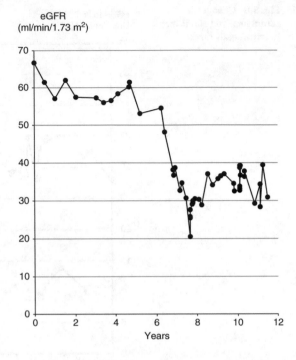

Fig. 3.10
Interpretation of the
eGFR graph as a
sequence of four
periods with different
pathological
processes

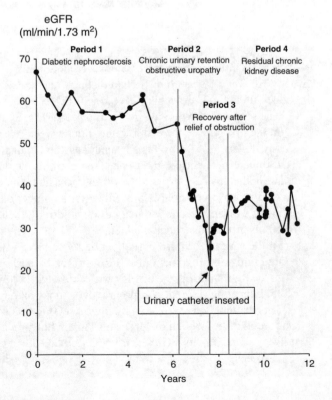

References

1. Morgan DB, Will EJ. Selection, presentation, and interpretation of biochemical data in renal failure. Kidney Int. 1983;24:438–45. http://www.nature.com/ki/journal/v24/n4/abs/ki1983180a.html.
2. Badrick T, Turner P. The uncertainty of the eGFR. Indian J Clin Biochem. 2013;28(3):242–7. http://link.springer.com/article/10.1007%2Fs12291-012-0280-1.
3. Rowe C, Sitch AJ, Barratt J, Brettell EA, Cockwell P, Dalton RN, Deeks JJ, Eaglestone G, Pellatt-Higgins T, Kalra PA, Khunti K, Loud FC, Morris FS, Ottridge RS, Stevens PE, Sharpe CC, Sutton AJ, Taal MW, Lamb EJ, eGFR-C Study Group. Biological variation of measured and estimated glomerular filtration rate in patients with chronic kidney disease. Kidney Int. 96(2):429–35. https://www.kidney-international.org/article/S0085-2538(19)30274-1/pdf.
4. Padala S, Tighiouart H, Inker LA, Contreras G, Beck GJ, Lewis J, Steffes M, Rodby RA, Schmid CH, Levey AS. Accuracy of a GFR estimating equation over time in people with a wide range of kidney function. Am J Kidney Dis. 2012;60(2):217–24. http://www.ncbi.nlm.nih.gov/pmc/articles/PMC3399947/.
5. NHS Improvement. Making data count. https://improvement.nhs.uk/resources/making-data-count/.
6. Tsai CW, Huang HC, Chiang HY, Chung CW, Chiu HT, Liang CC, Yu T, Kuo CC. First-year estimated glomerular filtration rate variability after pre-end-stage renal disease program enrollment and adverse outcomes of chronic kidney disease. Nephrol Dial Transplant. 2019;34(12):2066–78. https://doi.org/10.1093/ndt/gfy200. https://academic.oup.com/ndt/advance-article-abstract/doi/10.1093/ndt/gfy200/5049716?redirectedFrom=fulltext.

Kidney Function in Acute Illness and Acute Kidney Injury

4

Kidney Function in Acute Illness: Equilibrating Creatinine

The serum creatinine concentration is only a reliable marker of kidney function when it is in a steady state. Production and excretion of creatinine need to be in equilibrium. When the kidneys are affected by an acute illness, things are not in equilibrium.

If the GFR drops by half, the rate of creatinine excretion by filtration will fall by half. The fall in filtration leads to a rise in the serum creatinine concentration. The rise in the concentration increases the amount of creatinine contained in the smaller filtered volume. When the concentration reaches twice the previous level, the excretion rate of creatinine again matches the production rate and equilibrium is restored.

This is demonstrated by the surgical removal of a kidney for carcinoma. When the renal artery is clamped off there is an immediate step down in the patient's total GFR due to loss of the function of one kidney. At the moment the artery is clamped the serum creatinine concentration is unchanged but over the subsequent 24–48 h it progressively increases until a new equilibrium is reached (Fig. 4.1).

In some patients, the creatinine concentration falls over subsequent days as the remaining kidney's GFR increases through recruitment of nephrons and enlargement of glomeruli. In experimental rats, GFR starts to increase 24 h after nephrectomy [1]. The eGFR recovers to the pre-operative level over a median of 2 years in about half of patients undergoing a nephrectomy [2], due to this hypertrophic process.

The time that it takes for the serum creatinine to reach a new equilibrium depends upon the magnitude of the change in GFR. If the GFR falls suddenly to 5%, i.e. one twentieth of its previous level, equilibrium will only be restored when the serum creatinine is 20 times its previous concentration. A daily creatinine production of 8 mmol (930 mg) distributed in the 40 L of total body water would increase the serum creatinine by 200 µmol/L (2.3 mg/dL) per day. It would therefore be 6 days after a single acute event before serum creatinine reached a new equilibrium of 1200 µmol/L (13.6 mg/dL).

© Springer Nature Switzerland AG 2020
H. C. Rayner et al., *Understanding Kidney Diseases*,
https://doi.org/10.1007/978-3-030-43027-6_4

Fig. 4.1 Serum creatinine values following unilateral nephrectomy in six patients

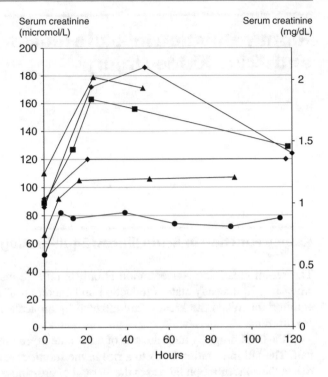

Table 4.1 Detection and staging of acute kidney injury in adults according to Kidney Disease Improving Global Outcomes (KDIGO)

Stage	Serum creatinine concentration	Urine volume
1	Rise of ≥26 µmol/L (0.3 mg/dL) within 48 h Or 50–99% rise from baseline within 7 days[a] (1.50–1.99 × baseline)	<0.5 mL/kg/h for more than 6 h
2	100–199% rise from baseline within 7 days (2.00–2.99 × baseline)	<0.5 mL/kg/h for more than 12 h
3	≥200% rise from baseline within 7 days (≥3 × baseline) Or current creatinine >354 µmol/L (4.0 mg/dL) with either: ≥26 µmol/L (0.3 mg/dL) rise within 48 h Or ≥50% rise from baseline within 7 days Or any requirement for kidney replacement therapy	<0.3 mL/kg/h for 24 h Or anuria for 12 h

[a]Where the rise is known (based on a prior blood test) or presumed (based on the patient's history) to have occurred within 7 days

Some acutely ill patients suffer sequential kidney insults, further lengthening the time before a new steady state is reached. The delay of days until the diagnosis of acute kidney injury can be made based on the rise in serum creatinine is why biomarkers of kidney injury may be added to the range of indicators used to detect kidney damage [3].

The magnitude of the rise in serum creatinine and the peak value reached are used to categorise acute kidney injury into three stages of severity, defined by their associated mortality risk (Table 4.1) [4].

The initial diagnosis of acute kidney injury is based upon a patient meeting any of the criteria for Stage 1. Staging of the clinical episode is carried out retrospectively when the episode is complete, and peak creatinine is known. Patients are classified according to the highest possible stage where any criterion is met, either by creatinine rise, or urine output, or need for dialysis.

Remember that serum creatinine can be acutely affected by changes other than in GFR, such as trimethoprim treatment, as discussed in Chap. 2. Sepsis can reduce the production of creatinine by skeletal muscle so the change in serum creatinine may underestimate the drop in GFR, especially if the patient also has a low muscle mass [5].

Dealing with Missing Data

Acute kidney injury is often unexpected and the patient may not have had their serum creatinine measured shortly before the illness. This can make it difficult to decide whether someone has AKI and to gauge its severity. One cannot assume the creatinine was previously in the normal range. Indeed, patients with AKI are more likely to have underlying chronic kidney disease.

Many ways have been explored to overcome this difficulty [4]. One option is to take an average of previous readings and use that number as the baseline to calculate the AKI stage. This is simple but potentially misleading. An average does not take into account the sequence of the values being averaged.

Figures 4.2 and 4.3 contain the same values of eGFR. The average of the first five results is shown as a horizontal dashed line. In the first chart (Fig. 4.2) the latest result has dropped compared to the average baseline. Using this definition, the

Fig. 4.2 Acute kidney injury—the latest eGFR measurement is below the previous range of variation. The average of the first five results is shown as a horizontal dashed line

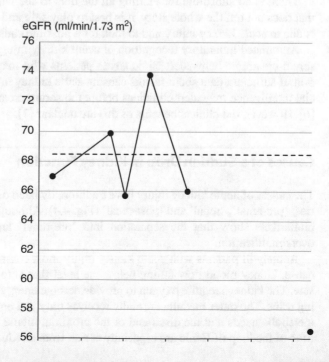

eGFR (ml/min/1.73 m^2)

Fig. 4.3 Progressive chronic kidney disease—the latest eGFR measurement is on the linear trendline projected from the previous values. The average of the first five results is shown as a horizontal dashed line

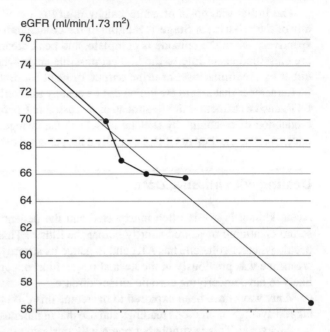

patient has suffered either acute kidney injury (defined as a decline occurring over ≤7 days) or acute kidney disease (defined as a decline occurring over 7–90 days).

In the second chart (Fig. 4.3), the average is the same but the baseline results show a declining trend. The latest result is in line with this trend. The patient has progressive chronic kidney disease rather than acute kidney injury or disease.

There is no substitute for plotting all the dots to see what is really going on. If that does not tell the whole story, it is best to play safe and assume that the decline is due to acute kidney injury and to look for a possible cause.

Automated laboratory recognition of acute kidney injury based upon the rise in serum creatinine helps alert clinicians to patients who may need further intervention. If sufficient data about factors causing acute kidney injury are available, artificial intelligence may alert clinicians before the serum creatinine has started to rise [6]. However, the clinical benefits of this are unclear [7].

Causes of a Sudden Drop in Kidney Function

The causes of acute kidney injury have traditionally been divided into three categories: 'pre-renal', 'renal' and 'post-renal' (Fig. 4.4). Although still useful, studies of biomarkers show that the separation into 'pre-renal' and 'renal' causes is an oversimplification.

Acutely ill patients with acute kidney injury most commonly have a 'pre-renal' cause, kidney blood flow falling below the level that autoregulation can compensate. The kidneys require oxygen to provide aerobic energy for the work of producing urine. The outer medulla normally receives only just enough oxygen to meet its metabolic needs and the distal end of the proximal tubule and the thick ascending limb of the loop of Henle are especially at risk from a reduction in blood flow.

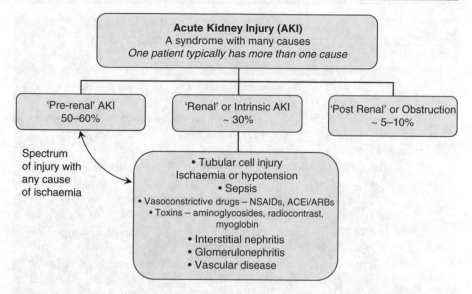

Fig. 4.4 The traditional categories of acute kidney injury (AKI). The spectrum of injury in pre-renal AKI ranges from minimal to severe tubular cell damage. *NSAID* Non-Steroidal Anti-Inflammatory Drug, *ACEi* Angiotensin Converting Enzyme inhibitor, *ARB* Angiotensin Receptor Blocker

Intraglomerular pressure to drive filtration is maintained by hormones, including vasodilatory prostaglandins that dilate the afferent arteriole and angiotensin II that constricts the efferent arteriole [8]. Blocking these hormones can lead to acute kidney injury.

Acute kidney injury is more likely when a number of factors that reduce GFR come together, such as hypovolaemia, sepsis and drug nephrotoxicity, especially when autoregulation of kidney blood flow is already impaired by hypertension, vascular disease or advanced age (Patient 4.1), and liver cirrhosis.

Patient 4.1 Physiological Measurements in Acute Kidney Injury
Mr. Thomas, an 83-year-old retired machine operator, was admitted to a cardiac ward for investigation of recurrent blackouts. He was a lifelong smoker and hypertensive, being treated with amlodipine.

On admission, urinalysis showed no blood or protein. U&E's and full blood count were normal.

During the night, about 24 h after admission, he complained of passing dark red urine in the toilet and became very anxious. Two hours later he became very unwell with a pulse rate of 170 beats per minute and collapsed to the floor, unresponsive and incontinent of faeces. Telemetry showed a prolonged period of supraventricular tachycardia.

His temperature was 40 °C, respiratory rate 44 breaths per minute, blood pressure 89/52 mmHg and pulse 150 beats per minute (Fig. 4.5).

Arterial blood gases on 15 L per minute of oxygen showed: pO_2 = 20 kPa (11–13), pCO_2 = 3.98 kPa (4.7–6.0).

There was a compensated metabolic acidosis: arterial pH = 7.403 (normal 7.34–7.44), base excess = −5.7 mmol/L (−2 to +2), venous $[HCO_3^-]$ = 9.6 mmol/L (22–26).

The serum anion gap was high (25 mmol/L) due to a lactic acidosis, serum lactate: arterial sample = 7.4 mmol/L (0.5–1.6) (explained in Chap. 15).

White blood count was normal, $7.7 \times 10^9/L$.

He was resuscitated with 3 L of IV normal (0.9%) saline over the following 24 h. A urinary catheter was inserted and he was given intravenous broad-spectrum antibiotics pending the results of urine and blood cultures.

The next day his white count had jumped to $26.6 \times 10^9/L$. C-reactive protein increased to 176 mg/L and serum albumin dropped from 38 to 29 g/L (3.8 to 2.9 g/dL)—an acute phase reaction. A mid-stream urine specimen contained 115 WBC/microL (normal range 0–80) but culture yielded no growth. However, blood culture yielded *Escherichia coli*, fully sensitive to antibiotics.

His serum creatinine rose from a baseline of 82 micromol/L (0.9 mg/dL) to a peak of 268 micromol/L (3.0 mg/dL), a 227% increase to 3.27 × baseline. Applying the KDIGO criteria, this is Stage 3 AKI.

During the first 24 h after the collapse his blood pressure was low, mean arterial pressure falling from 90 to 65 mmHg. During this period his kidney perfusion pressure fell below the level that could sustain glomerular filtration. He became oliguric for a period of 7 h.

Oliguria, defined as a urine volume of <400 mL per day or <0.5 mL/kg/h for more than 6 h, indicates an increased risk of mortality. Restoration of urine volume is a sign that GFR is recovering. As GFR increased, the slope of the serum creatinine graph switched from upwards to downwards (Fig. 4.6), until it eventually returned to his normal level.

Over 48 h Mr. Thomas received a total of 7 L of intravenous saline. The period of low blood pressure was short, the infection was treated promptly and his circulation returned to normal. Fluid given during resuscitation to restore the blood pressure was reabsorbed into the circulation and his urine volume increased—the diuretic phase.

Because kidney blood flow was restored within hours, damage to the tubules by ischaemia was limited.

Patients do not need to have very low blood pressure to develop acute kidney injury; a fall in systolic pressure from 135 to 120 mmHg can be sufficient in vulnerable patients [9]. So a systolic pressure of 100 mm Hg or less should not be regarded as the cutoff for shock or renal hypoperfusion. The latter can occur at higher blood pressures.

Persistently low kidney blood flow can cause irreversible damage to the tubular cells—acute tubular injury or necrosis—through a complex interplay of cellular and inflammatory processes [10]. So, a 'pre-renal' cause turns into a 'renal' cause.

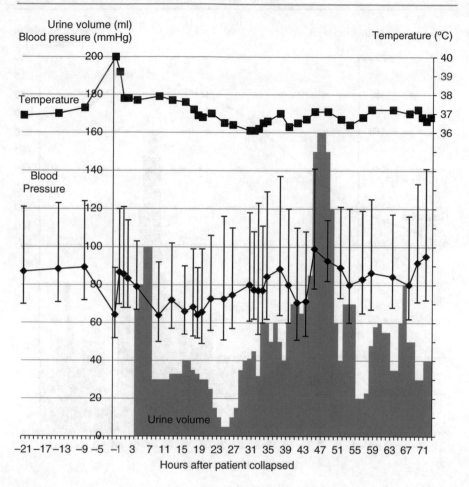

Fig. 4.5 Chart showing the vital signs for the 24 h before and 72 h after Mr. Thomas' collapse due to sepsis

'Renal' causes of acute kidney injury include inflammation of the glomeruli—glomerulonephritis—and of the interstitial tissue around the tubules—interstitial nephritis. Glomerulonephritis is usually an immune-mediated disease. Interstitial nephritis and direct tubular damage are usually caused by drugs.

'Post-renal' causes of acute kidney injury involve obstruction to the flow of urine from the kidney, anywhere from the renal pelvis to the urethra. Examples of conditions causing each of the three categories of acute kidney injury are given throughout the book and are listed in the index.

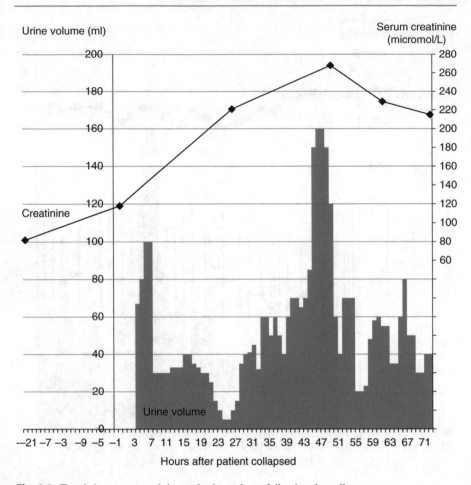

Fig. 4.6 Trends in serum creatinine and urine volume following the collapse

Fluid Balance in Acutely Ill Patients

Acute illness affects the excretion of salt and water and their distribution between body compartments:

- Cortisol production is increased leading to sodium and water retention
- Vasodilatation due to sepsis leads to low blood pressure
- Acute inflammation weakens the capillary endothelial barrier, so fluid leaks into the interstitial space
- Acute inflammation suppresses liver protein synthesis, so serum albumin concentration drops and tissue fluid is less easily reabsorbed into the circulation

When an acute illness occurs in someone who is already fluid overloaded, fluid balance is more difficult to assess. Blood pressure may be low due to reduced plasma volume despite there being peripheral oedema or ascites. Poor left ventricular function may contribute to the low blood pressure and giving intravenous fluid may risk causing pulmonary oedema.

Prompt treatment of sepsis with fluid and appropriate antibiotics can be lifesaving [11]. Tracking changes in vital signs and blood results helps when writing the fluid prescription (Patient 4.1).

Acute-on-Chronic Kidney Disease: Time in Two Dimensions

Kidney diseases have traditionally been divided into acute and chronic. This may be convenient for explaining different pathological processes but in practice the distinction is not so clear-cut.

There is a tendency, particularly in the hospital setting, to focus on the acute time dimension and overlook the chronic. If you plot the whole eGFR graph rather than reading only the last few results, you will see both dimensions of time (Fig. 4.7).

Fig. 4.7 eGFR graph from a man with diabetes who suffered an episode of severe gastroenteritis. The temporary drop in kidney function due to the gastroenteritis is superimposed upon a steady decline due to diabetic nephropathy

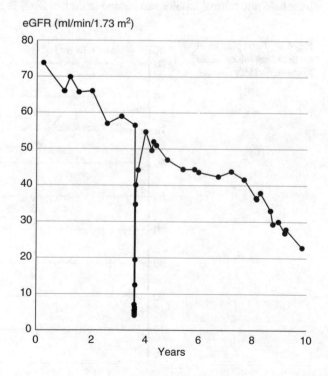

Acute and chronic kidney diseases are interlinked:

- Patients are more likely to suffer acute kidney injury if they already have chronic kidney disease or proteinuria [12]
- Kidney function is less likely to return to its previous level after an episode of acute kidney injury in patients with diabetes, chronic kidney disease or proteinuria [13]
- Patients who suffer multiple episodes of acute kidney injury are more likely to develop chronic kidney disease [14], progress to end-stage kidney failure and to die [15]

Figure 4.8 shows the eGFR graph from a 58-year-old female smoker with diabetes and hypertension. She suffered acute kidney injury at the time of her first myocardial infarction and was left with chronic kidney disease Stage G3. Two years later she suffered a second myocardial infarction that led to further acute and chronic loss of kidney function. She died suddenly at home 18 months later, presumably from another cardiac event.

The pathological link between acute and chronic kidney disease is the failure of tubules to regenerate fully after acute injury. The regenerating tubular cells do not differentiate into normal tubules and instead stimulate fibrosis in the interstitium. After a

Fig. 4.8 Two episodes of acute kidney injury leading to chronic kidney disease

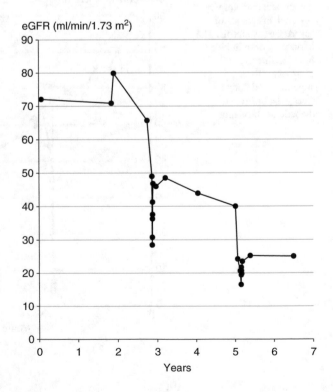

single injury, the fibrotic scar remains limited to the region of the damaged tubules. However, repeated acute injury on top of chronic damage stimulates progressive spreading fibrosis and glomerular damage [16].

Management of Acute Kidney Injury

The 'five Rs' are a helpful way to think about the management of acute kidney injury.

- **R**isk—is the patient at increased risk of AKI (reduced eGFR, proteinuria, diabetes, advanced age)?
- **R**ecognition—are there systems in place for checking serum creatinine, urine output, biomarkers?
- **R**espond rapidly—have all factors contributing to the AKI been identified (check urine for blood and protein to exclude glomerulonephritis) and been treated rapidly (stop inappropriate drugs, give fluid ± antibiotics)?
- **R**efer—should a nephrologist be involved [17]?
- **R**eview—has a follow up plan to monitor kidney function been made and communicated to the patient's primary care team?

Kidney replacement therapy is commonly started for someone with acute kidney injury who has [18]:

- Depressed consciousness due to uraemic encephalopathy
- Fluid overload that cannot be controlled by diuretic therapy
- Hyperkalaemia that cannot be controlled by medical therapy
- Severe metabolic acidosis

There is no benefit from starting dialysis based upon changes in serum creatinine or loss of urine output before these complications develop. Delaying the start allows time for kidney function to recover, potentially avoiding the need for dialysis [19]. Studies of earlier dialysis in acute kidney injury have produced conflicting results, so there is no clear evidence in favour of using early dialysis.

Various types of kidney replacement therapy are used for acutely ill patients with kidney failure. Continuous dialysis or haemofiltration is commonly used on an intensive care unit, especially when inotropic drugs such as noradrenaline (norepinephrine) are needed to maintain the circulation, as it causes less haemodynamic instability than intermittent haemodialysis [20].

In Asia and in less developed countries, acute peritoneal dialysis is more commonly used [21]. There is no good evidence that one form of therapy is inherently better than another.

References

1. Chamberlain RM, Shirley DG. Time course of the renal functional response to partial nephrectomy: measurements in conscious rats. Exp Physiol. 2007;92:251–62. http://onlinelibrary.wiley.com/doi/10.1113/expphysiol.2006.034751/full.
2. Zabor EC, Furberg H, Mashni J, Lee B, Jaimes EA, Russo P. Factors associated with recovery of renal function following radical nephrectomy for kidney neoplasms. Clin J Am Soc Nephrol. 2016;11(1):101–7. https://doi.org/10.2215/CJN.04070415. https://cjasn.asnjournals.org/content/11/1/101.
3. de Geus HR, Betjes MG, Bakker J. Biomarkers for the prediction of acute kidney injury: a narrative review on current status and future challenges. Clin Kidney J. 2012;5(2):102–8. https://doi.org/10.1093/ckj/sfs008. https://www.ncbi.nlm.nih.gov/pmc/articles/PMC3341843/.
4. Thomas ME, Blaine C, Dawnay A, Devonald MAJ, Ftouh S, Laing C, Latchem S, Lewington A, Milford DV, Ostermann M. The definition of acute kidney injury and its use in practice. Kidney Int. 2014;87(1):62–73. https://doi.org/10.1038/ki.2014.328. https://www.kidney-international.org/article/S0085-2538(15)30035-1/fulltext.
5. Doi K, Yuen PST, Eisner C, Hu X, Leelahavanichkul A, Schnermann J, Star RA. Reduced production of creatinine limits its use as marker of kidney injury in sepsis. J Am Soc Nephrol. 2009;20:1217–21. https://doi.org/10.1681/ASN.2008060617. http://jasn.asnjournals.org/content/20/6/1217.abstract.
6. Tomašev N, Glorot X, Rae JW, Zielinski M, Askham H, Saraiva A, Mottram A, Meyer C, Ravuri S, Protsyuk I, Connell A, Hughes CO, Karthikesalingam A, Cornebise J, Montgomery H, Rees G, Laing C, Baker CR, Peterson K, Reeves R, Hassabis D, King D, Suleyman M, Back T, Nielson C, Ledsam JR, Mohamed S. A clinically applicable approach to continuous prediction of future acute kidney injury. Nature. 2019;572:116–9. https://www.nature.com/articles/s41586-019-1390-1.
7. Van Biesen W, Vanmassenhove J, Decruyenaere J. Prediction of acute kidney injury using artificial intelligence: are we there yet? Nephrol Dial Transplant. 2020;35(2):204–5. https://doi.org/10.1093/ndt/gfz226. https://academic.oup.com/ndt/advance-article/doi/10.1093/ndt/gfz226/5647338.
8. Abuelo JG. Normotensive ischemic acute renal failure. N Engl J Med. 2007;357:797–805. http://www.nejm.org/doi/full/10.1056/NEJMra064398.
9. Liu YL, Prowle J, Licari E, Uchino S, Bellomo R. Changes in blood pressure before the development of nosocomial acute kidney injury. Nephrol Dial Transplant. 2009;24:504–11. https://doi.org/10.1093/ndt/gfn490. http://ndt.oxfordjournals.org/content/24/2/504.full.
10. Kanagasundaram NS. Pathophysiology of ischaemic acute kidney injury. Ann Clin Biochem. 2015;52(2):193–205. https://journals.sagepub.com/doi/10.1177/0004563214556820.
11. Mouncey PR, Osborn TM, Power GS, Harrison DA, Sadique MZ, Grieve RD, Jahan R, Harvey SE, Bell D, Bion JF, Coats TJ, Singer M, Young JD, Rowan KM, ProMISe Trial Investigators. Trial of early, goal-directed resuscitation for septic shock. New Eng J Med. 2015;372(14):1301–11. https://doi.org/10.1056/NEJMoa1500896. http://www.nejm.org/doi/pdf/10.1056/NEJMoa1500896
12. Hsu CY, Ordoñez JD, Chertow GM, Fan D, McCulloch CE, Go AS. The risk of acute renal failure in patients with chronic kidney disease. Kidney Int. 2008;74(1):101–7. https://doi.org/10.1038/ki.2008.107. https://www.ncbi.nlm.nih.gov/pmc/articles/PMC2673528/.
13. Lee BJ, Go AS, Parikh R, Leong TK, Tan TC, Walia S, Hsu RK, Liu KD, Hsu CY. Pre-admission proteinuria impacts risk of non-recovery after dialysis-requiring acute kidney injury. Kidney Int. 2018;93(4):968–76. https://doi.org/10.1016/j.kint.2017.10.017. Epub 2018 Jan 15. https://www.kidney-international.org/article/S0085-2538(17)30797-4/fulltext.
14. Thakar CV, Christianson A, Himmelfarb J, Leonard AC. Acute kidney injury episodes and chronic kidney disease risk in diabetes mellitus. Clin J Am Soc Nephrol. 2011;6(11):2567–72. https://doi.org/10.2215/CJN.01120211. https://cjasn.asnjournals.org/content/6/11/2567.

15. Horne KL, Packington R, Monaghan J, Reilly T, McIntyre CW, Selby NM. The effects of acute kidney injury on long-term renal function and proteinuria in a general hospitalised population. Nephron Clin Pract. 2014;128:192–200. https://doi.org/10.1159/000368243. http://www.karger.com/Article/Abstract/368243.

16. Liu BC, Tang TT, Lv LL, Lan HY. Renal tubule injury: a driving force toward chronic kidney disease. Kidney Int. 2018;93(3):568–79. https://doi.org/10.1016/j.kint.2017.09.033. Epub 2018 Jan 17. https://www.kidney-international.org/article/S0085-2538(17)30819-0/fulltext.

17. Ftouh S, Thomas M, Acute Kidney Injury Guideline Development Group. Acute kidney injury: summary of NICE guidance. BMJ. 2013;347:f4930. https://doi.org/10.1136/bmj.f4930. https://www.bmj.com/content/347/bmj.f4930.

18. KDIGO clinical practice guideline for acute kidney injury. Kidney Int Suppl. 2012;2:1. https://doi.org/10.1038/kisup.2012.1. https://kdigo.org/wp-content/uploads/2016/10/KDIGO-2012-AKI-Guideline-English.pdf.

19. Gaudry S, Hajage D, Schortgen F, Martin-Lefevre L, Pons B, Boulet E, Boyer A, Chevrel G, Lerolle N, Carpentier D, de Prost N, Lautrette A, Bretagnol A, Mayaux J, Nseir S, Megarbane B, Thirion M, Forel JM, Maizel J, Yonis H, Markowicz P, Thiery G, Tubach F, Ricard JD, Dreyfuss D, AKIKI Study Group. Initiation strategies for renal-replacement therapy in the intensive care unit. N Engl J Med. 2016;375:122–33. https://doi.org/10.1056/NEJMoa1603017. https://www.nejm.org/doi/full/10.1056/NEJMoa1603017.

20. Ahmed AR, Obilana A, Lappin D. Renal replacement therapy in the critical care setting. Crit Care Res Pract. 2019;2019:6948710. https://doi.org/10.1155/2019/6948710. https://www.hindawi.com/journals/ccrp/2019/6948710/.

21. Cullis B, Abdelraheem M, Abrahams G, Balbi A, Cruz DN, Frishberg Y, Koch V, McCulloch M, Numanoglu A, Nourse P, Pecoits-Filho R, Ponce D, Warady B, Yeates K, Finkelstein FO. Peritoneal dialysis for acute kidney injury. Perit Dial Int. 2014;34(5):494–517. https://doi.org/10.3747/pdi.2013.00222. http://www.pdiconnect.com/content/34/5/494.long.

How Are You Feeling? Symptoms of Kidney Disease

Symptoms Linked to the Kidneys and Urinary Tract

Most kidney diseases are silent—they do not cause symptoms linked directly to the kidneys. Exceptions include acute pyelonephritis, kidney stones, tumours, and polycystic kidney disease, which cause loin pain and haematuria, and retroperitoneal fibrosis, which causes back pain and can obstruct the ureters. An ultrasound san performed to investigate back pain may identify an asymptomatic kidney abnormality, such as a simple cyst. The pain may then be attributed inappropriately to that lesion.

Lower Urinary Tract Symptoms

Passing urine is the only physical sign that the kidneys are working, although the volume of urine bears no relation to the glomerular filtration rate. Symptoms related to the passage of urine are very common, especially in older adults and children, and are sometimes linked to loss of kidney function.

Lower urinary tract symptoms become increasingly common as people get older; up to 30% of men over the age of 65 years are bothered by them [1]. They can be categorised into voiding, storage or post-micturition symptoms. Voiding symptoms include a weak or intermittent urinary stream, straining, hesitancy, terminal dribbling and incomplete emptying. Storage symptoms include urgency, frequency, incontinence and nocturia. The most common post-micturition symptom is dribbling.

Urinary frequency refers to the frequent passing of small volumes of urine. It should be distinguished from the much less common symptom of polyuria, in which normal volumes are passed more often so that the total volume of urine is increased to over 3 L per day.

Polyuria is usually matched by excessive drinking, i.e. polydipsia. In psychogenic polydipsia, which occurs most often in adolescents, thirst and a compulsion to drink water are the main symptoms. The commonest causes of polyuria and polydipsia are hyperglycaemia due to diabetes mellitus, and diabetes insipidus, either

© Springer Nature Switzerland AG 2020
H. C. Rayner et al., *Understanding Kidney Diseases*,
https://doi.org/10.1007/978-3-030-43027-6_5

nephrogenic or cranial. Someone with diabetes insipidus may pass more than 10 L of urine per day.

The most common cause of lower urinary tract symptoms in men is benign prostatic enlargement. An initial assessment should seek out any symptoms and physical signs that suggest other pathology, such as bladder detrusor muscle weakness or overactivity, prostatitis, urinary tract infection, prostate cancer or neurological disease.

Prostate cancer is more likely in patients with a family history of prostate cancer, if symptoms suggest bladder outlet obstruction, or if the prostate gland feels abnormal on digital rectal examination. Measurement of serum prostate specific antigen (PSA) should be reserved for patients at higher risk of cancer rather than used as a screening test because it has a high false positive rate. The NHS Prostate Cancer Risk Management Programme provides information to help patients and clinicians decide whether to perform a PSA test [2].

You should measure kidney function (eGFR) in men with a history of urinary tract infection or kidney stones, incontinence at night or a palpable bladder. A portable bladder ultrasound scan is convenient way to confirm a possible palpable bladder.

Urinary Incontinence

Urinary incontinence means the unintentional passage of urine [3]. It is very common, especially in women. Most people with urinary incontinence have either stress or urge incontinence.

Stress incontinence is the leakage of urine when the bladder is put under sudden extra pressure, such as coughing or heavy lifting. It is usually associated with weakening of or damage to the pelvic floor muscles and urethral sphincter by pregnancy and vaginal birth, and is made worse by obesity.

Urge incontinence is the sudden and intense need to pass urine. This may be triggered by a change of position or the sound of running water and often occurs as part of an overactive bladder syndrome with frequency and nocturia. Stress and urge incontinence can occur together.

Overflow incontinence occurs with chronic urinary retention. The patient may frequently pass small trickles of urine and feel that their bladder cannot be emptied completely.

Total urinary incontinence is severe and continuous, with the passage of large amounts of urine, even at night, and occasional small leaks in between. It may be caused by a congenital bladder abnormality, a spinal injury, or a bladder fistula.

Bed Wetting: Enuresis

Most children can go through the night without wetting the bed by the age of 5 years. However, 15–20% of 5-year-old children wet the bed, as do 5% of 10-year-olds and

1–2% of 15-year-olds. Children who never achieve 6 months of dry nights have primary nocturnal enuresis. Children who achieve dryness but then have a recurrence of night-time wetting 6 or more months later have secondary nocturnal enuresis.

Primary nocturnal enuresis without daytime wetting is linked to one or more of the following factors: being a deep sleeper; having polyuria; and a delay in the maturation of bladder control. It is more likely to occur if there is a family history of bedwetting, in boys, and with obesity. About 30% of obese children wet the bed. Children with psychological and behavioural disorders such as attention deficit hyperactivity disorder (ADHD), autism spectrum disorder, anxiety, depression, and conduct disorders are more likely to be enuretic.

Children with primary nocturnal enuresis do not require urodynamic or radiological investigation. Enuresis due to a congenital abnormality is suggested by symptoms of daytime bladder dysfunction and abnormal bowel habit. The lower spine should be examined to look for developmental abnormalities, and the lower limbs for neurological problems. Two to four percent of children have a congenital dermal sinus, commonly called a pit or dimple, between the buttocks but these are not associated with a significant risk of spinal cord or intraspinal abnormality. They only require further investigation if there are other skin abnormalities or neurological symptoms [4].

Parents of children aged less than 5 years can be reassured that their child will probably eventually achieve night-time dryness. Parents of children who wet the bed beyond 5 years of age should be advised that bedwetting may resolve without treatment if it occurs less than twice a week. An adequate but not excessive daytime fluid intake helps develop normal bladder capacity and control; large volumes of fluid should be avoided in the evening. Children should be encouraged to void before bedtime and woken and taken to the toilet when the parent goes to bed. Caffeine-containing drinks should be avoided.

For children who wet the bed more frequently, it is best to delay treatment until 7–8 years of age. First-line treatment is to use an enuresis alarm that sounds to wake the child when the bed is wet, combined with positive rewards. Desmopressin (an analogue of vasopressin, aka antidiuretic hormone) reduces the volume of urine and is given at bedtime. It may be used if the alarm is unsuitable or if rapid or short-term control of bedwetting is needed.

Secondary nocturnal enuresis without daytime wetting may be caused by urine infection, diabetes mellitus, severe constipation or a response to family problems [5].

Daytime Wetting: Diurnal Enuresis

Children usually achieve daytime dryness before night-time dryness. Persistent daytime wetting is usually associated with symptoms such as urgency, frequency, abdominal straining or poor urinary stream, pain on passing urine, or passing urine fewer than four times a day. It is most commonly caused by an overactive bladder but may be linked to a congenital malformation or neurological disorder and occasionally to chronic constipation. Diurnal enuresis should be investigated and treated before nocturnal enuresis is addressed.

Useful information about bowel, bladder and toileting issues for children and families has been produced by ERIC, the Children's Bowel and Bladder Charity, and can be found at eric.org.uk.

Symptoms That Develop as Kidney Function Declines

As the GFR declines, symptoms and signs of kidney failure become more common and more severe (Fig. 5.1). To reflect that, CKD is graded into five stages by eGFR: G1 to G5.

Patients with eGFR >60 mL/min/1.73 m^2 need to have other evidence of kidney disease, such as proteinuria or a structural abnormality, to qualify as having Stage

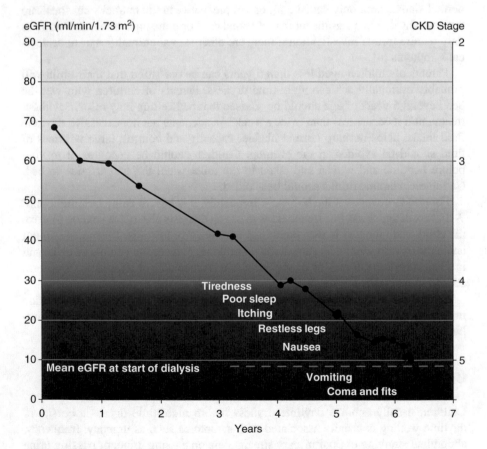

Fig. 5.1 The common symptoms experienced by patients at different stages of chronic kidney disease. Mean eGFR at start of dialysis refers to UK practice

G1 (eGFR > 90) or Stage G2 (eGFR 60–89). Stage G3 is divided into G3a (eGFR 45–60 mL/min/1.73 m^2) and G3b (eGFR 30–45). Stage G4 is eGFR 15–29 mL/min/1.73 m^2 and G5 is eGFR <15 mL/min/1.73 m^2.

The definition of CKD requires two reduced eGFR readings at least 3 months apart to confirm that the disease is chronic, and implications for health to justify the term 'disease'. The full classification of someone with CKD requires the underlying cause, the eGFR and the level of albuminuria [6].

Kidney failure does not make you feel ill until it is advanced, so taking a history from a patient with kidney disease is little help in judging kidney function. The severity of symptoms experienced at a given level of eGFR varies considerably between individuals, and some people remain asymptomatic despite very low function.

The duration of symptoms is not a reliable guide to how quickly kidney failure has developed. Patients with chronic kidney disease may present acutely after a long period of symptomless disease.

Uraemia and the Nervous System

As GFR falls below 45 the commonest symptom is fatigue, defined as extreme and persistent tiredness, weakness or exhaustion—either mental, physical or both [7]. Patients whose GFR declines very slowly and are otherwise well may adjust their lifestyle and expectations to minimize the effects of fatigue.

As GFR declines below 20, symptoms such as insomnia, restless legs and itching (uraemic pruritus) increase.

Restless legs syndrome is a curious unpleasant symptom that patients characteristically find hard to describe. They refer to throbbing, pulling or creeping sensations inside their legs and have an uncontrollable urge to move them. The symptoms are worse when the patient is relaxing and are often worst at night. Moving the legs temporarily eases the feeling.

Itching is common in patients with CKD stages G4 and 5 [8]. About one in five haemodialysis patients are very much or extremely bothered by itching [9]. Itching is much more than an irritation; it has a major effect on patients' work and social life. Its constant presence, especially at night, leads to exhaustion and depression (Patient 5.1). Severe itching is even associated with increased mortality [10].

Despite this, the symptoms are often poorly managed; 18% of severely affected patients use no treatment for itch and 17% do not report itching to health care staff [9], partly because they are unaware that it is linked to their kidney disease and have the impression it is something they have to live with [11].

Patient 5.1 Severe Uraemic Pruritus
Vanessa had been on dialysis for 12 years. Over recent months, she had suffered from severe itching that stopped her getting to sleep and disrupted her family life. The itching on her back was so bad that she used an old belt to scratch herself, making her skin bleed.

She describes her symptoms in a video interview at vimeo.com/49458473 (Fig. 5.2).

Fig. 5.2 Screenshot of video at http://vimeo.com/49458473

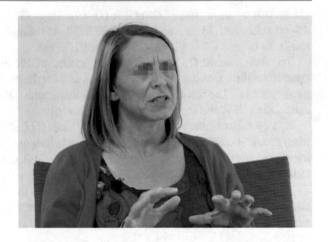

Fig. 5.3 Itchy nodules (nodular prurigo) and scratch marks due to uraemic pruritus

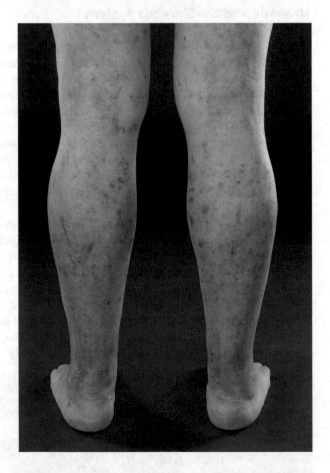

The itching may be associated with dry skin but there is usually no rash. Some patients have itchy nodules, called nodular prurigo (Fig. 5.3). Vigorous and prolonged scratching causes bleeding and scarring (Fig. 5.4).

Fig. 5.4 Bleeding caused by scratching due to uraemic pruritus

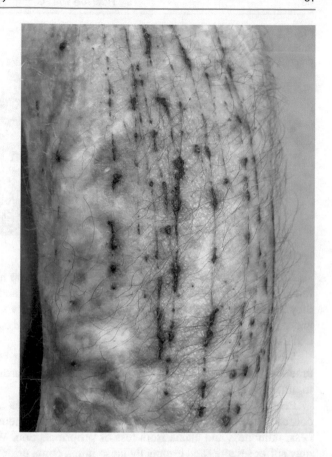

The pathophysiology of these symptoms is not fully understood. Itching is not caused by high serum phosphate levels, as is commonly believed [9]. Itching, insomnia and restless legs syndrome often occur together, making is likely that their cause lies in the effects of uraemia on the nervous system. Functional MRI scans of the brain in patients with itching show structural changes in grey matter and neuronal over-activity [12].

Treatment of severe insomnia, restless legs and itching requires careful use of drugs that modify neurotransmission. Gabapentin and pregabalin can be particularly helpful for all these symptoms [13, 14]. The effect of gabapentin on itching is often dramatic, a single tablet switching off the symptom (Patient 5.1 continued). These drugs are excreted by the kidneys and so must be given at a low dose and increased slowly [15].

Patient 5.1 Continued Treatment of Uraemic Pruritus with Gabapentin
Vanessa was offered treatment with gabapentin. After the first tablet the itching stopped almost completely.

She describes the effect of the treatment and the impact this had on her life in a video interview at vimeo.com/49455976 (Fig. 5.5).

Fig. 5.5 Screenshot of
video at http://vimeo.
com/49455976

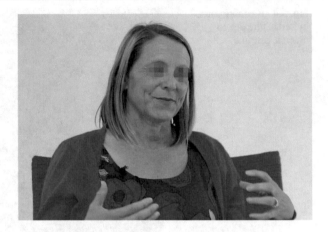

As GFR declines below 15, the fatigue becomes more marked and people often
fall asleep during the day. They may lose their appetite and feel sick, particularly if
they have a diet high in protein. The sickness is typically worse in the mornings
and there may be a bad taste in the mouth. Poor appetite can lead to weight loss
and eventually malnutrition.

When GFR reaches very low levels, patients suffer recurrent vomiting and a
uraemic smell may be detected on their breath. A pericardial rub may be heard due
to uraemic pericarditis.

People with underlying brain disease such as dementia become more drowsy and
confused due to metabolic encephalopathy. Peripheral neuropathy can cause weakness, numbness and ataxia from loss of proprioception. Without dialysis, patients
may suffer seizures and eventually lapse into a coma prior to death.

These neurological complications can be exacerbated by dialysis. Rapid changes
in the biochemistry of the blood cause disequilibrium across the blood-brain barrier.
The reduction in the osmotic pressure in the blood causes fluid to cross the blood-
brain barrier into the brain leading to cerebral oedema.

In the UK, the mean eGFR when people start dialysis is 8.5 mL/min/1.73 m^2,
although some feel well despite having an eGFR below this. An extreme example
(Patient 5.2) was a man who only presented to hospital when his eGFR reached
1.4 mL/min/1.73 m^2!

Patient 5.2 Extreme Results

Amar, a 20-year-old computer science student, had become increasing unwell
over the previous 2 months with loss of appetite, weight loss, weakness, pain
in the legs and tremors. His walking had become increasingly unsteady. He
had continued his studies until this recent illness.

On admission, his blood pressure was 150/87, a loud pericardial rub was
heard and he had bilateral leg oedema. An echocardiogram showed severe left
ventricular hypertrophy with systolic and diastolic dysfunction.

There were signs of peripheral neuropathy in his legs with numbness, an ataxic gait and bilateral foot drop. Subsequent neurophysiology tests showed severe axonal sensory and motor polyneuropathy.

Both kidneys were grossly atrophic and difficult to see on an ultrasound scan. The right measured 5.5 cm and the left 5.0 cm in length. The cortices were extremely thin.

Here are his blood results (Table 5.1).

He was started on haemodialysis, initially via a femoral vein haemodialysis catheter. His first session was for 3 h at a relatively slow blood pump speed of 150 mL/min. This was to reduce the risk of disequilibrium syndrome caused by the first dialysis.

The dose of dialysis delivered can be estimated from the percentage by which urea is reduced during the treatment, the Urea Reduction Ratio (URR):

$$URR = \frac{Pre \ dialysis \ urea \ concentration - Post \ dialysis \ urea \ concentration}{Pre \ dialysis \ urea \ concentration} \%$$

The goal for a regular dialysis treatment is >65%. The first treatment achieved only 40.8% but Amar suffered a generalised tonic-clonic seizure near the end of dialysis.

He was severely anaemic, haemoglobin = 49 g/L (4.9 g/dL), so was given a blood transfusion and started on erythropoietin. The pain from the peripheral neuropathy was treated with amitriptyline and gabapentin and he wore foot drop supports.

With daily dialysis for the first 2 weeks then three times a week, Amar steadily improved. After 6 months he could walk without assistance. After 9 months an echocardiogram showed normal left ventricular function.

A year after first presenting, Amar received a successful kidney transplant from his father.

Table 5.1 Blood results at the time Amar presented to hospital

		Normal range	Non-SI units
Sodium	125 mmol/L	133–146	125 mEq/L
Potassium	5.8 mmol/L	3.5–5.3	5.8 mEq/L
Urea	104.9 mmol/L	2.5–7.8	BUN 294 mg/dL
Creatinine	3378 micromol/L	64–111	38.2 mg/dL
eGFR	1.4 mL/min/1.73 m²		
Bicarbonate	7.2 mmol/L	22.0–29.0	Total CO_2 7.2 mEq/L
Albumin	33 g/L	35–50	3.3 g/dL
Calcium (corrected for serum albumin)	1.44 mmol/L	2.20–2.60	5.8 mg/dL
Phosphate	5.17 mmol/L	0.80–1.50	Phosphorus 16.0 mg/dL
Alkaline phosphatase	63 IU/L	30–130	

Fig. 5.6 Tophus on second toe due to chronic gout in a lady with chronic kidney disease. Note the shiny red skin overlying the cream coloured deposits around the joint. The toe was very tender to touch

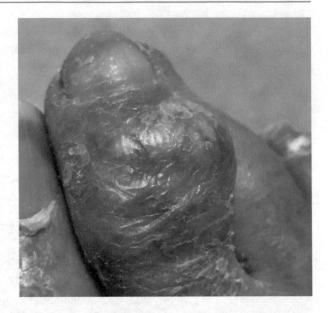

Gout

Gout is caused by the deposition of monosodium urate crystals. Two-thirds of urate excretion is by the kidneys and so serum uric acid levels are increased in chronic kidney disease. This leads to an increased risk of gout, made worse by treatment with diuretics. Various joints may be involved, not just the typical acutely painful big toe (podagra) (Fig. 5.6).

Precipitation of uric acid in tubules can cause acute kidney injury in patients with a very high serum uric acid concentration. Massive amounts of uric acid are released by cell breakdown in tumour lysis syndrome and crush injury. However, it is not clear whether chronic deposition of monosodium urate crystals in the medulla contributes to the progression of kidney disease [16] and raised uric acid levels are not usually treated unless the patient has clinical signs of gout.

References

1. National Institute for Health and Care Excellence. Lower urinary tract symptoms in men: management. Clinical guideline [CG97]. https://www.nice.org.uk/Guidance/CG97.
2. Public Health England. Prostate cancer risk management programme: overview. Last updated 29 March 2016. https://www.gov.uk/guidance/prostate-cancer-risk-management-programme-overview.
3. National Health Service. Urinary incontinence. https://www.nhs.uk/conditions/urinary-incontinence/symptoms/.
4. Weprin BE, Oakes WJ. Coccygeal pits. Pediatrics. 2000;105(5):E69. https://pediatrics.aappublications.org/content/105/5/e69.
5. National Institute for Health and Care Excellence. Clinical knowledge summary. Bedwetting (enuresis). https://cks.nice.org.uk/bedwetting-enuresis.

6. Kidney Disease: Improving Global Outcomes (KDIGO) CKD Work Group. KDIGO 2012 clinical practice guideline for the evaluation and management of chronic kidney disease. Kidney Int Suppl. 2013;3:1–150. http://kdigo.org/home/guidelines/ckd-evaluation-management.

7. Artom M, Moss-Morris R, Caskey F, Chilcot J. Fatigue in advanced kidney disease. Kidney Int. 2014;86:497–505. https://doi.org/10.1038/ki.2014.86. https://www.kidney-international.org/article/S0085-2538(15)30331-8/fulltext.

8. Sukul N, Speyer E, Tu C, Bieber BA, Li Y, Lopes AA, Asahi K, Mariani L, Laville M, Rayner HC, Stengel B, Robinson BM, Pisoni RL, CKDopps and CKD-REIN Investigators. Pruritus and patient reported outcomes in non-dialysis CKD. Clin J Am Soc Nephrol. 2019;14(5):673–81. https://doi.org/10.2215/CJN.09600818. Epub 2019 Apr 11. https://cjasn.asnjournals.org/content/14/5/673.long.

9. Rayner HC, Larkina M, Wang M, Graham-Brown M, van der Veer SN, Ecder T, Hasegawa T, Kleophas W, Bieber BA, Tentori F, Robinson BM, Pisoni RL. International comparisons of prevalence, awareness, and treatment of pruritus in people on hemodialysis. Clin J Am Soc Nephrol. 2017;12(12):2000–7. https://doi.org/10.2215/CJN.03280317. https://cjasn.asnjournals.org/content/clinjasn/12/12/2000.full.pdf.

10. Pisoni RL, Wikstrom B, Elder SJ, et al. Pruritus in haemodialysis patients: international result from the Dialysis Outcomes and Practice Patterns Study (DOPPS). Nephrol Dial Transplant. 2006;21:3495–505. http://ndt.oxfordjournals.org/content/21/12/3495.full.

11. Aresi G, Rayner HC, Hassan L, Burton JO, Mitra S, Sanders C, van der Veer S. Reasons for underreporting of uremic pruritus in people with chronic kidney disease: a qualitative study. J Pain Symptom Manage. 2019;58(4):578–586.e2. https://doi.org/10.1016/j.jpainsymman.2019.06.010. https://www.jpsmjournal.com/article/S0885-3924(19)30343-4/fulltext.

12. Papoiu AD, Emerson NM, Patel TS, Kraft RA, Valdes-Rodriguez R, Nattkemper LA, Coghill RC, Yosipovitch G. Voxel-based morphometry and arterial spin labeling fMRI reveal neuropathic and neuroplastic features of brain processing of itch in end-stage renal disease. J Neurophysiol. 2014;112(7):1729–38. https://doi.org/10.1152/jn.00827.2013. Epub 2014 Jun 18. https://www.physiology.org/doi/pdf/10.1152/jn.00827.2013.

13. Gunal AI, Ozalp G, Yoldas TK, Gunal SY, Kirciman E, Celiker H. Gabapentin therapy for pruritus in haemodialysis patients: a randomized, placebo-controlled, double-blind trial. Nephrol Dial Transplant. 2004;19:3137–9. http://ndt.oxfordjournals.org/content/19/12/3137.full.pdf.

14. Yue J, Jiao S, Xiao Y, Ren W, Zhao T, Meng J. Comparison of pregabalin with ondansetron in treatment of uraemic pruritus in dialysis patients: a prospective, randomized, double-blind study. Int Urol Nephrol. 2015;47(1):161–7. https://doi.org/10.1007/s11255-014-0795-x. http://download.springer.com/static/pdf/823/art%253A10.1007%252Fs11255-014-0795-x.pdf?auth66=1425491040_c2475cbe1d116e09fa6998febcb2b056&ext=.pdf.

15. Rayner H, Baharani J, Smith S, Suresh V, Dasgupta I. Uraemic pruritus: relief of itching by gabapentin and pregabalin. Nephron Clin Pract. 2013;122(3–4):75–9. https://doi.org/10.1159/000349943. https://www.karger.com/Article/FullText/349943.

16. Vargas-Santos AB, Neogi T. Management of gout and hyperuricemia in CKD. Am J Kidney Dis. 2017;70(3):422–39. https://www.ncbi.nlm.nih.gov/pmc/articles/PMC5572666.

Do You Have Any Risk Factors or Long-Term Health Conditions? How Environment, Lifestyle and Other Medical Conditions Are Linked to Kidney Disease

6

In this chapter we discuss factors in a patient's environment and lifestyle that can be associated with kidney disease. High blood pressure is such an important factor that it has its own chapter (Chap. 11).

We then focus on the most common long-term conditions that affect the kidneys—diabetes, atherosclerosis, liver cirrhosis, and chronic infection and inflammation. The kidneys may be damaged as one part of a multisystem disease. Examples of such conditions are included throughout the book and can be located using the index. Immune-mediated diseases are described in Chap. 17.

Risk Factors for Kidney Disease

A variety of environmental and lifestyle factors have been linked with an increased risk of developing kidney disease or with worse outcomes in people who have kidney disease. These factors have been identified from epidemiological studies of large populations of patients. Such 'observational' studies use statistical tests to find significant associations between different factors and patients' outcomes. For example, being exposed to air pollution containing fine particulate matter is associated with the development of chronic kidney disease [1].

It is important to remember that observational studies cannot prove that a factor is the cause of the outcome, even if this seems very plausible. Both the factor and the outcome may be caused by some other unidentified factor, so called 'confounding'. Proof of causation comes from interventional clinical trials. Unfortunately, it is impossible or unethical to carry out trials of many environmental or lifestyle factors, so observational studies may be the best evidence we can get.

© Springer Nature Switzerland AG 2020
H. C. Rayner et al., *Understanding Kidney Diseases*,
https://doi.org/10.1007/978-3-030-43027-6_6

Many studies have shown an association between eating red meat and the development of chronic kidney disease [2], and increased mortality in people with chronic kidney disease [3]. Conversely, plant-based diets are associated with a lower risk of chronic kidney disease developing [4] and progressing [5], and of subsequent mortality [3].

Drinks containing caffeine [6], particularly coffee [7], are associated with a reduced risk of mortality in patients with chronic kidney disease. Conversely, soda drinks are associated with a greater risk of end stage kidney disease [8].

Having a good night's sleep goes with good kidney health, as well as with better general health and wellbeing. Having too little sleep and a disrupted sleep pattern are associated with a higher risk of progression in patients with chronic kidney disease [9].

Long term exposure to high temperatures is thought to be a major factor causing chronic kidney disease in people working in the sugarcane industry in Central America, so called Mesoamerican nephropathy [10]. These workers harvest five to six tons of sugarcane per day while heavily clothed, in temperatures that frequently exceed 40 °C (104 °F). The heat exposure may cause daily subclinical acute kidney injury through ischemia, temperature-induced oxidative stress, and decreased intracellular energy stores. As global warming progresses, such heat-related chronic kidney disease is likely to become a global problem.

Diabetes Mellitus

Diabetes mellitus is the commonest cause of chronic kidney disease; in some countries such as the United States and Germany, up to half of patients with chronic kidney disease attending nephrology clinics have diabetes.

The prevalence of diabetes worldwide is growing at an alarming rate. In 2014, 422 million people had diabetes—8.5% of the adult population. The rise has been almost exponential in the UK and the prevalence is likely to increase as the obesity epidemic continues (Fig. 6.1).

Kidney involvement in diabetes is common; about 25% of people with diabetes in England have proteinuria [11]. Although only 0.5% has end-stage kidney failure, this percentage more than doubled between 2004 and 2010.

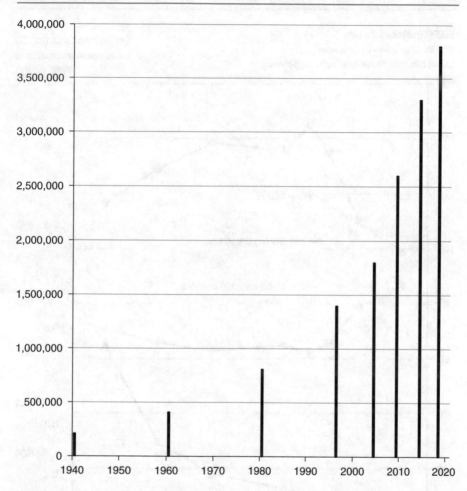

Fig. 6.1 The rising prevalence of diabetes in the UK over the last 78 years. (Data from various sources)

The natural history of diabetic nephropathy typically progresses from microalbuminuria to macroalbuminuria and then to a decline in GFR [12]. eGFR may be high initially (Fig. 6.2) but this is not associated with a higher risk of later glomerular damage [13]. This seems inconsistent with the traditional theory that hyperfiltration in individual nephrons causes glomerular damage [14]. It may be that the high eGFR indicates a high number of functioning nephrons, which reduces the risk of kidney disease [15].

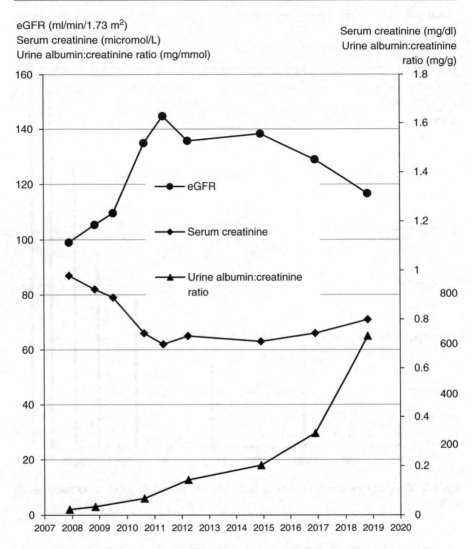

Fig. 6.2 The natural history of early diabetic nephropathy. There is steadily increasing albuminuria before eGFR declines

In more advanced disease, there is progressive sclerosis of glomeruli and the GFR declines. The decline is almost always linear in type 1 diabetes [16] and usually linear in type 2 diabetes. Its slope varies, tending to be steeper in patients with heavy proteinuria [17] (Fig. 6.3).

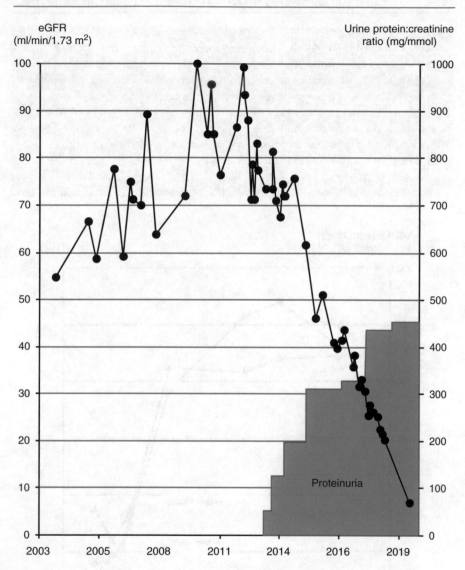

Fig. 6.3 The natural history of diabetic nephropathy showing hyperfiltration followed by heavy proteinuria and a decline in GFR to end stage kidney failure

Risk Factors for Diabetic Nephropathy

Two clinical factors increase the risk of someone with diabetes developing nephropathy—poor glucose control and high blood pressure.

Patient 6.1 Controlling Glucose Does Not Protect Against Loss of GFR Once Nephropathy Is Present
Andrea had type 1 diabetes since she was 8 years old and struggled for many years to control her blood glucose. In 2017, aged 23 years, she attended a diabetes education course where she learned how to estimate her insulin needs and adjust the dose accordingly.

Her blood glucose control improved dramatically, as shown by the fall in glycated haemoglobin (HbA1c). Despite this, her GFR continued to decline (Fig. 6.4).

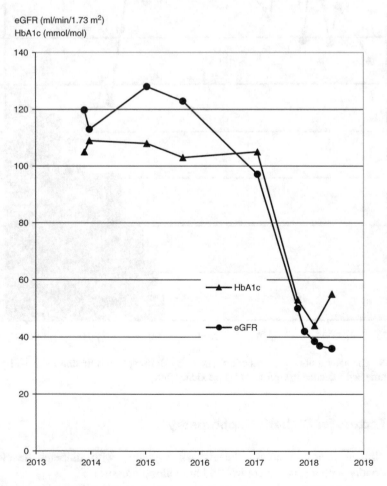

Fig. 6.4 Decline in GFR despite marked improvement in glucose control (HbA1c)

Achieving good glucose control is particularly important in the first few years after diagnosis as this can leave a legacy of reduced risk in future years, the 'metabolic memory'. Control needs to be achieved before albuminuria is established. In type 1 diabetes, tight glucose control in the early years halves the risk of reduced kidney function [18].

However, glucose control does not correlate closely with kidney damage. One third of people with type 1 diabetes develop nephropathy despite adequate glucose control, while others maintain normal renal function despite severe chronic hyperglycemia.

The risk of developing nephropathy in type 1 diabetes is partly inherited and a large genome-wide association study has found a strong link to a gene that codes for type IV collagen and the width of glomerular basement membranes (*COL4A3*) [19]. This is the same gene that is involved in the autosomal recessive form of Alport syndrome and in thin glomerular basement membrane disease, suggesting that the susceptibility of glomerular membranes to damage in diabetes is partly inherited.

In type 2 diabetes, controlling blood glucose delays the development of albuminuria and reduces the risk of end-stage kidney disease [20–22] but once nephropathy is established it has no effect on the rate of decline in GFR [23] or the risk of mortality [24]. Over-aggressive glucose control may even be harmful. Intensive glucose treatment in people with kidney disease, including CKD stage 1, increases the risk of mortality by 30% [25].

Treatment with Renin-Angiotensin-Aldosterone System (RAAS) Inhibitors

Treatment with inhibitors of the renin-angiotensin-aldosterone system improves outcomes in diabetic nephropathy [26]. Albuminuria can often be reduced, with microalbuminuria sometimes clearing completely [27]. Even patients with nephrotic-range proteinuria can benefit considerably from these drugs (Patient 6.2).

Patient 6.2 The Effect of ACE Inhibition on Diabetic Nephropathy
Mr. Archer had neglected his type 1 diabetes over many years and had failed to attend the diabetic clinic for long periods. He had developed peripheral and autonomic neuropathy, and suffered from postural hypotension and severe nocturnal and gustatory sweating.

He was persuaded to attend clinic by his partner who was increasingly concerned about his health. His blood pressure was high when seated (164/84 mmHg) but low when he stood up (90/54). He had very swollen legs, nephrotic-range proteinuria; protein:creatinine ratio = 1148 mg/mmol (11,000 mg/g), and hypoalbuminaemia (21 g/L; 2.1 g/dL). In other words, he had the nephrotic syndrome. His eGFR had dropped considerably compared to the result 2 years earlier (Fig. 6.5).

Because of the apparent suddenness of the loss of kidney function, a renal biopsy was performed. It showed typical features of diabetic nephropathy (Figs. 6.6 and 6.7).

The ACE inhibitor ramipril was started, at a modest dose of 5 mg daily. He had not previously taken this class of drug.

Over the following month, the rate of loss of albumin in his urine reduced to levels that could be matched by synthesis in his liver. As a result, his serum albumin concentration returned to normal, i.e. he was no longer nephrotic.

The rate of decline in his eGFR slowed dramatically, from 30 mL/min/1.73 m^2 per year to 8 mL/min/1.73 m^2 per year (Fig. 6.8).

He eventually reached end-stage kidney failure and had a combined kidney and pancreas transplant, which transformed his health.

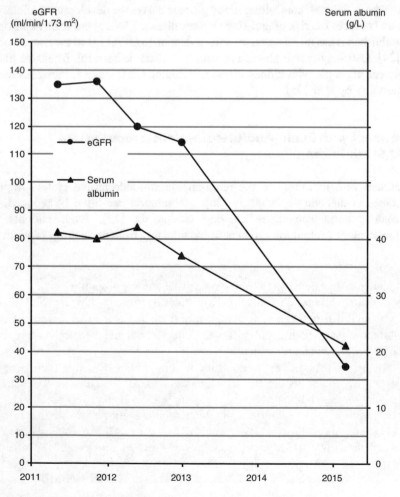

Fig. 6.5 Rapid decline in GFR, 30 mL/min/1.73 m^2 per year, and drop in serum albumin due to diabetic nephropathy with nephrotic syndrome

Fig. 6.6 Typical changes of diabetic nephropathy: diffuse glomerulosclerosis and hyalinosis. The walls of the glomerular capillaries are thickened and the mesangium is expanded. There is a nodular deposit of hyaline material at the vascular pole of the glomerulus (*arrow*). Haematoxylin and eosin ×200

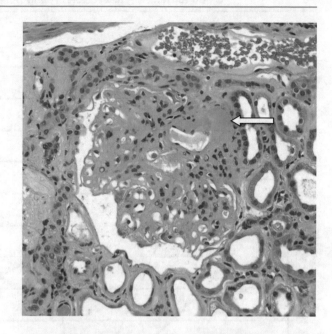

Fig. 6.7 Diffuse glomerular sclerosis of diabetes with Kimmelstiel-Wilson nodules, thickening of the glomerular basement membrane and focal hyalinosis. Silver ×200

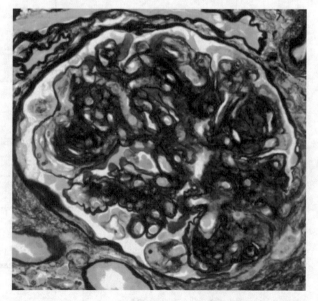

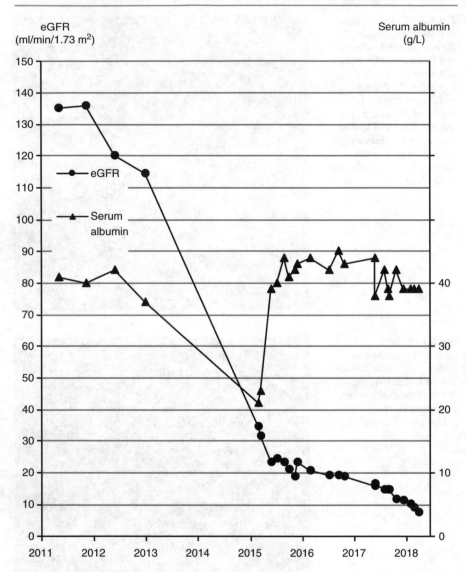

Fig. 6.8 Slowing in the rate of decline in eGFR to 8 mL/min/1.73 m² per year with restoration in serum albumin to normal following ACE inhibitor treatment, started in 2015

Treatment with Sodium–Glucose Cotransporter-2 (SGLT2) Inhibitors

Ninety-eight percent of glucose in the glomerular filtrate is reabsorbed by sodium–glucose cotransporter-2 (SGLT2) in proximal tubular cells. Inhibitors of SGLT2, identified by the name '-agliflozin', lower blood glucose by inhibiting its reabsorption in the proximal tubule. The threshold concentration at which glucose reabsorption is saturated and hence lost into the urine is reduced from 10 mmol/L

(180 mg/dL) to 2–7 mmol/L (40–120 mg/dL). Blood glucose concentration therefore falls towards this lower threshold level. Body weight also falls [28].

When SGLT2 is inhibited, increased amounts of both glucose and sodium flow into the distal convoluted tubule. The juxtaglomerular apparatus interprets this as indicating that glomerular perfusion has increased and so causes vasoconstriction of the afferent arteriole through autoregulation. This reduces intraglomerular pressure and leads to a short term drop in GFR. In addition, levels of angiotensin II and atrial natriuretic peptide drop, and there is a decrease in inflammation and an increase in oxygenation of the kidney, which may reduce tissue fibrosis.

Whatever their exact mechanism, SGLT2 inhibitors lead to big improvements in cardiovascular and kidney outcomes, over and above the effect of RAAS inhibitors. Using canagliflozin, the rate of adverse outcomes is reduced by about a third and the number of patients needed to be treated for 2.5 years to prevent one reaching either end-stage kidney disease, a doubling of serum creatinine, or a kidney or cardiovascular death is only 22 [29].

Atherosclerosis

Atherosclerotic cardiovascular disease, such as angina, myocardial infarction or stroke, is strongly associated with the development of kidney disease. Similarly, patients with kidney disease are much more likely to develop cardiovascular disease.

When atherosclerosis affects the renal arterial circulation, there may be diffuse narrowing of the intrarenal arterial tree and/or a stenosis of one or more renal arteries (Figs. 6.9 and 6.10).

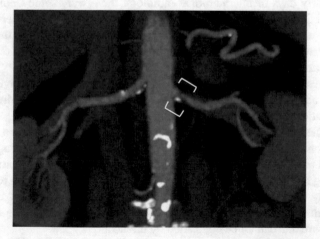

Fig. 6.9 CT angiogram of the abdominal vessels showing a left renal artery stenosis—image taken in the arterial phase. Contrast reveals the blood flowing in the arteries and veins. There are calcified atherosclerotic plaques in the aorta, renal arteries and other vessels. The calcium is in the wall of the arteries that are otherwise not seen and so appears outside the blood in the lumen. There is a narrowing in the lumen near the origin of the left renal artery at the site of a calcified plaque (*brackets*). The left kidney appears smaller than the right

Fig. 6.10 3D
reconstruction of the CT
scan in Fig. 6.9 showing
the stenosis more clearly
(*brackets*). The column of
blood in the left renal
artery is narrower than in
the right

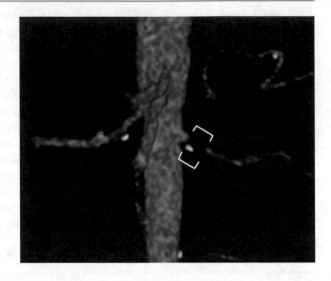

Renal Artery Stenosis

Renal artery stenosis usually causes high blood pressure and reduced kidney function. Less commonly it causes sudden pulmonary oedema despite left ventricular function being well preserved. This is called flash pulmonary oedema.

The loss of kidney function is not proportional to the degree of narrowing of the renal artery. However, as the artery becomes completely occluded, GFR declines (Fig. 6.11).

In the early days of interventional radiology there were some impressive case reports of patients with sudden occlusion of the renal arteries who underwent angioplasty and recovered their kidney function (Fig. 6.12). This led to the hope that angioplasty and stenting of narrowed but not occluded renal arteries would improve blood pressure and halt the decline in kidney function.

Unfortunately, a number of clinical trials have since shown that angioplasty and stenting of atherosclerotic renal artery stenosis does not improve kidney function and most patients continue to require antihypertensive drugs [30].

Atherosclerosis of the renal artery is usually associated with more widespread disease of smaller renal arteries and with glomerulosclerosis. Widening of the stenosed renal artery does not improve the more distal disease. It also carries the risk of damaging the arterial wall, causing cholesterol crystal embolisation to the kidney or occluding the artery completely (Patient 6.3). Angioplasty is now reserved for patients with flash pulmonary oedema, rapidly worsening kidney function or high blood pressure that cannot be controlled by medication.

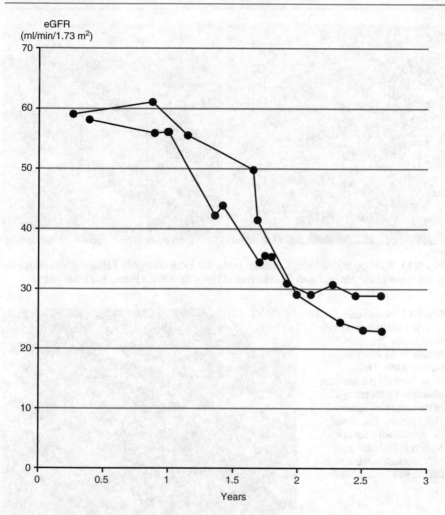

Fig. 6.11 eGFR graphs from two patients with peripheral vascular disease affecting their lower limbs. Their eGFR fell by half over 1 year. In both patients, imaging showed that one kidney had atrophied due to complete occlusion of the renal artery

The renal arteries can be narrowed by a non-atherosclerotic disease—fibromuscular dysplasia. This is much less common, affects women between 40 and 60 years of age and often involves the carotid arteries [31]. It usually presents with headache and hypertension that cannot be controlled with medication. It rarely causes loss of kidney function. Unlike atherosclerotic disease, it responds well to angioplasty or surgery.

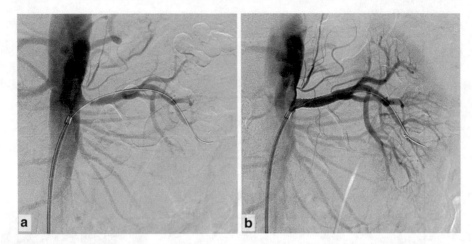

Fig. 6.12 Arteriograms showing a catheter in the left renal artery (**a**). Following balloon angioplasty, a stent has been deployed (**b**). The arterial blood flow to the kidney has improved

Fig. 6.13 A cholesterol crystal embolism in a small renal artery. The elastic lamina of the artery is stained black. The cholesterol crystal has been dissolved by the processing of the specimen, leaving a cleft (*arrow*). The crystal has stimulated a foreign body reaction with giant cells, occluding the artery. Elastic Van Gieson ×200

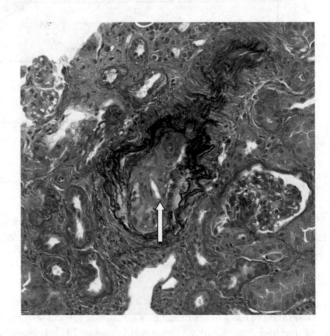

Cholesterol Crystal Embolisation

Passing a catheter along an atheromatous artery, such as during a coronary angiogram, carries the risk of destabilising atheromatous plaques. If they lie above the renal arteries, cholesterol crystals are carried downstream to the kidneys where they lodge in the glomeruli. The kidney damage this causes progresses over a few weeks or months as cholesterol crystals are repeatedly released into the circulation, and a foreign body reaction to the crystals causes further occlusion of the vessel lumen (Fig. 6.13). Less often, massive embolism causes acute kidney injury due to renal infarction (Fig. 18.24).

Patient 6.3 Cholesterol Crystal Embolisation

Mrs. Simpson, aged 86, was admitted as an emergency with chest pain. An ECG showed ST elevation in the inferior leads. Coronary angiography via the right femoral artery showed a stenosis of the left circumflex artery which was stented. Two days later she had another episode of chest pain with ST elevation in leads I, II and V6. Repeat coronary angiography showed a sub-acute stent thrombosis. This was treated with balloon angioplasty and dual antiplatelet therapy using aspirin and ticagrelor. A CT scan showed an atheromatous aorta with a 4.5 cm diameter infrarenal aneurysm.

Over the following 3 months her eGFR declined and the full blood count showed varying degrees of eosinophilia (Fig. 6.14).

Serum complement C3 was low (0.61 g/L, normal range 0.83–1.93); C4 was normal. CRP was modestly elevated (maximum 68 mg/L), in parallel with the eosinophil count. Autoantibodies were not present. Her urine contained no protein, blood, white cells or casts. All these features are consistent with cholesterol crystal embolisation to the kidneys.

She developed an extremely painful dusky rash over her feet and a necrotic little toe (Fig. 6.15). Peripheral pulses were normal. The appearances are characteristic of cholesterol embolisation—so called 'trash feet' with 'blue toe syndrome' and livedo reticularis, a blue network-like discolouration.

The very high eosinophil count and low complement C3 suggests that the kidney disease was linked to an inflammatory response to the crystals, occluding the renal arterioles.

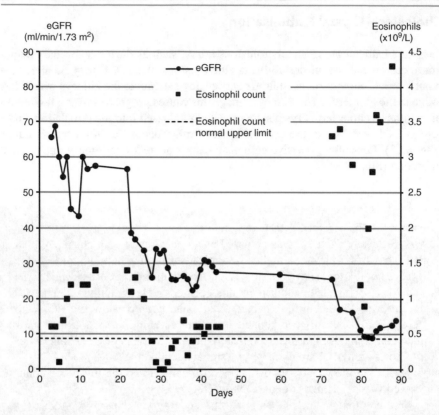

Fig. 6.14 Changes in eGFR and eosinophil count following two coronary angiography procedures

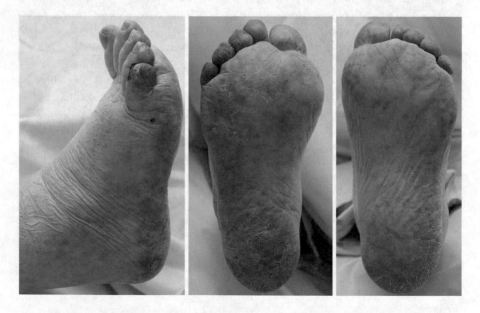

Fig. 6.15 Typical appearances of 'trash feet' due to cholesterol crystal embolisation

Liver Disease: Hepatorenal Syndrome

Patients with liver cirrhosis and portal hypertension have vasodilation of the splanchnic arteries, mediated by vasodilatory factors such as prostaglandins and nitric oxide. In the early stages of cirrhosis, cardiac output is increased because of the decrease in cardiac afterload due to this vasodilatation and to stimulation of the sympathetic nervous system. However, as the disease progresses, cardiac output cannot increase sufficiently, leading to a decline in blood pressure and kidney blood flow.

Cirrhosis is also an inflammatory state, mainly due to alteration in the permeability of the intestinal mucosa allowing bacteria and genes that encode inflammatory molecules to enter the circulation. The inflammation further stimulates vasodilatation.

Low arterial pressure stimulates the sympathetic nervous system, the renin-angiotensin-aldosterone system, and production of antidiuretic hormone (vasopressin). This leads to vasoconstriction, especially within the kidneys, a fall in GFR, salt and water retention, and ascites—the hepatorenal syndrome [32].

Treatment in the early stages of the hepatorenal syndrome aims to reverse the effects of vasodilation using vasoconstrictor agents, in particular terlipressin, and albumin. It is important, although not always easy, to make a correct diagnosis of the cause of acute kidney injury in someone with cirrhosis as vasoconstrictor treatment may make acute tubular necrosis worse.

The only cure for the hepatorenal syndrome is a liver transplant.

Chronic Infection and Inflammation

Long-term stimulation of the immune system can lead to a range of glomerular diseases. Chronic bacterial infections (e.g. tuberculosis, bronchiectasis and osteomyelitis) and inflammatory diseases (e.g. rheumatoid arthritis and Crohn's disease) stimulate the production of acute-phase proteins including serum amyloid A protein. Over years, this protein can accumulate in tissues such as blood vessels, nerves and kidneys to cause AA-amyloidosis. Deposition in glomerular membranes causes heavy proteinuria or the nephrotic syndrome.

Chronic viral infections can cause specific glomerular diseases. Chronic hepatitis B infection is associated with membranous nephropathy and mesangiocapillary glomerulonephritis (also called membranoproliferative glomerulonephritis) [33]. Persistence of hepatitis C virus can stimulate B-lymphocytes to produce mixed cryoglobulins that are deposited in capillaries including the glomerulus. This is associated with a vasculitic skin rash and the nephritic syndrome, with fibrinoid necrosis of glomeruli [34].

HIV-associated nephropathy (HIVAN) can present with nephrotic syndrome or renal failure. Renal biopsy usually shows focal segmental glomerulosclerosis (FSGS) although other histological changes have been reported [35]. The mechanism differs from hepatitis viruses in that the HIV damages the podocytes causing proteinuria, nephrotic syndrome and glomerulosclerosis, and the tubular cells causing kidney failure.

Before highly active antiretroviral therapy became available, HIVAN progressed rapidly to end-stage kidney disease. This is now much less common outside sub-Saharan Africa, and the risk of kidney failure is more closely linked to metabolic and cardiovascular risk factors. Patients with genetic risk factors such as the APOL1 gene have a worse prognosis.

Tenofovir disoproxil fumarate (TDF), a commonly used antiretroviral drug, is associated with a decline in GFR and with proximal tubular damage, causing a type of Fanconi syndrome [36].

References

1. Bowe B, Xie Y, Li T, Yan Y, Xian H, Al-Aly Z. Particulate matter air pollution and the risk of incident CKD and progression to ESRD. J Am Soc Nephrol. 2018;29(1):218–30. https://doi.org/10.1681/ASN.2017030253. Epub 2017 Sep 21. https://jasn.asnjournals.org/content/jnephrol/29/1/218.full.pdf.
2. Lew QJ, Jafar TH, Koh HW, Jin A, Chow KY, Yuan JM, Koh WP. Red meat intake and risk of ESRD. J Am Soc Nephrol. 2017;28(1):304–12. https://doi.org/10.1681/ASN.2016030248. https://jasn.asnjournals.org/content/28/1/304.long.
3. Kelly JT, Palmer SC, Wai SN, Ruospo M, Carrero JJ, Campbell KL, Strippoli GF. Healthy dietary patterns and risk of mortality and ESRD in CKD: a meta-analysis of cohort studies. Clin J Am Soc Nephrol. 2017;12(2):272–9. https://doi.org/10.2215/CJN.06190616. Epub 2016 Dec 8. https://cjasn.asnjournals.org/content/12/2/272.long.
4. Bach KE, Kelly JT, Palmer SC, Khalesi S, Strippoli GFM, Campbell KL. Healthy dietary patterns and incidence of CKD—a meta-analysis of cohort studies. Clin J Am Soc Nephrol. 2019;14(10):1441–9. https://doi.org/10.2215/CJN.00530119. https://cjasn.asnjournals.org/content/early/2019/09/23/CJN.00530119.full.
5. Kim H, Caulfield LE, Garcia-Larsen V, Steffen LM, Grams ME, Coresh J, Rebholz CM. Plant-based diets and incident CKD and kidney function. Clin J Am Soc Nephrol. 2019;14(5):682–91. https://doi.org/10.2215/CJN.12391018. Epub 2019 Apr 25. https://cjasn.asnjournals.org/content/clinjasn/14/5/682.full.pdf.
6. Bigotte Vieira M, Magriço R, Viegas Dias C, Leitão L, Neves JS. Caffeine consumption and mortality in chronic kidney disease: a nationally representative analysis. Nephrol Dial Transplant. 2019;34(6):974–80. https://doi.org/10.1093/ndt/gfy234. https://academic.oup.com/ndt/article/34/6/974/5063554.
7. Hu EA, Selvin E, Grams ME, Steffen LM, Coresh J, Rebholz CM. Coffee consumption and incident kidney disease: results from the Atherosclerosis Risk in Communities (ARIC) Study. Am J Kidney Dis. 2018;72(2):214–22. https://doi.org/10.1053/j.ajkd.2018.01.030. https://www.ajkd.org/article/S0272-6386(18)30109-4/fulltext.
8. Rebholz CM, Grams ME, Steffen LM, Crews DC, Anderson CA, Bazzano LA, Coresh J, Appel LJ. Diet soda consumption and risk of incident end stage renal disease. Clin J Am Soc Nephrol. 2017;12(1):79–86. https://doi.org/10.2215/CJN.03390316. https://cjasn.asnjournals.org/content/12/1/79.long.
9. Ricardo AC, Knutson K, Chen J, Appel LJ, Bazzano L, Carmona-Powell E, Cohan J, Kurella Tamura M, Steigerwalt S, Thornton JD, Weir M, Turek NF, Rahman M, Van Cauter E, Lash JP, Chronic Renal Insufficiency Cohort (CRIC) Study Investigators. The association of sleep duration and quality with CKD progression. J Am Soc Nephrol. 2017;28(12):3708–15. https://doi.org/10.1681/ASN.2016121288. https://jasn.asnjournals.org/content/28/12/3708.long.
10. Sorensen C, Garcia-Trabanino R. A new era of climate medicine—addressing heat-triggered renal disease. N Engl J Med. 2019;381:693–6. https://doi.org/10.1056/NEJMp1907859. https://www.nejm.org/doi/full/10.1056/NEJMp1907859?query=TOC.

11. Raymond NT, Paul O'Hare J, Bellary S, Kumar S, Jones A, Barnett AH, UKADS Study Group. Comparative risk of microalbuminuria and proteinuria in UK residents of south Asian and white European ethnic background with type 2 diabetes: a report from UKADS. Curr Med Res Opin. 2011;27(Suppl 3):47–55. https://doi.org/10.1185/03007995.2011.614937. http://informahealthcare.com/doi/abs/10.1185/03007995.2011.614937.

12. Alicic RZ, Rooney MT, Tuttle KR. Diabetic kidney disease. Challenges, progress, and possibilities. Clin J Am Soc Nephrol. 2017;12(12):2032–45. https://www.ncbi.nlm.nih.gov/pmc/articles/PMC5718284/.

13. Molitch ME, Gao X, Bebu I, de Boer IH, Lachin J, Paterson A, Perkins B, Saenger AK, Steffes M, Zinman B, Diabetes Control and Complications Trial/Epidemiology of Diabetes Interventions and Complications (DCCT/EDIC) Research Group. Early glomerular hyperfiltration and long-term kidney outcomes in Type 1 diabetes: the DCCT/EDIC experience. Clin J Am Soc Nephrol. 2019;14(6):854–61. https://doi.org/10.2215/CJN.14831218. https://cjasn.asnjournals.org/content/clinjasn/early/2019/05/22/CJN.14831218.full.pdf.

14. Tonneijck L, Muskiet MH, Smits MM, van Bommel EJ, Heerspink HJ, van Raalte DH, Joles JA. Glomerular hyperfiltration in diabetes: mechanisms, clinical significance, and treatment. J Am Soc Nephrol. 2017;28(4):1023–39. https://doi.org/10.1681/ASN.2016060666. Epub 2017 Jan 31. https://www.ncbi.nlm.nih.gov/pmc/articles/PMC5373460/.

15. Tummalapalli SL, Shlipak MG. Hyperfiltration. Clin J Am Soc Nephrol. 2019. https://doi.org/10.2215/CJN.05330419. https://cjasn.asnjournals.org/content/clinjasn/early/2019/05/22/CJN.05330419.full.pdf.

16. Skupien J, Warram JH, Smiles AM, Stanton RC, Krolewski AS. Patterns of estimated glomerular filtration rate decline leading to end-stage renal disease in Type 1 diabetes. Diabetes Care. 2016;39(12):2262–9. Epub 2016 Sep 19. https://www.ncbi.nlm.nih.gov/pmc/articles/PMC5127236/.

17. Krolewski AS, Skupien J, Rossing P, Warram JH. Fast renal decline to ESRD: an unrecognized feature of nephropathy in diabetes. Kidney Int. 2017;91(6):1300–11. https://www.ncbi.nlm.nih.gov/pmc/articles/PMC5429989/.

18. de Boer IH, DCCT/EDIC Research Group. Kidney disease and related findings in the diabetes control and complications trial/epidemiology of diabetes interventions and complications study. Diabetes Care. 2014;37(1):24–30. https://doi.org/10.2337/dc13-2113. http://care.diabetesjournals.org/content/37/1/24.full.

19. Salem RM, Todd JN, Sandholm N, et al. SUMMIT Consortium, DCCT/EDIC Research Group, GENIE Consortium. Genome-wide association study of diabetic kidney disease highlights biology involved in glomerular basement membrane collagen. J Am Soc Nephrol. 2019;30(10):2000–16. https://doi.org/10.1681/ASN.2019030218. https://jasn.asnjournals.org/content/jnephrol/early/2019/09/18/ASN.2019030218.full.pdf.

20. Coca SG, Ismail-Beigi F, Haq N, Krumholz HM, Parikh CR. Role of intensive glucose control in development of renal end points in type 2 diabetes mellitus: systematic review and meta-analysis intensive glucose control in type 2 diabetes. Arch Intern Med. 2012;172(10):761–9. https://doi.org/10.1001/archinternmed.2011.2230. http://archinte.jamanetwork.com/article.aspx?articleid=1170041.

21. Wong MG, Perkovic V, Chalmers J, Woodward M, Li Q, Cooper ME, Hamet P, Harrap S, Heller S, MacMahon S, Mancia G, Marre M, Matthews D, Neal B, Poulter N, Rodgers A, Williams B, Zoungas S, ADVANCE-ON Collaborative Group. Long-term benefits of intensive glucose control for preventing end-stage kidney disease: ADVANCE-ON. Diabetes Care. 2016;39(5):694–700. https://doi.org/10.2337/dc15-2322. Epub 2016 Mar 22. http://care.diabetesjournals.org/content/39/5/694.long.

22. Mottl AK, Buse JB, Ismail-Beigi F, Sigal RJ, Pedley CF, Papademetriou V, Simmons DL, Katz L, Mychaleckyj JC, Craven TE. Long-term effects of intensive glycemic and blood pressure control and fenofibrate use on kidney outcomes. Clin J Am Soc Nephrol. 2018;13(11):1693–702. https://doi.org/10.2215/CJN.06200518. Epub 2018 Oct 25. https://cjasn.asnjournals.org/content/13/11/1693.long.

23. Ruospo M, Saglimbene VM, Palmer SC, et al. Glucose targets for preventing diabetic kidney disease and its progression. Cochrane Database Syst Rev. 2017;6:CD010137. https://www. cochranelibrary.com/cdsr/doi/10.1002/14651858.CD010137.pub2/full.

24. Reaven PD, Emanuele NV, Wiitala WL, Bahn GD, Reda DJ, McCarren M, Duckworth WC, Hayward RA, VADT Investigators. Intensive glucose control in patients with Type 2 diabetes—15-year follow-up. N Engl J Med. 2019;380(23):2215–24. https://doi.org/10.1056/ NEJMoa1806802. https://www.nejm.org/doi/full/10.1056/NEJMoa1806802?url_ver=Z39.88-2003&rfr_id=ori:rid:crossref.org&rfr_dat=cr_pub%3dpubmed.

25. Papademetriou V, Lovato L, Doumas M, Nylen E, Mottl A, Cohen RM, Applegate WB, Puntakee Z, Yale JF, Cushman WC, ACCORD Study Group. Chronic kidney disease and intensive glycemic control increase cardiovascular risk in patients with type 2 diabetes. Kidney Int. 2015;87:649–59. https://doi.org/10.1038/ki.2014.296. http://www.nature.com/ki/journal/v87/ n3/full/ki2014296a.html.

26. Gregg EW, Li Y, Wang J, Burrows NR, Ali MK, Rolka D, Williams DE, Geiss L. Changes in diabetes-related complications in the United States, 1990–2010. N Engl J Med. 2014;370:1514–23. https://doi.org/10.1056/NEJMoa1310799. http://www.nejm.org/doi/ full/10.1056/NEJMx140023.

27. Andrésdóttir G, Jensen ML, Carstensen B, Parving HH, Hovind P, Hansen TW, Rossing P. Improved prognosis of diabetic nephropathy in type 1 diabetes. Kidney Int. 2015;87(2):417–26. https://doi.org/10.1038/ki.2014.206. http://www.nature.com/ki/journal/ v87/n2/abs/ki2014206a.html.

28. Ingelfinger JR, Rosen CJ. Clinical credence—SGLT2 inhibitors, diabetes, and chronic kidney disease. N Engl J Med. 2019;380(24):2371–3. https://doi.org/10.1056/NEJMe1904740. https://www.nejm.org/doi/full/10.1056/NEJMe1904740?url_ver=Z39.88-2003&rfr_ id=ori:rid:crossref.org&rfr_dat=cr_pub%3dpubmed.

29. Perkovic V, Jardine MJ, Neal B, Bompoint S, Heerspink HJL, Charytan DM, Edwards R, Agarwal R, Bakris G, Bull S, Cannon CP, Capuano G, Chu PL, de Zeeuw D, Greene T, Levin A, Pollock C, Wheeler DC, Yavin Y, Zhang H, Zinman B, Meininger G, Brenner BM, Mahaffey KW, CREDENCE Trial Investigators. Canagliflozin and renal outcomes in Type 2 diabetes and nephropathy. N Engl J Med. 2019;380(24):2295–306. https://www.nejm.org/doi/full/10.1056/ NEJMoa1811744.

30. Jennings CG, Houston JG, Severn A, Bell S, Mackenzie IS, MacDonald TM. Renal artery stenosis—when to screen, what to stent? Curr Atheroscler Rep. 2014;16(6):416. https://doi.org/10.1007/s11883-014-0416-2.   http://link.springer.com/article/10.1007/ s11883-014-0416-2/fulltext.html.

31. Escárcega RO, Mathur M, Franco JJ, Alkhouli M, Patel C, Singh K, Bashir R, Patil P. Nonatherosclerotic obstructive vascular diseases of the mesenteric and renal arteries. Clin Cardiol. 2014;37(11):700–6. https://doi.org/10.1002/clc.22305. Epub 2014 Aug 6. http:// onlinelibrary.wiley.com/doi/10.1002/clc.22305/pdf.

32. Francoz C, Durand F, Kahn JA, Genyk YS, Nadim MK. Hepatorenal syndrome. Clin J Am Soc Nephrol. 2019;14(5):774–81. https://doi.org/10.2215/CJN.12451018. https://cjasn.asnjour- nals.org/content/14/5/774.

33. Kupin WL. Viral-associated GN: hepatitis B and other viral infections. Clin J Am Soc Nephrol. 2017;12(9):1529–33. https://doi.org/10.2215/CJN.09180816. Epub 2016 Oct 18. https://cjasn. asnjournals.org/content/12/9/1529.long.

34. Kupin WL. Viral-associated GN: hepatitis C and HIV. Clin J Am Soc Nephrol. 2017;12(8):1337–42. https://doi.org/10.2215/CJN.04320416. Epub 2016 Oct 24. https://cjasn. asnjournals.org/content/12/8/1337.long.

35. Phair J, Palella F. Renal disease in HIV-infected individuals. Curr Opin HIV AIDS. 2011;6(4):285–9. https://doi.org/10.1097/COH.0b013e3283476bc3. http://www.ncbi. nlm.nih.gov/pmc/articles/PMC3266688/.

36. de Seigneux S, Lucas GM. Renal injury and human immunodeficiency virus: what remains after 30 years? Nephrol Dial Transplant. 2019:gfz162. https://doi.org/10.1093/ndt/gfz162. https://academic.oup.com/ndt/advance-article/doi/10.1093/ndt/gfz162/5549238.

Are You Pregnant or Planning a Pregnancy? How Pregnancy Affects the Kidneys and Vice Versa

7

Pregnancy in a woman who has or has had kidney disease poses risks to both the baby and the mother [1]. These issues can be a significant emotional burden [2]. If, after consideration of the risks, a woman decides that she does not wish to become pregnant, it is important that contraceptive advice tailored to her circumstances and kidney disease is given [3].

Risks to the Baby

Overall, the risk of a worse outcome for the baby is more than doubled in women: with chronic kidney disease [1]; who are born with only one kidney [4]; or who have recovered from a previous episode of acute kidney injury [5]. Uncontrolled hypertension can slow the growth of the foetus and result in an infant that is small for gestational age.

Before a planned pregnancy, drugs that may damage a developing foetus should be reviewed. Drugs commonly used in patients with kidney disease that may be teratogenic include angiotensin-converting enzyme inhibitors, angiotensin II receptor blockers, and immunosuppressive drugs such as mycophenolate.

Angiotensin converting enzyme inhibitors and angiotensin receptor blockers can cause renal tubular agenesis and other abnormalities if taken during the second or third trimester and should be stopped as soon as possible after conception [6]. The risk of teratogenicity must be weighed against the risk posed to the mother by stopping the drug.

© Springer Nature Switzerland AG 2020
H. C. Rayner et al., *Understanding Kidney Diseases*,
https://doi.org/10.1007/978-3-030-43027-6_7

Risks to the Mother

The GFR of normal kidneys increases by 50% over the first 3 months of a pregnancy (Fig. 7.1). In someone with a well-functioning kidney transplant the GFR will increase by up to this amount, proving that this effect is not mediated by the kidney's nerve supply. When a pregnant woman shows no fall in serum creatinine, this is a sign that her nephrons are unable to 'hyperfilter' and she is likely to have underlying chronic kidney disease.

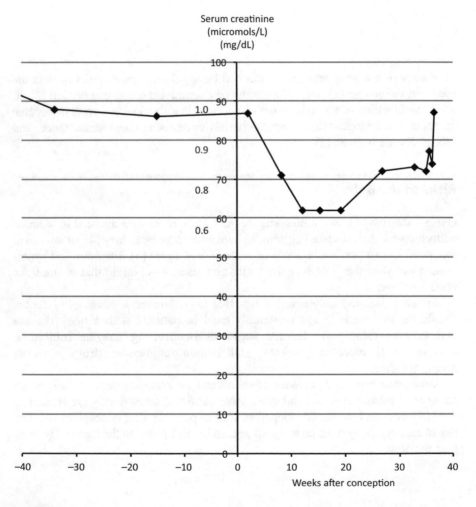

Fig. 7.1 Changes in serum creatinine during pregnancy in a woman with a kidney transplant. The baby was delivered by caesarean section. The last data point is the serum creatinine measured the day after delivery

Hyperfiltration due to pregnancy can damage already diseased glomeruli. The risk increases in proportion to the stage of CKD before pregnancy, whatever the cause of the kidney disease.

If the eGFR is more than 60 mL/min/1.73 m² the outlook is good, including with a kidney transplant. If the patient has hypertension or proteinuria there is an increased risk of pre-eclampsia and loss of kidney function. Women with vesico-ureteric reflux have an increased risk of urinary tract infections during pregnancy and may benefit from daily prophylactic antibiotics.

If the eGFR is less than 40 mL/min/1.73 m² or there is heavy proteinuria—more than 1 g per day, i.e. protein:creatinine ratio >100 mg/mmol (1000 mg/g)—the rate of decline in GFR is accelerated by pregnancy, and the time to end-stage kidney failure is shortened [7].

With CKD stages 4 and 5, the likelihood of becoming pregnant is significantly reduced as ovulation is irregular or absent. If conception does occur, the foetus usually does not grow at the normal rate and is either born prematurely or stillborn. Successful pregnancy is a rare but wonderful event for a woman on dialysis.

Pre-eclampsia

Pregnancy itself can cause kidney disease; a condition called pre-eclampsia [8]. This presents with hypertension, peripheral oedema and proteinuria, usually in the last 6 weeks of pregnancy. If it occurs earlier than 34 weeks the outcomes are worse. The clinical severity of the kidney disease can vary from just hypertension and proteinuria to severe acute kidney injury requiring dialysis due to thrombotic thrombocytopaenic purpura (TTP).

The primary cause of pre-eclampsia is a dysfunctional placenta that releases anti-angiogenic factors into the mother's circulation. These factors damage vascular endothelial cells. The ratio between the anti-angiogenic factor sFlt-1 (soluble FMS-like tyrosine kinase-1) and the angiogenic factor PGF (placental growth factor) increases before the onset of the pre-eclampsia. This ratio can help distinguish between preeclampsia and other causes of proteinuria and hypertension, and guide when to intervene in the pregnancy [9].

The risk of pre-eclampsia is higher in first and twin pregnancies, where the level of anti-angiogenic factors is higher, and in women with hypertension, diabetes and obesity, where the endothelial cells are more susceptible to these factors. The risk is increased by about 5 times in women who have recovered from a previous episode of acute kidney injury [5]. Antiplatelet therapy with low-dose aspirin (75 mg daily) protects the endothelium and reduces the risk of pre-eclampsia by 10% [10].

In women who have had pre-eclampsia in a previous pregnancy the risk of it recurring is at least 15%. This increases to over 50% with increasing severity of the previous episode.

Proteinuria due to pre-eclampsia usually clears after the pregnancy. If it is still present after 3 months, another kidney disease may be present.

Pre-eclampsia increases the risk of long-term hypertension by up to four times, doubles the risk of ischaemic heart disease, stroke and venous thromboembolism, and increases the risk of chronic kidney disease [11].

Patient 7.1 Assessing the Risk of Pregnancy in a Woman with Chronic Kidney Disease

Christine attended the renal clinic with her new partner at the age of 25. She was under follow up for reflux nephropathy, which she had inherited from her mother. She was desperate to have another baby.

In her first pregnancy 5 years previously she had had pre-eclampsia requiring an emergency caesarian section. During that pregnancy, her GFR had increased only slightly and had dropped during the episode of pre-eclampsia (Fig. 7.2).

Since then it had recovered and the proteinuria had returned to trace on dipstick testing. She was feeling well, not diabetic and had a body mass index of 22 kg/m^2. She was taking the calcium channel blocker amlodipine for high blood pressure that was well controlled.

The following factors that increase the risk of pre-eclampsia were discussed:

- Age older than 40
- First pregnancy
- History of pre-eclampsia
- New paternity
- Interval between pregnancies of less than 2 years or more than 10 years
- Multiple pregnancy e.g. twins
- Obesity
- Chronic conditions—high blood pressure, migraine, diabetes, kidney disease, thrombophilia, SLE

Everyone agreed that the risks to her and her baby were acceptable. A urine specimen was sent for culture and she was referred to the renal-antenatal clinic for follow up. She was delighted.

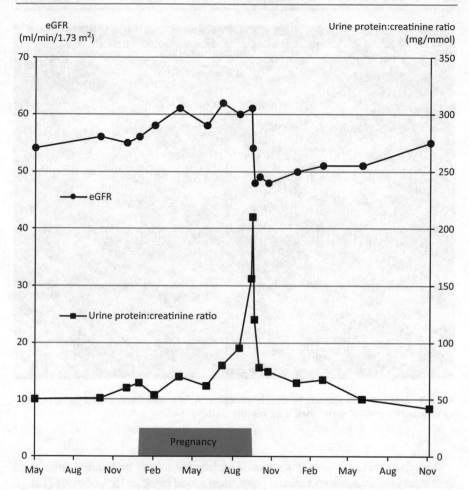

Fig. 7.2 The effect of pregnancy on eGFR and urine protein excretion in a lady with reflux nephropathy. Increasing proteinuria culminated in pre-eclampsia

Antenatal Diagnosis of Kidney and Urinary Tract Abnormalities

The introduction of routine ultrasound scanning during pregnancy has led to the diagnosis of kidney and urinary tract abnormalities in the foetus (Fig. 7.3). The incidence of these varies between 3 and 6 per 1000 pregnancies. Findings include transient or persistent dilatation of the urinary tract, cystic kidney abnormalities, agenesis of one or both kidneys, ectopic placement of kidneys, and bladder abnormalities.

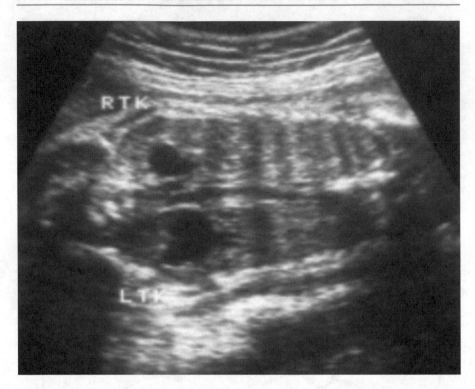

Fig. 7.3 Antenatal scan showing bilateral hydronephrosis. In a male foetus this raises the possibility of posterior urethral valves even if the bladder is empty

The abnormality is usually a sporadic finding but it may be familial, autosomal dominant inheritance with variable penetrance found in up to 15% of cases [12].

After birth, a neonate who is known to have had antenatal urinary tract dilatation must be examined carefully and checked to make sure they pass urine. Kidney function should be tested and an ultrasound scan formed within the first 2 days. If the first scan shows no dilatation, another scan should be done at 1 week of age as dilatation can be delayed due to the urine volume being low in the early days after birth (Patient 8.2). In male infants with hydronephrosis, the most important diagnosis to consider is posterior urethral valves (Fig. 7.4).

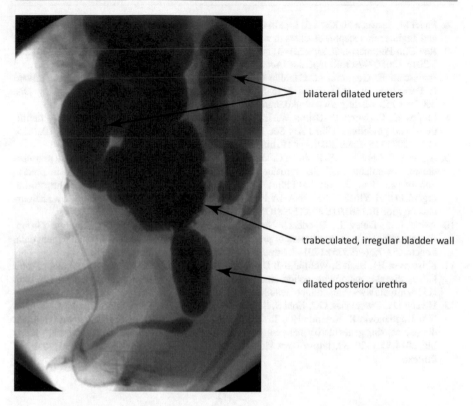

bilateral dilated ureters

trabeculated, irregular bladder wall

dilated posterior urethra

Fig. 7.4 Cystogram of an infant with showing grossly dilated ureters, a trabeculated bladder and a dilated posterior urethra, diagnostic of posterior urethral valves

References

1. Wiles KS, Nelson-Piercy C, Bramham K. Reproductive health and pregnancy in women with chronic kidney disease. Nat Rev Nephrol. 2018;14(3):165–84. https://doi.org/10.1038/nrneph.2017.187. Epub 2018 Jan 22. https://www.nature.com/articles/nrneph.2017.187.
2. Tong A, Jesudason S, Craig JC, Winkelmayer WC. Perspectives on pregnancy in women with chronic kidney disease: systematic review of qualitative studies. Nephrol Dial Transplant. 2015;30(4):652–61. https://doi.org/10.1093/ndt/gfu378. http://ndt.oxfordjournals.org/content/30/4/652.abstract.
3. Burgner A, Hladunewich MA. Contraception and CKD. Clin J Am Soc Nephrol. 2019. https://doi.org/10.2215/CJN.09770819. https://cjasn.asnjournals.org/content/clinjasn/early/2019/11/15/CJN.09770819.full.pdf.
4. Kendrick J, Holmen J, You Z, Smits G, Chonchol M. Association of unilateral renal agenesis with adverse outcomes in pregnancy: a matched cohort study. Am J Kidney Dis. 2017;70(4):506–11. https://www.ajkd.org/article/S0272-6386(17)30562-0/fulltext.
5. Tangren JS, Powe CE, Ankers E, Ecker J, Bramham K, Hladunewich MA, Karumanchi SA, Thadhani R. Pregnancy outcomes after clinical recovery from AKI. J Am Soc Nephrol. 2017;28(5):1566–74. https://doi.org/10.1681/ASN.2016070806. Epub 2016 Dec 22. https://jasn.asnjournals.org/content/28/5/1566.long.

6. Pucci M, Sarween N, Knox E, Lipkin G, Martin U. Angiotensin-converting enzyme inhibitors and angiotensin receptor blockers in women of childbearing age: risks versus benefits. Expert Rev Clin Pharmacol. 2015;8:221–31. https://www.tandfonline.com/doi/full/10.1586/1751243 3.2015.1005074?scroll=top&needAccess=true.
7. Imbasciati E, Gregorini G, Cabiddu G, Gammaro L, Ambroso G, Del Giudice A, Ravani P. Pregnancy in CKD stages 3 to 5: fetal and maternal outcomes. Am J Kidney Dis. 2007;49:753–62. http://www.ajkd.org/article/S0272-6386(07)00692-0/abstract.
8. Phipps E, Prasanna D, Brima W, Jim B. Preeclampsia: updates in pathogenesis, definitions, and guidelines. Clin J Am Soc Nephrol. 2016;11(6):1102–13. https://doi.org/10.2215/CJN.12081115. Epub 2016 Apr 19. https://cjasn.asnjournals.org/content/11/6/1102.
9. Agrawal S, Cerdeira AS, Redman C, Vatish M. Meta-analysis and systematic review to assess the role of soluble FMS-like tyrosine kinase-1 and placenta growth factor ratio in prediction of preeclampsia: the SaPPPhirE study. Hypertension. 2018;71(2):306–16. https://doi.org/10.1161/HYPERTENSIONAHA.117.10182. Epub 2017 Dec 11. https://www.ahajournals.org/doi/10.1161/HYPERTENSIONAHA.117.10182.
10. Askie LM, Duley L, Henderson-Smart DJ, Stewart LA, PARIS Collaborative Group. Antiplatelet agents for prevention of pre-eclampsia: a meta-analysis of individual patient data. Lancet. 2007;369(9575):1791–8. http://www.ncbi.nlm.nih.gov/pubmed/17512048.
11. Kristensen JH, Basit S, Wohlfahrt J, Damholt MB, Boyd HA. Pre-eclampsia and risk of later kidney disease: nationwide cohort study. BMJ. 2019;365:l1516. https://doi.org/10.1136/bmj.l1516. https://www.bmj.com/content/365/bmj.l1516.long.
12. Hwang DY, Dworschak GC, Kohl S, Saisawat P, Vivante A, Hilger AC, Reutter HM, Soliman NA, Bogdanovic R, Kehinde EO, Tasic V, Hildebrandt F. Mutations in 12 known dominant disease-causing genes clarify many congenital anomalies of the kidney and urinary tract. Kidney Int. 2014;85:1429–33. https://www.kidney-international.org/article/S0085-2538(15)56367-9/fulltext.

What Is Your Family History? The Molecular Genetics of Inherited Kidney Diseases

It is well known that some kidney diseases are inherited. It is less well known that someone with a family history of kidney failure has double the risk of kidney disease from a different cause and six times the risk of developing chronic kidney disease between 10 and 19 years of age [1]. So, it is important to ask about any family history of kidney disease and to document the family in a pedigree chart.

Parents with a positive family history should receive genetic counselling before conception to help them consider the risk of having an affected child. Counselling may be more difficult if the parents are unaffected carriers and also if there are cultural or language barriers. Mothers who are carriers of X-linked conditions generally have a mild phenotype and may be unaware of the risk to a male child. Autosomal recessive diseases are more common in consanguineous parents.

Our understanding of the environmental and genetic factors that lead to the increased risk is advancing rapidly. With modern molecular techniques, genetic testing is relatively simple [2]. However, interpretation of the results and the implications they have for someone's physical and psychological health can be more complex.

Knowing that you have inherited a kidney condition may allow you to prepare psychologically and physically for kidney failure. Alternatively it may cause prolonged anxiety about an uncertain prognosis. It may affect your ability to obtain insurance or a mortgage. Informing other family members that they may be at risk and advising whether or not they should be genetically tested is a delicate matter.

If someone has a disease caused by a mutation in a single gene, the predictive value of the mutation, the penetrance, is nearly 100%. However, the disease may appear at different ages and with differing severity. Furthermore, some single-gene diseases vary due to interaction between the abnormal gene and a mutation in a modifier gene.

In the United States, blacks have a nearly four times higher lifetime risk of end-stage kidney disease than whites [3]. This is partly due to variants in the gene coding for apolipoprotein L1 (APOL1). 13% of blacks have two copies of the APOL1 autosomal recessive variants G1 and G2, and genotypes G1/G1, G2/G2, and G1/G2 are

© Springer Nature Switzerland AG 2020
H. C. Rayner et al., *Understanding Kidney Diseases*,
https://doi.org/10.1007/978-3-030-43027-6_8

associated with end-stage kidney disease in people of African descent. These genotypes are uncommon in whites and have been conserved in evolution by providing increased resistance against *Trypanosoma brucei rhodesiense*.

Diseases caused by multiple mutations on different genes are much more common. They have a variable phenotype and are more affected by environmental factors. Genome-wide association studies have identified genes that confer an increased risk of hypertension and diabetic nephropathy, as well as vesico-ureteric reflux, focal segmental glomerulosclerosis (FSGS) and atypical haemolytic uraemic syndrome (aHUS) [4]. However, common genetic polymorphisms are not suitable for use as screening, diagnostic, or prognostic tools because the increased risk associated with having the genetic marker is very small compared with the underlying risk of kidney disease in the general population [5].

Genetic abnormalities are like experiments of nature. They have helped us understand how the kidneys work at a molecular level. We will describe the more common disorders in sequence along the nephron from the glomerulus to the ureter.

The Glomerulus

Alport Syndrome

Cecil Alport described a syndrome of hereditary nephritis with haematuria and deafness in a British family in 1927 [6]. He thought the nephritis was due to an infection but we now know that it and the deafness are due to a mutation of one of the type IV collagen genes. The abnormal collagen disrupts the structure of membranes in the glomerulus (Fig. 8.1) and in the organ of Corti in the cochlea of the ear.

Alport reported that: "The male members of a family tend to develop nephritis and deafness and do not as a rule survive. The females have deafness and haematuria and live to old age." Males are more severely affected than females because the type IV alpha 5 collagen gene is located on the X-chromosome and women are heterozygotes. Because women have two X-chromosomes, twice as many are affected. Affected women are commonly undiagnosed but 15–30% develop end-stage kidney failure by 60 years of age and often have hearing loss by middle age [7].

The presentation in males varies. As Alport reported: "The last couple of cases are interesting evidence of the variations in the course of nephritis. The kidneys of two members of the same family were attacked, apparently by the same organism, at the same time, and under exactly the same conditions. The elder brother contracted acute nephritis, which cleared up completely; the younger developed parenchymatous nephritis, passing into small white kidney, and ending in death."

Alport did not refer to the eye abnormalities that can accompany the syndrome: a misshapen lens (anterior lenticonus) and abnormal colouration of the retina. These rarely lead to loss of vision [8].

A number of conditions have been described within the Alport syndrome family, involving mutations of genes coding for different protein chains that together form

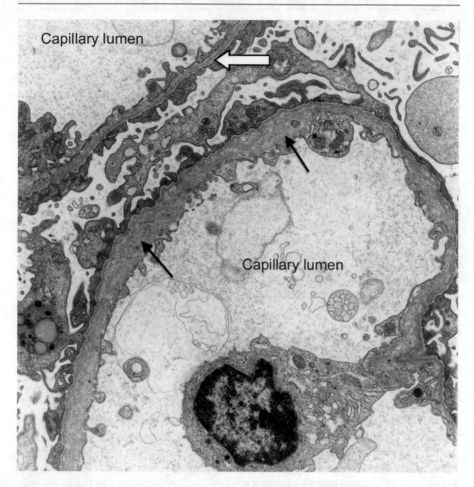

Fig. 8.1 Electron micrograph of a section through two glomerular capillaries in a child with Alport syndrome. The glomerular basement membrane in one capillary is abnormally thin (*white arrow*). The other is abnormally thick and the arrangement of collagen fibres is disorganised (*black arrows*) showing a 'basket-weave' pattern

type IV collagen. Eighty-five percent are X-linked recessive. Fifteen percent have autosomal recessive inheritance—homozygotes have the syndrome whereas heterozygote carriers are unaffected or have thin glomerular basement membrane nephropathy. A small number show autosomal dominant inheritance, heterozygotes being affected.

Congenital Nephrotic Syndrome

Numerous genetic abnormalities, both dominant and recessive, have been described in children with congenital nephrotic syndrome. The age of onset depends upon the

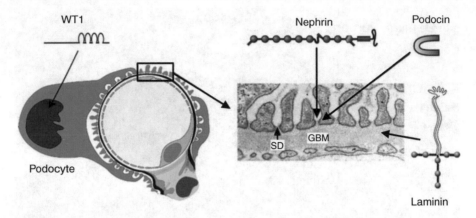

Fig. 8.2 Cross-section of a glomerular capillary (*left*) and electron microscopy image of a normal capillary wall (*right*). WT1 is a transcription factor important for podocyte function. Nephrin is a major component of the slit diaphragm (SD) connecting podocyte foot processes. Podocin is an adapter protein located intracellularly in the SD area. Laminin is a major structural protein of the glomerular basement membrane (GBM). Genetic mutations in these proteins lead to congenital nephrotic syndrome. (From [9])

gene affected and whether one or both alleles are affected. If the presentation is before 3 months of age, the cause is invariably genetic [9]. The nephrotic syndrome is steroid-resistant and often progresses to kidney failure. Unlike non-genetic causes, genetic steroid-resistant nephrotic syndrome does not recur after kidney transplantation [10].

The gene mutations lead to abnormal proteins in the basement membrane or the podocytes and have helped identify the role of these proteins in the glomerular filtration barrier. For example, in the Finnish type of congenital nephrotic syndrome there is an abnormality of nephrin, a transmembrane protein in the slit diaphragm between the podocyte foot processes. Other causes are mutations in the genes coding for laminin and podocin (Fig. 8.2).

Fabry or Anderson–Fabry Disease

The German dermatologist Johannes Fabry and English surgeon William Anderson independently described this disease in 1898. It is one of the lysosomal storage diseases caused by a mutation of the alpha-galactosidase A (*GLA*) gene. This enzyme normally breaks down glycosphingolipids, particularly globotriaosylceramide (Gb3). Deficiency or absence of this enzyme leads to accumulation of Gb3 in cells throughout the body, including the glomeruli (Fig. 8.3) and kidney tubules, the skin, brain, gut, peripheral nerves, cornea and heart.

Males are affected earlier and more severely than females due to the X-linked inheritance. Patients often present early in childhood with neuropathic pain

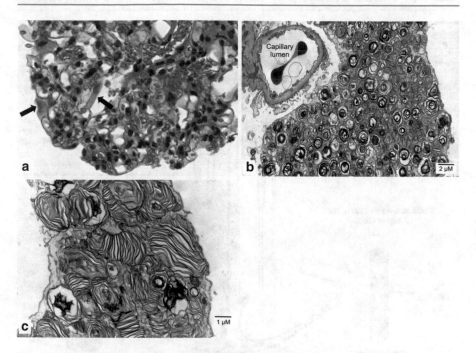

Fig. 8.3 (a) Light microscopy, showing vacuolation (oval bodies) in podocytes (arrows) cause by deposition of glycosphingolipid. Haematoxylin and eosin ×400. (**b, c**) Electron microscopy, showing inclusions of glycosphingolipid in lysosomes—round myelin figures (**b**) and parallel layered zebra bodies in a podocyte, detached from the glomerular capillary (**c**). These are not pathognomonic of Fabry disease so genetic testing is need for confirmation. EM ×3000 and ×7000

(acroparaesthesia) in the extremities, and may be intolerant of extreme heat or cold. They may have angiokeratomas, like tiny blood blisters, around the umbilicus and in the 'underpants area', and the feet may be unable to sweat. Other symptoms include premature cardio- and cerebrovascular disease, heart block and restrictive cardiomyopathy. The variety of symptoms and atypical forms of the disease can make diagnosis very difficult.

Up to 20% of females and 50% of males develop kidney disease, leading to end-stage kidney failure under the age of 60 years in males [11]. Deposition in glomeruli can cause proteinuria (Fig. 8.3) but progressive kidney failure can occur with only haematuria or normal urine and hypertension. Tubular cell damage can cause nephrogenic diabetes insipidus. The finding of multiple parapelvic cysts on a kidney scan suggests Fabry disease.

Diagnosis is made in males by measuring the serum level of alpha-galactosidase A. Some males and most females have near normal levels so genetic testing for abnormal variants of the *GLA* gene is needed if the level of alpha-galactosidase A is normal. Early diagnosis is important as treatment with fortnightly intravenous enzyme replacement therapy can slow or prevent disease progression [12].

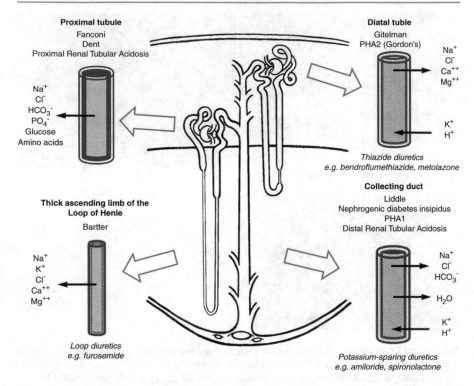

Fig. 8.4 Genetic diseases of the nephron, the normal transport functions that are affected and the sites of action of the main classes of diuretics [13]

The Tubules

Figure 8.4 summarises the main genetic diseases affecting the nephron.

The Proximal Tubule

The majority of reabsorption and secretion of solutes occurs in the proximal tubule [14]. The surface area of the tubule is maximised by the brush border microvilli on the epithelial cell surface. The main features of the genetic disorders that disrupt solute transport are polyuria and the loss of electrolytes, sugar or amino acids into the urine. Table 8.1 describes some of the more common disorders.

The Loop of Henle

The loop of Henle is the part of the nephron that creates the environment for the urine to be concentrated [15]. In the thick ascending limb, sodium, potassium and chloride ions are reabsorbed by transporter proteins but water cannot follow [16].

Table 8.1 Genetic disorders of the proximal tubule, their mode of inheritance and clinical consequences

Solute	Gene symbol	Gene product(s)	Inheritance	Disorder	Consequence
Glucose	SLC5A1 SLC5A2	Na/Glu cotransporter SGLT1 SGLT2	AR	Renal glycosuria	Positive urine dipstick test for glucose
Amino acids e.g. cystine	CSNU1 SLC7A9	Amino acid transporter	AR	Cystinuria	Cysteine stones
Bicarbonate	CA2 SLCA4A	Carbonic anhydrase NaHCO$_3$ cotransporter	AR	Proximal (type 2)	Metabolic acidosis
Multiple solutes	CLCN5	Cl⁻ channel	XR	Dent type 1 disease: Fanconi syndrome (uricosuria, glycosuria, phosphaturia, aminoaciduria, low molecular weight proteinuria) and proximal renal tubular acidosis	Nephrocalcinosis, Stones, Osteomalacia, rickets
Phosphate	PHEX SLC34A3	Endopeptidase which regulates FGF23 NaP-cotransporter	XD AR	Hypophosphataemic rickets	Phosphaturia, Vitamin D resistant rickets

AR autosomal recessive, *AD* autosomal dominant, *XR* X-linked recessive, *XD* X-linked dominant

Ions are trapped within the interstitium of the medulla, creating a concentration gradient. The hyperosmolar environment in the deep medulla draws water out of the collecting duct.

Mutations of the genes that code for transporter proteins lead to a condition called Bartter syndrome. The effects are similar to the action of loop diuretics such as furosemide, which blocks the transport of sodium, potassium and chloride into the cells of the thick ascending limb.

Abnormally large amounts of sodium ions flow from the loop of Henle into the distal tubule where they are reabsorbed in exchange for potassium and hydrogen ions. Hence the patient, usually a child, has polyuria, hypovolaemia, hypokalaemia, hypochloraemia and metabolic alkalosis [17]. Because calcium and magnesium are normally reabsorbed with sodium and chloride in the thick ascending limb, urinary calcium and magnesium excretion are increased and nephrocalcinosis can develop.

There are five types of Bartter syndrome with varying renal and extrarenal manifestations [18].

The Distal Tubule

The main function of the distal convoluted tubule is the reabsorption of sodium and chloride, as well as some calcium and magnesium [19]. The sodium/chloride transporter is blocked by thiazide diuretics such as bendroflumethiazide. An autosomal recessive mutation that leads to loss of this protein's function causes similar effects; a condition called Gitelman syndrome [18]. Compared to Bartter syndrome, the salt loss and volume contraction is less severe. The condition usually presents in older children and adults when hypokalaemia and metabolic alkalosis are detected incidentally. In contrast to Bartter syndrome and in line with the effect of thiazides, urinary calcium excretion is reduced [18].

The opposite of Gitelman syndrome is Gordon's syndrome (pseudohypoaldosteronism type 2, PHA2), an autosomal dominant condition in which the sodium/chloride transporter is overactive. Excessive sodium reabsorption results in high blood pressure. Reduced potassium and hydrogen ion excretion leads to hyperkalaemia and metabolic acidosis. Thiazide diuretics counteract the abnormalities in Gordon's syndrome.

The Collecting Duct

The collecting duct has two cell types:

- principal cells which reabsorb salt and water, secrete potassium, and control the concentration of the urine [20]

- intercalated cells which regulate acid-base balance by secreting hydrogen ions and adjusting bicarbonate [21]

The principal cells contain membrane channels in the epithelial membrane (ENaC) that selectively allow sodium and water to enter the cell and potassium to leave. Sodium is then pumped out through the basal membrane by the Na/K ATPase. An autosomal dominant mutation prevents the epithelial sodium channel being removed from the cell membrane, leading to increased absorption of sodium and excretion of potassium and H^+. This results in high blood pressure, hypokalaemia and metabolic alkalosis, a condition called Liddle syndrome. This is counteracted by amiloride, a potassium-sparing diuretic that blocks ENaC.

The epithelial sodium and potassium channels and the Na/K ATPase in the basal membrane are regulated by aldosterone through the mineralocorticoid receptor. Its overall effect is to increase sodium reabsorption and potassium excretion. Mutations of the gene coding for the sodium channel make it unable to respond to aldosterone—pseudohypoaldosteronism type 1 (PHA1). This results in the opposite of Liddle syndrome—salt wasting, hyperkalaemia and acidosis, like Addison's disease.

The water channel (aquaporin 2) is controlled by the antidiuretic hormone, vasopressin. Mutations in the genes that code for the vasopressin receptor or for the water channel lead to hereditary nephrogenic diabetes insipidus. Because the ability to concentrate the urine is lost, patients have polyuria and nocturia. Urine osmolality is low and plasma osmolality inappropriately raised. This stimulates thirst leading to polydipsia, which prevents severe hypernatraemia.

The intercalated cells break down carbonic acid to H^+ and bicarbonate via a reaction catalyzed by carbonic anhydrase. The H^+ ions are actively pumped into the urine by a H^+ ATPase. The bicarbonate ions are carried to the blood by a Cl^-/HCO_3^- anion exchanger. Genetic mutations causing loss of function of either of these mechanisms lead to distal renal tubular acidosis (type 1 RTA). The H^+ ATPase is also present in the inner ear, hence autosomal recessive mutations cause distal RTA with congenital sensorineural deafness.

The inappropriately alkaline urine in distal RTA leads to the precipitation of calcium in the urine as stones, or within the kidney tissue as nephrocalcinosis. In adults, this syndrome is usually an acquired defect associated with autoimmune diseases. RTA and other tubular transport mechanisms are discussed in more detail in Chap. 15.

Uromodulin

Formerly known as Tamm-Horsfall protein, uromodulin is the most abundant protein in normal urine. Its function is not well understood [22]. It is secreted by the thick ascending limb of the loop of Henle and the distal tubule, where it modulates the sodium and potassium channels.

Genetic variants of the UMOD gene that lead to increased levels of uromodulin in the urine are associated with salt retention, hypertension and kidney damage. However, they are also associated with a reduced risk of urinary tract infection, which may explain their persistence in human evolution [23].

Autosomal-dominant mutations in the uromodulin (UMOD) gene alter the structure of uromodulin, preventing its release from the kidney cells and allowing leakage back into the interstitial space around the tubules. Here, uromodulin has an inflammatory effect leading to interstitial nephritis and fibrosis—Uromodulin Kidney Disease. End-stage kidney failure is reached between 30 and 60 years of age (Patient 8.1).

Uromodulin helps sodium to be reabsorbed in the thick ascending limb of the loop of Henle. In patients with UMOD, sodium reabsorption in this part of the tubule is reduced. To compensate for this, reabsorption of sodium in the proximal tubule is increased. In this part of the tubule, sodium and urate reabsorption are linked and so patients have hyperuricaemia and gout [24].

Patient 8.1 Uromodulin Kidney Disease

Nick had a kidney transplant 15 years ago. At that time the cause his kidney failure was unclear. He had severe hypertension throughout his 20s.

His late mother had gout from the age of 16 followed by severe hypertension, kidney failure and a transplant. His mother's kidney biopsy had shown normal glomeruli, hypertensive changes in the vessels and some atrophy of the collecting tubules. Nick's sister also had severe hypertension and kidney failure and had sadly died from complications after a kidney transplant. Neither Nick nor his sister had gout.

On this occasion, Nick attended clinic with his son, aged 19, who was having occasional attacks of gout. His blood pressure was 159/107 mmHg and his eGFR was 53 mL/min/1.73 m². His urine contained no blood or protein. His serum urate was 769 micromol/L (normal range 200–430).

The familial association of teenage gout, hypertension and reduced GFR pointed to uromodulin kidney disease. The family had samples taken for genetic testing, which confirmed that Nick and his son and daughter had all inherited a mutation of the uromodulin gene.

Nick's family pedigree chart is shown in Fig. 8.5.

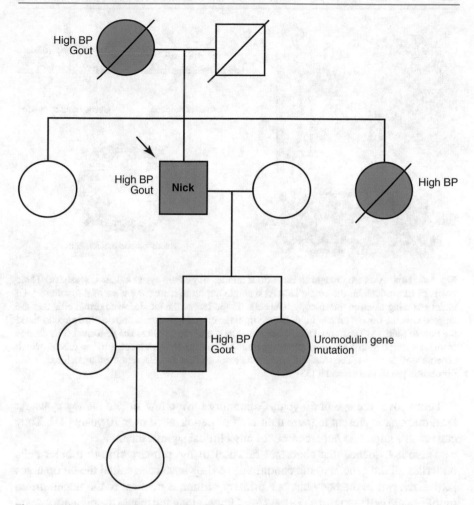

Fig. 8.5 Nick's uromodulin kidney disease family pedigree

Cystic Kidney Diseases

Cysts feature in a range of genetic disorders and can develop from all segments of the nephron. They vary in size from small, e.g. medullary sponge kidney [25, 26], to large, e.g. autosomal dominant polycystic kidney disease.

The cysts develop from the proliferation of tubular cells forming a bulge in the normal tubule. The bulge breaks off from the lumen to form a cyst surrounded by fibrous tissue. Instead of absorbing solutes, the cells lining the cyst secrete fluid into the lumen, making it enlarge.

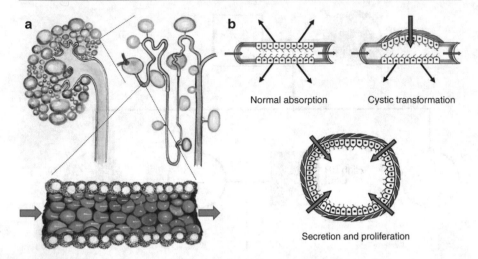

Normal absorption   Cystic transformation

Secretion and proliferation

Fig. 8.6 How cysts are thought to form from tubules in genetic cystic kidney disease. (**a**) Three levels of magnification: the whole kidney; a single nephron; a cutaway view of a tubule as seen under scanning electron microscopy. The cells on the left of the tubule have normal cilia that are aligned with the flow of tubular fluid. On the right the cilia are abnormal and do not correctly sense the flow of fluid. (**b**) The normal tubule reabsorbs fluid and electrolytes. The abnormal cells change from an absorptive to a secretory phenotype and proliferate to form a bulge in the tubule, which separates off as a cyst. The remaining nephron ceases to function. Secretion enlarges the cyst and fibroblasts proliferate around it [33]

People over the age of 50 years commonly have a few simple kidney cysts. At least one cyst is present in more than 20% of people aged over 70 years [27]. They can reach a large size but are rarely of any clinical significance.

There is evidence that abnormal function of the primary cilia in tubular cells underlies all the genetic cystic conditions, so they have been called the ciliopathies [28]. Each cell in the body has one primary cilium, equivalent to the flagellum on motile single cell organisms [29]. As fluid flows along the tubule the cilia are moved and the epithelial cell senses the direction and rate of flow. They may also sense the chemical composition of the tubular fluid.

Movement of the cilia triggers the release of chemical messengers that control the transport functions of tubular epithelial cells. Malfunction of the cilia stops the epithelial cells detecting flow and removes the control of cell division, allowing them to proliferate and dilate the tubule. The membrane transport processes are disrupted and the cells secrete fluid into the lumen to enlarge the cyst (Fig. 8.6).

The three commonest inherited cystic kidney diseases are nephronophthisis, autosomal recessive (ARPKD) and autosomal dominant polycystic kidney disease (ADPKD). Nephronophthisis is the commonest genetic cause of kidney failure in children. The kidneys are normal sized or small and cysts form near the border of the cortex and medulla. It is caused by mutations in a range of recessive genes and can be associated with extra-renal abnormalities, such as in Bardet-Biedl syndrome [30].

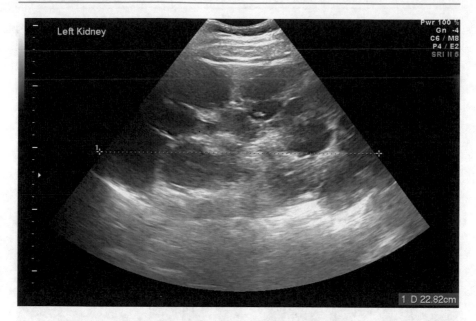

Fig. 8.7 Ultrasound scan in ADPKD—the kidney is enlarged and contains multiple simple cysts

ARPKD is due to mutations in a large gene that codes for the protein fibrocystin/polyductin. This protein is located on the primary cilium of the tubular epithelial cell and plays a critical role in controlling the division of cells into two rather than into multiple daughter cells [31]. Despite having the same mutation, the clinical presentation may vary—cysts forming in utero or in the neonatal period. The protein is also found in the cilia of bile duct cholangiocytes and some older children present with symptoms caused by liver disease.

ADPKD is due to a mutation in one of the genes PKD1 or PKD2; 85% of affected patients have the PKD1 mutation [32]. PKD1 mutations cause more severe disease than PKD2 [34].

The PKD genes code for polycystin, a protein that controls the function of cilia. It is thought that in early life the normal PKD allele of the heterozygote controls cell division. In adulthood, the normal allele may undergo a somatic mutation—a 'second hit'—and a clone of cells divides to form a cyst (Fig. 8.5). Alternatively, the production of polycystin by some cells may fall below the threshold level required to control cilia, allowing unregulated cell proliferation.

Criteria have been agreed to help distinguish incidental simple cysts found on ultrasound from the early stages of ADPKD (Fig. 8.7) [35].

Cysts can also develop in the liver, pancreas and spleen (Fig. 8.8), and there is an increased risk of complications due to biliary tract disease [36].

Weakness of the heart valve apparatus can cause mitral valve prolapse. Weakness of the arterial walls of intracranial arteries can lead to berry aneurysms and subarachnoid haemorrhage. The 10% risk of intracranial aneurysms is four-times higher than in the general population. Other risk factors are hypertension, smoking and alcohol [37].

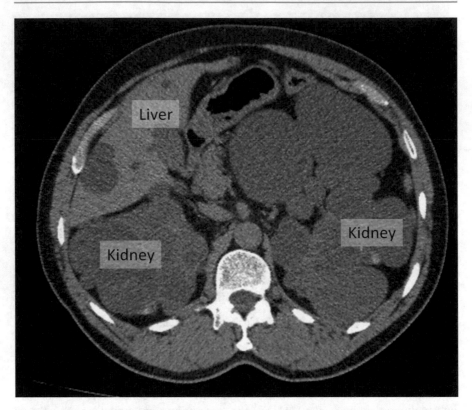

Fig. 8.8 CT scan with intravenous contrast from the same patient as in Fig. 8.6. The kidneys are grossly enlarged by multiple cysts, which are also present in the liver

Traditional practice has been to screen patients who have a positive family history of cerebral aneurysm as the risk is three times greater with a positive family history [37]. It is unclear if screening all ADPKD patients with magnetic resonance angiography is cost-effective [37, 38]. If the first study is normal, repeat screening every 5 years has been recommended. Patients with intracranial aneurysm should be studied annually and treatment considered for enlarging, high-risk aneurysms [37, 39].

The progression of kidney failure in ADPKD is related to the growth of cysts. When the cyst breaks off, the remaining nephron ceases to function. As the cysts enlarge, surrounding nephrons are compressed and obstructed. Interventions such as blood pressure control have a less beneficial effect on the decline in kidney function than in glomerular diseases where there is proteinuria. However, hypertension often develops early in the disease and warrants treatment for its cardiovascular benefits.

A patient's prognosis can be estimated from the size of the kidneys. If they are longer than 16.5 cm on an ultrasound scan the patient is more likely to develop kidney failure [40]. The rates of growth of cysts and decline in kidney function are faster in obese patients [40].

Treatment of adults with the vasopressin antagonist tolvaptan slows the growth of cysts and reduces the risk of haematuria, urinary infection and kidney pain [41].

The rate of decline in kidney function in patients with an eGFR less than 60 mL/min/1.73 m^2 is slowed by about one third [42] to an average of 1 mL/min/1.73 m^2 per year [43]. Vasopressin is the same as antidiuretic hormone and so tolvaptan causes a marked diuresis. The large volume of fluid that patients must drink makes this treatment hard to tolerate for some patients.

It is uncertain whether it is beneficial to screen children for ADPKD and start treatment early to prevent complications [44].

Kidney Tumours

A number of autosomal dominant mutations lead to the formation of benign and malignant kidney tumours. Familial papillary cell carcinomas result from a mutation causing overactivity of the MET proto-oncogene. The kidney tumours may be one part of a characteristic syndrome of abnormalities caused by mutations of tumour suppressor genes; for example tuberous sclerosis [45], von Hippel-Lindau disease [46] and Wilms tumour-aniridia syndrome, also known as WAGR syndrome—Wilms tumour of the kidney, Aniridia (absence of the iris), Genitourinary anomalies, and mental Retardation [47].

The Lower Urinary Tract

The junction between the ureter and bladder normally acts as a valve, preventing the flow of urine back up the ureter during micturition when the pressure within the bladder increases. If this valve is incompetent, vesico-ureteric reflux (VUR) occurs [48]. If this causes hydronephrosis it may be detected on a routine ultrasound scan during pregnancy (Chap. 7).

The embryological development of the junction between the ureter and bladder is a complex process involving chemical signaling to control the differentiation and organization of cells. This process may be affected by genetic abnormalities and by mechanical forces acting on the developing structures.

In a study of 211 pregnant women with a family history of VUR, 186 infants had a micturating cystogram and 38 (20%) showed VUR [49]. The majority of index cases were the pregnant woman's mother or sibling.

When VUR is familial, inheritance is usually autosomal dominant, although recessive and X-linked inheritances have been reported. The wide range in the severity of the damage, from asymptomatic to end-stage kidney disease, suggests that a variety of underlying abnormalities can lead to VUR.

VUR can be an isolated finding or associated with abnormalities such as posterior urethral valves or ureterocele. VUR can also be part of a multiorgan malformation syndrome—congenital abnormalities of the kidney and ureteric tract (CAKUT) [50]. For example, the urogenital sinus may persist in females so that the urethra and vagina do not have separate openings. The vagina or uterus becomes distended and compresses the urethra, increasing pressure in the bladder and causing VUR.

Ureteric obstruction in the developing embryo in utero causes hydronephrosis and dysplasia of the kidneys with a reduced number of functioning nephrons at birth. As much of the kidney parenchymal damage occurs in utero, end-stage kidney disease is not easily prevented (Patient 8.2). About 40% of people who reach end-stage kidney disease within the first three decades of life have CAKUT.

Patient 8.2 Complex Vesico-Ureteric Reflux (VUR)

Aisha was the first of twin girls born by emergency caesarean section at 28 weeks gestation because her mother had pre-eclampsia. An antenatal ultrasound scan had shown bilateral renal pelvic dilatation. A scan soon after birth was normal because urine volume is low in the first few days.

Aisha was treated with prophylactic trimethoprim. Despite this, during the first 3 months she had septicaemia from an *Enterococcus faecalis* urine infection. Later, a suprapubic urine specimen cultured a pure growth of *Escherichia coli*. She responded well to antibiotics.

Her serum creatinine was 144 micromol/L (1.63 mg/dL) compared to the normal range for her age of 18–51 micromol/L. A DMSA isotope scan was performed at 3 months of age to measure the relative function of her two kidneys. It showed 75% of total function in the right kidney, 25% in the left (Fig. 8.9).

A micturating cystogram was performed at 5 months of age to image the anatomy of her ureters and bladder. It showed severe bilateral vesico-ureteric reflux (Fig. 8.10).

A MAG 3 renogram was performed to track the flow of urine down the urinary tract. It showed very poor ureteric drainage from both kidneys (Fig. 8.11).

An ultrasound scan showed both kidneys to be echogenic. There was bilateral hydronephrosis and hydroureter with a very dilated right lower ureter (Fig. 8.12). The bladder was trabeculated indicating muscle hypertrophy due to bladder outlet obstruction.

Cystoscopy revealed a urogenital sinus and bilateral paraureteric diverticulae caused by the pressure from bladder outlet obstruction. To relieve the obstruction, the bladder was opened to the anterior abdominal wall—a vesicostomy. At age 8 the vesicostomy was closed, the bladder enlarged using redundant ureteric tissue and a Mitrofanoff fistula fashioned using her appendix to allow the bladder to be catheterized directly (Fig. 8.13).

Aisha's blood pressure was raised from the age of 4 years. Despite treatment with the ACE inhibitor enalapril, her GFR progressively declined due to hyperfiltration of the remaining nephrons. She received a kidney transplant at age 11.

Fig. 8.9 DMSA scan from three viewing angles—posterior, left posterior-oblique (*LPO*) and right posterior-oblique (*RPO*). The right kidney has taken up much more isotope than the left

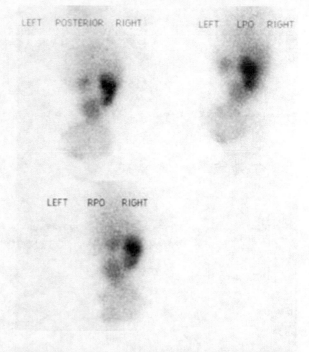

Fig. 8.10 Micturating cystogram showing severe bilateral vesico-ureteric reflux

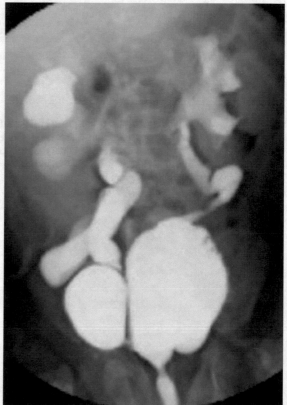

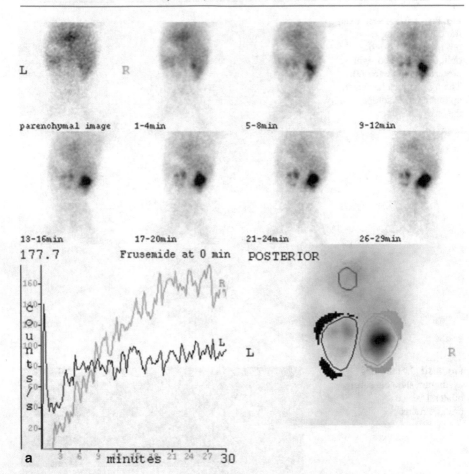

Fig. 8.11 (**a**) MAG3 renogram from Aisha. There is delayed uptake of isotope by the kidneys, measured as counts/second of radioactivity. The right kidney trace peaks at 27 min (normal <6 min). The left kidney reaches a lower level than the right due to its relatively worse function. There is no decline from either kidney within 30 min indicating obstruction to urinary flow (normal T1/2 <15 min). (**b**) A normal renogram for comparison showing symmetrical uptake and excretion of the isotope; TMax = 2 min, T1/2 left = 6 min, T1/2 right = 7 min

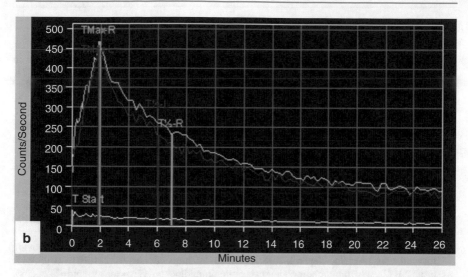

Fig. 8.11 (continued)

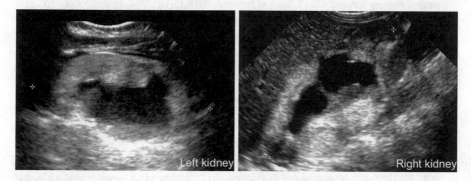

Fig. 8.12 Ultrasound scan of the kidneys showing echogenic kidneys with bilateral hydronephrosis and hydroureter

Fig. 8.13 Diagrammatic representation of a Mitrofanoff fistula with a catheter in place

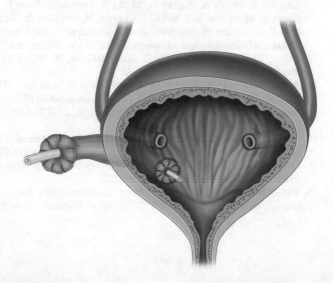

References

1. Akrawi DS, Li X, Sundquist J, Sundquist K, Zöller B. Familial risks of kidney failure in Sweden: a nationwide family study. PLoS One. 2014;9(11):e113353. https://doi.org/10.1371/journal.pone.0113353. eCollection 2014. http://www.ncbi.nlm.nih.gov/pmc/articles/PMC4244139/.
2. Bullich G, Domingo-Gallego A, Vargas I, Ruiz P, Lorente-Grandoso L, Furlano M, Fraga G, Madrid Á, Ariceta G, Borregán M, Piñero-Fernández JA, Rodríguez-Peña L, Ballesta-Martínez MJ, Llano-Rivas I, Meñica MA, Ballarín J, Torrents D, Torra R, Ars E. A kidney-disease gene panel allows a comprehensive genetic diagnosis of cystic and glomerular inherited kidney diseases. Kidney Int. 2018;94(2):363–71. https://doi.org/10.1016/j.kint.2018.02.027. Epub 2018 May 22. https://www.kidney-international.org/article/S0085-2538(18)30241-2/fulltext.
3. Foster MC, Coresh J, Fornage M, Astor BC, Grams M, Franceschini N, et al. APOL1 variants associate with increased risk of CKD among African Americans. J Am Soc Nephrol. 2013;24:1484–91. https://jasn.asnjournals.org/content/24/9/1484?ijkey=54889dc3e604d0494df82b706806737736802c32&keytype2=tf_ipsecsha.
4. Limou S, Vince N, Parsa A. Lessons from CKD-related genetic association studies-moving forward. Clin J Am Soc Nephrol. 2018;13(1):140–52. https://doi.org/10.2215/CJN.09030817. Epub 2017 Dec 14. http://cjasn.asnjournals.org/cgi/pmidlookup?view=long&pmid=29242368.
5. Kestenbaum B, Seliger SL. Commentary on lessons from CKD-related genetic association studies-moving forward. Clin J Am Soc Nephrol. 2018;13(1):153–4. https://doi.org/10.2215/CJN.12421117. Epub 2017 Dec 14. https://cjasn.asnjournals.org/content/13/1/153.long.
6. Alport AC. Hereditary familial congenital haemorrhagic nephritis. BMJ. 1927;1(3454):504–6. https://doi.org/10.1136/bmj.1.3454.504. http://www.ncbi.nlm.nih.gov/pmc/articles/PMC2454341/.
7. Savige J, Colville D, Rheault M, Gear S, Lennon R, Lagas S, Finlay M, Flinter F. Alport syndrome in women and girls. Clin J Am Soc Nephrol. 2016;11(9):1713–20. https://doi.org/10.2215/CJN.00580116. https://cjasn.asnjournals.org/content/11/9/1713.
8. Savige J, Sheth S, Leys A, Nicholson A, Mack HG, Colville D. Ocular features in Alport syndrome: pathogenesis and clinical significance. Clin J Am Soc Nephrol. 2015;10(4):703–9. https://doi.org/10.2215/CJN.10581014. http://cjasn.asnjournals.org/cgi/pmidlookup?view=long&pmid=25649157.
9. Ha TS. Genetics of hereditary nephrotic syndrome: a clinical review. Korean J Pediatr. 2017;60(3):55–63. https://doi.org/10.3345/kjp.2017.60.3.55. https://www.ncbi.nlm.nih.gov/pmc/articles/PMC5383633/.
10. Bierzynska A, McCarthy HJ, Soderquest K, Sen ES, Colby E, Ding WY, Nabhan MM, Kerecuk L, Hegde S, Hughes D, Marks S, Feather S, Jones C, Webb NJ, Ognjanovic M, Christian M, Gilbert RD, Sinha MD, Lord GM, Simpson M, Koziell AB, Welsh GI, Saleem MA. Genomic and clinical profiling of a national nephrotic syndrome cohort advocates a precision medicine approach to disease management. Kidney Int. 2017;91(4):937–47. https://doi.org/10.1016/j.kint.2016.10.013. Epub 2017 Jan 20. https://www.kidney-international.org/article/S0085-2538(16)30612-3/fulltext.
11. Arends M, Wanner C, Hughes D, Mehta A, Oder D, Watkinson OT, Elliott PM, Linthorst GE, Wijburg FA, Biegstraaten M, Hollak CE. Characterization of classical and nonclassical Fabry disease: a multicenter study. J Am Soc Nephrol. 2017;28:1631–41. https://doi.org/10.1681/ASN.2016090964.
12. El Dib R, Gomaa H, Carvalho RP, Camargo SE, Bazan R, Barretti P, Barreto FC. Enzyme replacement therapy for Anderson-Fabry disease. Cochrane Database Syst Rev. 2016;7:CD006663. https://doi.org/10.1002/14651858.CD006663.pub4. https://www.cochranelibrary.com/cdsr/doi/10.1002/14651858.CD006663.pub3/full.
13. Walsh SB, Unwin RJ. Renal tubular disorders. Clin Med. 2012;12:476–9. https://doi.org/10.7861/clinmedicine.12-5-476. http://www.clinmed.rcpjournal.org/content/12/5/476.full.

14. Curthoys NP, Moe OW. Proximal tubule function and response to acidosis. CJASN. 2014;9(9):1627–38. https://doi.org/10.2215/CJN.10391012. http://cjasn.asnjournals.org/content/9/9/1627.full.

15. Dantzler WH, Layton AT, Layton HE, Pannabecker TL. Urine-concentrating mechanism in the inner medulla: function of the thin limbs of the loops of Henle. CJASN. 2014;9(10):1781–9. https://doi.org/10.2215/CJN.08750812. http://cjasn.asnjournals.org/content/9/10/1781.full.

16. Kleta R, Bockenhauer D. Salt-losing tubulopathies in children: what's new, what's controversial? J Am Soc Nephrol. 2018;29(3):727–39. https://doi.org/10.1681/ASN.2017060600. Epub 2017 Dec 13. https://jasn.asnjournals.org/content/29/3/727.long.

17. Mount DB. Thick ascending limb of the loop of Henle. CJASN. 2014;9(11):1974–86. https://doi.org/10.2215/CJN.04480413. http://cjasn.asnjournals.org/content/9/11/1974.full.

18. Fremont OT, Chan JC. Understanding Bartter syndrome and Gitelman syndrome. World J Pediatr. 2012;8(1):25–30. https://doi.org/10.1007/s12519-012-0333-9. Epub 2012 Jan 27. http://link.springer.com/article/10.1007%2Fs12519-012-0333-9.

19. Subramanya AR, Ellison DH. Distal convoluted tubule. CJASN. 2014;9(12):2147–63. https://doi.org/10.2215/CJN.05920613. http://cjasn.asnjournals.org/content/9/12/2147.full.

20. Pearce D, Soundararajan R, Trimpert C, Kashlan OB, Deen PMT, Kohan DE. Collecting duct principal cell transport processes and their regulation. Clin J Am Soc Nephrol. 2015;10(1):135–46. https://doi.org/10.2215/CJN.05760513. http://cjasn.asnjournals.org/cgi/pmidlookup?view=long&pmid=24875192.

21. Roy A, Al-bataineh MM, Pastor-Soler NM. Collecting duct intercalated cell function and regulation. Clin J Am Soc Nephrol. 2015;10(2):305–24. https://doi.org/10.2215/CJN.08880914. http://cjasn.asnjournals.org/cgi/pmidlookup?view=long&pmid=25632105.

22. Rampoldi L, Scolari F, Amoroso A, Ghiggeri G, Devuyst O. The rediscovery of uromodulin (Tamm-Horsfall protein): from tubulointerstitial nephropathy to chronic kidney disease. Kidney Int. 2011;80(4):338–47. https://doi.org/10.1038/ki.2011.134. Epub 2011 Jun 8. http://www.ncbi.nlm.nih.gov/pubmed/21654721.

23. Ghirotto S, Tassi F, Barbujani G, Pattini L, Hayward C, Vollenweider P, Bochud M, Rampoldi L, Devuyst O. The uromodulin gene locus shows evidence of pathogen adaptation through human evolution. J Am Soc Nephrol. 2016;27(10):2983–96. Epub 2016 Mar 10. https://jasn.asnjournals.org/content/27/10/2983.

24. Bleyer AJ, Kmoch S. Tamm Horsfall glycoprotein and uromodulin: it is all about the tubules! Clin J Am Soc Nephrol. 2016;11(1):6–8. https://doi.org/10.2215/CJN.12201115. https://cjasn.asnjournals.org/content/11/1/6.long.

25. Goldfarb DS. Evidence for inheritance of medullary sponge kidney. Kidney Int. 2013;83:193–6. https://doi.org/10.1038/ki.2012.417. http://www.nature.com/ki/journal/v83/n2/full/ki2012417a.html.

26. Fabris A, Lupo A, Ferraro PM, Anglani F, Pei Y, Danza FM, Gambaro G. Familial clustering of medullary sponge kidney is autosomal dominant with reduced penetrance and variable expressivity. Kidney Int. 2013;83:272–7. https://doi.org/10.1038/ki.2012.378. http://www.nature.com/ki/journal/v83/n2/full/ki2012378a.html.

27. Ravine D, Gibson RN, Donlan J, Sheffield LJ. An ultrasound renal cyst prevalence survey: specificity data for inherited renal cystic diseases. Am J Kidney Dis. 1993;22(6):803–7. http://www.ncbi.nlm.nih.gov/pubmed/8250026.

28. Davenport JR, Yoder BK. An incredible decade for the primary cilium: a look at a once-forgotten organelle. Am J Physiol Renal Physiol. 2005;289(6):F1159–69. https://doi.org/10.1152/ajprenal.00118.2005. http://ajprenal.physiology.org/content/289/6/F1159.

29. Pluznick JL, Caplan MJ. Chemical and physical sensors in the regulation of renal function. Clin J Am Soc Nephrol. 2015;10(9):1626–35. https://doi.org/10.2215/CJN.00730114. http://cjasn.asnjournals.org/cgi/pmidlookup?view=long&pmid=25280495.

30. Forsythe E, Sparks K, Best S, Borrows S, Hoskins B, Sabir A, Barrett T, Williams D, Mohammed S, Goldsmith D, Milford DV, Bockenhauer D, Foggensteiner L, Beales PL. Risk factors for severe renal disease in Bardet-Biedl syndrome. J Am Soc Nephrol. 2017;28(3):963–70. https://doi.org/10.1681/ASN.2015091029. https://jasn.asnjournals.org/content/28/3/963.long.

31. Zhang J, Wu M, Wang S, Shah JV, Wilson PD, Zhou J. Polycystic kidney disease protein fibrocystin localizes to the mitotic spindle and regulates spindle bipolarity. Hum Mol Genet. 2010;19(17):3306–19. https://doi.org/10.1093/hmg/ddq233. First published online June 16, 2010; http://hmg.oxfordjournals.org/content/19/17/3306.full.

32. Cornec-Le Gall E, Torres VE, Harris PC. Genetic complexity of autosomal dominant polycystic kidney and liver diseases. J Am Soc Nephrol. 2018;29(1):13–23. https://doi.org/10.1681/ASN.2017050483. Epub 2017 Oct 16. https://jasn.asnjournals.org/content/29/1/13.

33. Avner ED, McDonough AA, Sweeney WE. Transport, cilia, and PKD: must we in (cyst) on interrelationships? Am J Physiol Cell Physiol. 2012;302(10):C1434–5. https://doi.org/10.1152/ajpcell.00070.2012. http://www.ncbi.nlm.nih.gov/pmc/articles/PMC3362002/.

34. Cornec-Le Gall E, Audrézet MP, Renaudineau E, Hourmant M, Charasse C, Michez E, Frouget T, Vigneau C, Dantal J, Siohan P, Longuet H, Gatault P, Ecotière L, Bridoux F, Mandart L, Hanrotel-Saliou C, Stanescu C, Depraetre P, Gie S, Massad M, Kersalé A, Séret G, Augusto JF, Saliou P, Maestri S, Chen JM, Harris PC, Férec C, Le Meur Y. PKD2-related autosomal dominant polycystic kidney disease: prevalence, clinical presentation, mutation spectrum, and prognosis. Am J Kidney Dis. 2017;70(4):476–85. https://doi.org/10.1053/j.ajkd.2017.01.046. Epub 2017 Mar 27. https://www.ncbi.nlm.nih.gov/pmc/articles/PMC5610929/.

35. Pei Y, Obaji J, Dupuis A, Paterson AD, Magistroni R, Dicks E, Ravine D. Unified criteria for ultrasonographic diagnosis of ADPKD. J Am Soc Nephrol. 2009;20(1):205–12. https://doi.org/10.1681/ASN.2008050507. http://www.ncbi.nlm.nih.gov/pmc/articles/PMC2615723.

36. Judge PK, Harper CHS, Storey BC, Haynes R, Wilcock MJ, Staplin N, Goldacre R, Baigent C, Collier J, Goldacre M, Landray MJ, Winearls CG, Herrington WG. Biliary tract and liver complications in polycystic kidney disease. J Am Soc Nephrol. 2017;28(9):2738–48. https://doi.org/10.1681/ASN.2017010084. Epub 2017 May 2. https://jasn.asnjournals.org/content/28/9/2738.long.

37. Sanchis IM, Shukoor S, Irazabal MV, Madsen CD, Chebib FT, Hogan MC, El-Zoghby Z, Harris PC, Huston J, Brown RD, Torres VE. Pre-symptomatic screening for intracranial aneurysms in patients with autosomal dominant polycystic kidney disease. CJASN. 2019;14(8):1151–60. https://doi.org/10.2215/CJN.14691218. https://cjasn.asnjournals.org/content/14/8/1151.

38. Flahault A, Trystram D, Nataf F, Fouchard M, Knebelmann B, Grünfeld JP, Joly D. Screening for intracranial aneurysms in autosomal dominant polycystic kidney disease is cost-effective. Kidney Int. 2018;93(3):716–26. https://doi.org/10.1016/j.kint.2017.08.016. https://www.kidney-international.org/article/S0085-2538%2817%2930613-0/fulltext.

39. Malhotra A, Wu X, Matouk CC, Forman HP, Gandhi D, Sanelli P. MR angiography screening and surveillance for intracranial aneurysms in autosomal dominant polycystic kidney disease: a cost-effectiveness analysis. Radiology. 2019;291(2):400–8. https://doi.org/10.1148/radiol.2019181399. Epub 2019 Feb 19. https://pubs.rsna.org/doi/full/10.1148/radiol.2019181399.

40. Bhutani H, Smith V, Rahbari-Oskoui F, Mittal A, Grantham JJ, Torres VE, Mrug M, Bae KT, Wu Z, Ge Y, Landslittel D, Gibbs P, O'Neill WC, Chapman AB. A comparison of ultrasound and magnetic resonance imaging shows that kidney length predicts chronic kidney disease in autosomal dominant polycystic kidney disease. Kidney Int. 2015;88(1):146–51. https://doi.org/10.1038/ki.2015.71. Epub 2015 Apr. http://www.nature.com/ki/journal/v88/n1/full/ki201571a.html.

41. Torres VE, Higashihara E, Devuyst O, Chapman AB, Gansevoort RT, Grantham JJ, Perrone RD, Ouyang J, Blais JD, Czerwiec FS, TEMPO 3:4 Trial Investigators. Effect of tolvaptan in autosomal dominant polycystic kidney disease by CKD stage: results from the TEMPO 3:4 trial. Clin J Am Soc Nephrol. 2016;11(5):803–11. https://doi.org/10.2215/CJN.06300615. https://cjasn.asnjournals.org/content/11/5/803.

42. Torres VE, Chapman AB, Devuyst O, Gansevoort RT, Perrone RD, Koch G, Ouyang J, McQuade RD, Blais JD, Czerwiec FS, Sergeyeva O, REPRISE Trial Investigators. Tolvaptan in later-stage autosomal dominant polycystic kidney disease. N Engl J Med. 2017;377(20):1930–42. https://doi.org/10.1056/NEJMoa1710030. https://www.nejm.org/doi/10.1056/NEJMoa1710030?url_ver=Z39.88-2003&rfr_id=ori:rid:crossref.org&rfr_dat=cr_pub%3dwww.ncbi.nlm.nih.gov.

43. Edwards ME, Chebib FT, Irazabal MV, Ofstie TG, Bungum LA, Metzger AJ, Senum SR, Hogan MC, El-Zoghby ZM, Kline TL, Harris PC, Czerwiec FS, Torres VE. Long-term administration of tolvaptan in autosomal dominant polycystic kidney disease. Clin J Am Soc Nephrol. 2018;13(8):1153–61. https://doi.org/10.2215/CJN.01520218. Epub 2018 Jul 19. https://cjasn.asnjournals.org/content/13/8/1153.

44. De Rechter S, Bammens B, Schaefer F, Liebau MC, Mekahli D. Unmet needs and challenges for follow-up and treatment of autosomal dominant polycystic kidney disease: the paediatric perspective. Clin Kidney J. 2018;11(Suppl 1):i14–26. https://doi.org/10.1093/ckj/sfy088. Epub 2018 Dec 17. https://www.ncbi.nlm.nih.gov/pmc/articles/PMC6295604/.

45. http://www.tuberous-sclerosis.org.

46. http://www.patient.co.uk/doctor/von-hippel-lindau-disease.

47. http://www.wagr.org.

48. Williams G, Fletcher JT, Alexander SI, Craig JC. Vesicoureteral reflux. JASN. 2008;19:847–62. https://doi.org/10.1681/ASN.2007020245. Published ahead of print March 5, 2008. http://jasn.asnjournals.org/content/19/5/847.abstract.

49. Scott JE, Swallow V, Coulthard MG, Lambert HJ, Lee RE. Screening of newborn babies for familial ureteric reflux. Lancet. 1997;350(9075):396–400. https://www.thelancet.com/journals/lancet/article/PIIS0140-6736(97)01515-8/fulltext.

50. van der Ven AT, Vivante A, Hildebrandt F. Novel insights into the pathogenesis of monogenic congenital anomalies of the kidney and urinary tract. J Am Soc Nephrol. 2018;29(1):36–50. https://doi.org/10.1681/ASN.2017050561. Epub 2017 Oct 27. https://jasn.asnjournals.org/content/29/1/36.

What Have You Been Taking? Nephrotoxicity from Medications and Other Chemicals

A detailed drug history is a crucial part of the assessment of any patient, especially when kidney disease is suspected. The history must cover any drugs taken, prescribed or otherwise.

In patients with chronic kidney disease, the use of illicit hard drugs is associated with faster loss of kidney function and death. Tobacco smoking is associated with a higher risk of death. Conversely, alcohol intake is associated with a lower risk of death [1]. The use of alternative remedies derived from plants and animals is associated with acute kidney injury [2].

Details of each drug, when it was started and stopped, and the doses prescribed and taken should be compared with changes in the patient's kidney function. If more than a third of the excretion of a drug or its metabolites is by the kidneys, loss of kidney function can have important effects on the drug's pharmacokinetics, that is the changes in drug concentration after the dose is given. If kidney disease reduces drug clearance by more than half, the effects can be clinically important [3].

Some commonly used drugs can affect kidney function and/or structure, in other words can be nephrotoxic. There are three main mechanisms of injury: ischaemia, tubular toxicity and interstitial inflammation [4]. Injury to the glomerulus is less common [5, 6].

© Springer Nature Switzerland AG 2020
H. C. Rayner et al., *Understanding Kidney Diseases*,
https://doi.org/10.1007/978-3-030-43027-6_9

Vasoactive Drugs

For glomerular filtration to occur, blood needs to flow into the glomeruli at an adequate rate and under sufficient pressure to force filtrate through the glomerular filtration barrier. Vasoactive drugs can affect this by changing vascular resistance and glomerular blood flow.

ACEI and ARBs

Angiotensin-II (A-II) constricts the efferent arterioles, which increases glomerular filtration pressure by restricting the flow of blood out of the glomeruli. The renin-angiotensin-aldosterone system (RAAS) is inhibited by Angiotensin Converting Enzyme (ACE) inhibitors, which block the synthesis of A-II, and Angiotensin Receptor Blockers (ARBs), which inhibit the action of A-II on its receptor (Fig. 9.1). Both classes of drug allow the efferent arterioles to dilate and so lower the glomerular filtration pressure. The drop in GFR is usually small and the reduction in intraglomerular pressure can be beneficial by reducing hydrostatic damage.

If the pressure going into the glomerulus in the afferent arteriole is low, glomerular filtration is dependent upon vasoconstriction of the efferent arteriole to maintain intraglomerular pressure. This is the case in someone with poor left ventricular function and low systolic blood pressure, or with atherosclerosis of the renal arteries.

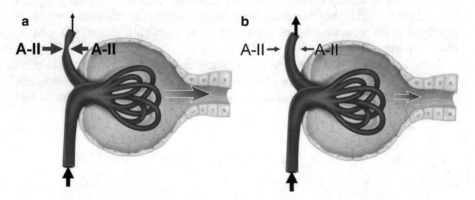

Fig. 9.1 (**a**) The effect of angiotensin II on glomerular filtration. AII causes vasoconstriction of the efferent arteriole and increases glomerular filtration pressure and rate. (**b**) Inhibition of AII leads to dilatation of the efferent arteriole, releasing the intra-glomerular pressure and reducing glomerular filtration rate

If such a person is given an ACE inhibitor or an ARB, there is a risk that the drop in intraglomerular pressure will be clinically significant (Patient 9.1). There is a typical pattern of changes in the laboratory results that helps to identify this effect:

- ↓ eGFR—low glomerular filtration pressure
- ↑ potassium—reduced AII stimulation of aldosterone production, leading to reduced potassium excretion
- ↑ urea-to-creatinine ratio—slow flow of filtrate along the nephron allowing diffusion of urea back into the blood

The changes almost always reverse after stopping the drug, which can be used as a diagnostic test for the effect. A drop in GFR with RAAS inhibitors does not necessarily mean that these drugs need to be stopped. For example, in patients with heart failure due to reduced left ventricular function, they have proven benefits and should be continued if possible [7].

Patient 9.1 Recurrent ACE Inhibitor Nephrotoxicity
Mrs. Blake, aged 72 years, had high blood pressure, proteinuria and diabetes. She was started on the ACE inhibitor lisinopril and her blood pressure was well controlled. Over the following year her eGFR steadily declined and the serum urea and potassium levels rose, suggesting that the ACE inhibitor was the cause (Fig. 9.2). The lisinopril was stopped and her eGFR returned to its previous level. The high blood pressure was controlled with a calcium channel blocker.

Four years later, a doctor unfamiliar with her history reviewed Mrs. Blake in the diabetes clinic. This doctor was concerned about the heavy proteinuria and so started ramipril.

Changes in eGFR, urea and potassium repeated the pattern of 4 years previously, this time to more extreme values as her underlying kidney function had worsened (Fig. 9.2).

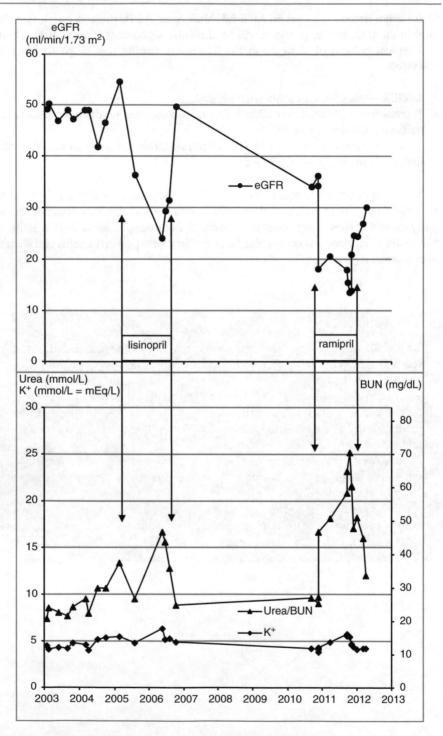

Fig. 9.2 Changes in eGFR, serum urea and serum potassium during repeated periods of ACE inhibitor treatment

NSAIDs

Prostaglandins help to maintain kidney blood flow by dilating the kidney arterioles. Non-steroidal anti-inflammatory drugs (NSAIDs) inhibit cyclo-oxygenase enzymes and reduce the production of prostaglandins. Removing the vasodilator effect of prostaglandins leads to vasoconstriction and a drop in renal blood flow and GFR.

An overdose of NSAIDs can cause acute kidney injury (Patient 9.2). Normal doses given repeatedly over a long period of time can lead to permanent damage due to ischaemia.

Patient 9.2 NSAID Overdose

John, an 18-year-old musician who suffered from depression, was admitted having taken an overdose of 300 mg seroxat, 700 mg diclofenac and 3.5 g naproxen. His U&E's were normal: creatinine = 103 micromols/L (1.2 mg/dL), eGFR = 87 mL/min/1.73 m^2. After a psychiatric assessment, he went home.

Over the next 2 days he became unwell with vomiting and pain in the loins and so returned to hospital. His eGFR had dropped to 50 and continued to decline over the following 3 days (Fig. 9.3). In retrospect, the initial creatinine result had indicated acute kidney injury as 2 years previously it had been 77 micromols/L (0.9 mg/dL). The peak serum creatinine was 287 micromols/L (3.2 mg/dL), making this episode AKI stage 3.

Fig. 9.3 Changes in eGFR with time after overdose of NSAIDs

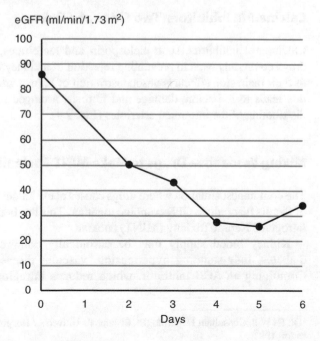

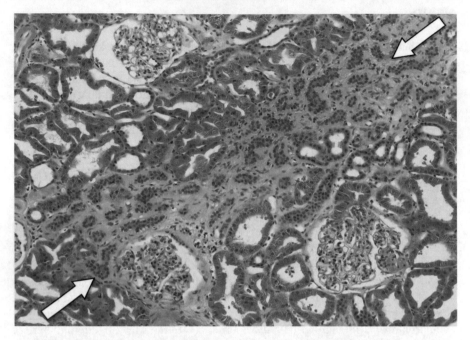

Fig. 9.4 A transplant kidney biopsy showing a band of fibrosis through the interstitium caused by long-term ciclosporin therapy (*arrows*). The glomeruli are normal. Haematoxylin and eosin ×200

Calcineurin Inhibitors: Two Sides of a Coin

Calcineurin inhibitors, such ciclosporin and tacrolimus, are immunosuppressive drugs commonly used to preventing rejection of a kidney transplant. Ironically, one of their main side effects is vasoconstriction of kidney arterioles. With chronic use, this leads to ischaemic damage and fibrosis, arranged in stripes along the radial distribution of the intrarenal arterioles (Fig. 9.4).

Mixing Vasoactive Drugs to Make MINT Cocktails

The commonest situation where drugs causes acute kidney injury is where a number of factors that reduce GFR combine together. This has been termed a Multifactorial Iatrogenic NephroToxicity (MINT) cocktail.[1]

Kidney blood supply may be chronically compromised in patients with diabetes, long-standing hypertension, vascular disease or advanced age [8]. Combining an ACE inhibitor, which reduces intraglomerular pressure, and a

---

[1] Dr. Es Will, Consultant Nephrologist, St James's University Hospital, Leeds, personal communication 1992.

diuretic, which drops plasma volume and thereby renal blood flow, can lead to a marked drop in GFR (Patient 9.1). Patients with normal kidneys can still suffer acute kidney injury if a number of nephrotoxic factors are combined (Patient 9.3).

Patient 9.3 A MINT Cocktail

Mrs. Kent was admitted as an emergency on 31st October having had a painful swollen right knee for 3 weeks. She had had no fever but her C-reactive protein (CRP) was very high, 237 mg/L, suggesting a septic arthritis. Her urine contained + protein on dipstick testing. Her serum creatinine was 57 micromol/L (0.6 mg/dL).

The large effusion in her knee was aspirated. The fluid was turbid with pus cells but no crystals or organisms. On the afternoon of 1st November she was taken to the operating theatre for a knee arthroscopy and washout.

Her blood pressure on admission was 126/74 mmHg with a pulse rate of 109 beats per minute but this fell to an average of 100/65 over the 12 h before the operation. Her blood pressure averaged 80/50 during the 30-min anaesthetic and 100/60 over the 12 h following the operation, then returned to normal.

Her usual medications were continued, including losartan 50 mg once daily for hypertension, and pregabalin 150 mg twice daily and naproxen 500 mg twice daily for pain. She was started on intravenous benzyl penicillin and flucloxacillin.

Here is her medication chart (Fig. 9.5).

The next day she felt better and began physiotherapy. Routine blood tests taken on the morning after the operation showed acute kidney injury, serum creatinine = 271 micromols/L (3.1 mg/dL). The next day this had risen to a peak of 459 micromols/L (5.2 mg/dL), that is AKI stage 3.

Despite a normal blood pressure of 135/78, Mrs. Kent felt dizzy and had visual hallucinations in her peripheral vision. This was attributed to the accumulation of pregabalin and codeine, which are normally excreted by the kidneys.

The following medications were stopped: losartan, naproxen, codeine, pregabalin and omeprazole. Intravenous fluids were given, urine volume increased and Mrs. Kent went on to make a good recovery. By the time of discharge from hospital, serum creatinine was 108 micromols/L (1.2 mg/dL), eGFR = 48 mL/min/1.73 m^2, indicating a 50% drop in GFR compared to before the illness.

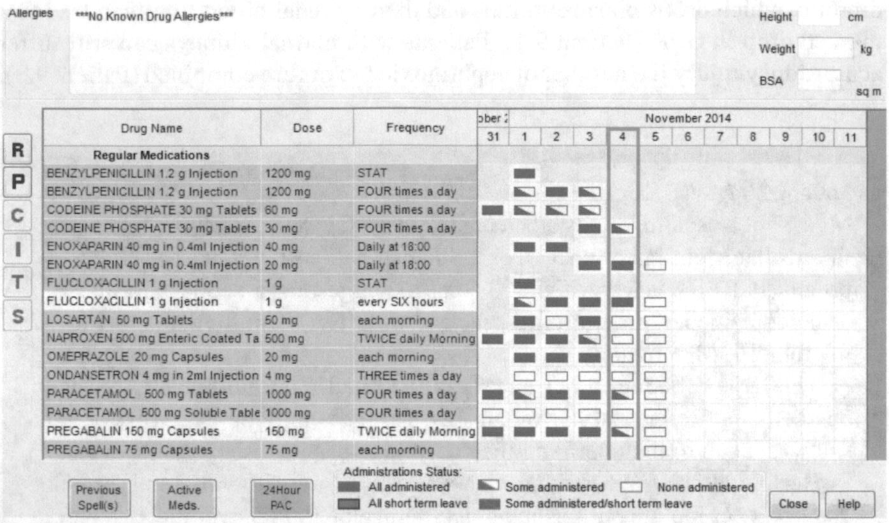

| Allergies | ***No Known Drug Allergies*** | | | | | | | | | | | | | Height | | cm |

Weight   kg

BSA   sq m

	Drug Name	Dose	Frequency	ober 2 31	November 2014 1	2	3	4	5	6	7	8	9	10	11
R	**Regular Medications**														
P	BENZYLPENICILLIN 1.2 g Injection	1200 mg	STAT	■											
C	BENZYLPENICILLIN 1.2 g Injection	1200 mg	FOUR times a day		◣	◣	◣								
	CODEINE PHOSPHATE 30 mg Tablets	60 mg	FOUR times a day	■	◣	◣	◣								
I	CODEINE PHOSPHATE 30 mg Tablets	30 mg	FOUR times a day					■	◣						
T	ENOXAPARIN 40 mg in 0.4ml Injection	40 mg	Daily at 18:00	■	■										
S	ENOXAPARIN 40 mg in 0.4ml Injection	20 mg	Daily at 18:00				■	■	□						
	FLUCLOXACILLIN 1 g Injection	1 g	STAT	■											
	FLUCLOXACILLIN 1 g Injection	1 g	every SIX hours		◣	■	■	■							
	LOSARTAN 50 mg Tablets	50 mg	each morning		■	□	■	□	□						
	NAPROXEN 500 mg Enteric Coated Ta	500 mg	TWICE daily Morning	■	■	■	◣	□	□						
	OMEPRAZOLE 20 mg Capsules	20 mg	each morning		■	■	■	□	□						
	ONDANSETRON 4 mg in 2ml Injection	4 mg	THREE times a day		□	□	□	□	□						
	PARACETAMOL 500 mg Tablets	1000 mg	FOUR times a day	■	◣	■	■	◣	□						
	PARACETAMOL 500 mg Soluble Table	1000 mg	FOUR times a day	□	□	□	□	□	□						
	PREGABALIN 150 mg Capsules	150 mg	TWICE daily Morning	■	■	■	■	◣	□						
	PREGABALIN 75 mg Capsules	75 mg	each morning						□						

Administrations Status:
■ All administered   ◣ Some administered   □ None administered
■ All short term leave   ■ Some administered/short term leave

| Previous Spell(s) | Active Meds. | 24Hour PAC | | Close | Help |

Fig. 9.5 Medication chart for Mrs. Kent documenting the drugs administered following her admission to hospital

Anticoagulant-Related Nephropathy

Anticoagulant-related nephropathy is an uncommon cause of acute kidney injury in patients with chronic kidney disease and an INR >3 [9]. The combination of increased glomerular pressure and impaired clotting causes bleeding into the glomeruli and hematuria. Kidney function usually does not fully recover due to residual glomerular damage (Patient 9.4).

> **Patient 9.4 Anticoagulant-Related Nephropathy**
> Mr. Edwards had CKD stage 3 with hypertension and heavy proteinuria, PCR = 194 mg/mmol (2000 mg/g). He was taking long-term warfarin prophylaxis for a prosthetic aortic valve replacement. The INR was unstable, especially when taking antibiotics for recurrent cellulitis.
>
> In 2018 he was admitted to hospital the day after a phlebotomy because of a swollen, painful, bruised right arm. Over the previous 2 weeks he had had nose bleeds, subconjunctival haemorrhages, abdominal wall bruising and visible haematuria.
>
> INR on admission was 6.8. The eGFR dropped acutely (Fig. 9.6). An ultrasound scan excluded urinary tract obstruction. The INR remained erratic and his kidney function declined for a period before both gradually improved.

eGFR
(ml/min/1.73 m²)   INR

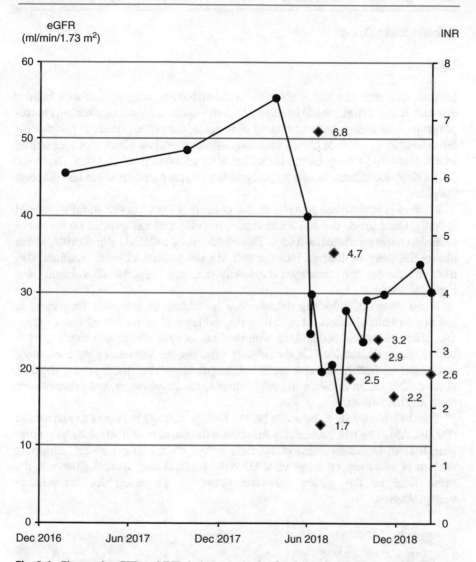

Fig. 9.6 Changes in eGFR and INR during an episode of anticoagulant-related nephropathy

Tubulotoxic Drugs

Lithium

Lithium carbonate is a highly effective mood-stabilising drug used to treat bipolar disorder. It can restore mental health without the sedative effects of other psychotropic drugs. Unfortunately, in a minority of patients, chronic use leads to progressive tubulotoxicity and loss of kidney function despite careful monitoring of serum drug levels. End-stage kidney failure is reached after an average of 20 years' treatment [10]. Other side effects include hypothyroidism, hyperparathyroidism and diabetes insipidus.

Lithium is reabsorbed by cells in the collecting duct via the sodium channel (ENaC). Once inside the cell it can inhibit the effect of vasopressin on the water channel, causing diabetes insipidus. This effect can be reduced by amiloride, which blocks the entry of lithium into the cell via the sodium channel. Lithium also has effects on the parathyroid glands, causing hyperparathyroidism and hypercalcaemia.

When progressive kidney damage due to lithium is detected, the patient is posed a difficult dilemma. Should they stop taking it to avoid further kidney damage, take alternative medications with unpleasant side effects and risk a relapse into mania or depression? Or should they continue the lithium, enjoy continuing stable mental health and risk further damage? Resolving these issues requires close collaboration between the nephrologist, the psychiatrist, the primary care team and the patient.

The decision needs to be made before kidney damage becomes too advanced (Patient 9.5). The risk that kidney function will continue to decline despite stopping lithium increases when eGFR falls below 45 mL/min/1.73 m^2. Stopping lithium at an advanced stage of CKD risks precipitating mental illness at the same time as the patient has the stress of preparing for dialysis or transplantation.

Patient 9.5 Lithium Nephrotoxicity

Mrs. Ballard had suffered multiple episodes of mania and depression since the age of 25. She started lithium in 1989. It was stopped in 1991 but she relapsed into mania so it was restarted. Her mood then stabilized and she felt well. Serum lithium levels were consistently within the therapeutic range.

By 2008 it was clear her kidney function was declining (Fig. 9.7). Despite the risk of another relapse in her bipolar disorder, she decided to stop lithium and use other antipsychotic and mood stabilizing drugs. The rate of decline in eGFR slowed significantly.

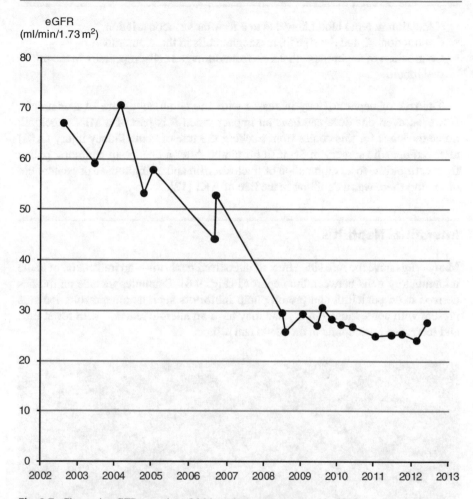

Fig. 9.7 Change in eGFR over time. Lithium therapy was stopped in 2000

Aminoglycoside Antibiotics: Gentamicin

The antibiotic gentamicin is tubulotoxic as well as ototoxic [11]. Sodium and water reabsorption are affected, especially in the proximal part of the nephron that is exposed to the drug. Urine volume is usually normal or increased and increased amounts of tubular enzymes, amino acids, glucose, calcium and magnesium are excreted.

Glomerular filtration is reduced by:

- Increased tubulo-glomerular feedback—reduced absorption in the proximal tubule allows more filtrate to reach the distal tubule and the macula densa. This stimulates the release of vasoconstrictors which reduce glomerular filtration and protect against excessive salt and water loss

- Reduction in renal blood flow due to arteriolar vasoconstriction
- Contraction of, and damage to, mesangial cells in the glomeruli
- Obstruction of nephrons with debris from damaged cells, especially in the proximal tubule

The risk of nephrotoxicity increases with the cumulative dose of gentamicin. However, even one dose can have an impact when it is part of a MINT cocktail. Some evidence for this comes from tracking the rate of acute kidney injury (AKI) after orthopaedic surgery in Scottish hospitals. After a change in antibiotic policy from cefuroxime to a combination of flucloxacillin and a single-dose of gentamicin (4 mg/kg) there was a doubling in the rate of AKI [12].

Interstitial Nephritis

Many drugs have the rare side effect of interstitial nephritis—an infiltration of acute inflammatory cells between the nephrons (Fig. 9.8). Examples include antibiotics derived from penicillin and proton pump inhibitors such as omeprazole. Patients present with acute kidney injury and may have an allergic reaction with fever, rash and increased eosinophils in the blood and urine.

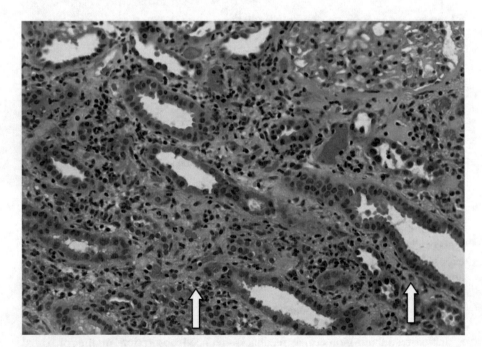

Fig. 9.8 Section of a kidney biopsy from a patient who had been taking omeprazole, showing typical appearances of interstitial nephritis. There is an infiltration of inflammatory cells between the tubules, mainly lymphocytes with some eosinophils (*arrows*). The glomerulus (*top right*) is normal. Haematoxylin and eosin ×200

Proton pump inhibitors (PPIs) can cause both acute kidney injury due to interstitial nephritis and chronic kidney disease. The risk of acute kidney injury is doubled in patients taking a PPI and, although the absolute risk for each user is low, the number of people affected is high because PPI use is so common [13]. A survey has found that 7.8% of US adults had used prescription PPIs in the previous 30 days [14] and the drugs may also be available without prescription.

PPI-induced acute interstitial nephritis is hard to detect clinically as most patients do not have systemic allergic symptoms or signs, or any urinary abnormality. This means that diagnosis is often delayed, allowing chronic damage to develop. Patients taking a PPI are 20–50% more likely to develop chronic kidney disease than those taking a histamine 2 receptor antagonist, such as ranitidine [15] and twice as likely to develop end-stage kidney disease [16]. The chronic damage does not necessarily follow an episode of acute kidney injury [17] and may be mediated by damage to vascular endothelial cells [18].

Metformin: Villain or Victim?

Metformin is a first-line hypoglycaemic drug used to treat diabetes. Its use is associated with lower all-cause mortality in patients with diabetes and chronic kidney, heart and liver diseases, and so it should not be stopped without good reason [19].

One of the actions of metformin is to reduce pyruvate dehydrogenase activity in the liver, which leads to an increase in pyruvate and lactic acid. In advanced kidney failure metformin accumulates, leading to potentially severe lactic acidosis. Guidelines recommend reducing the dose of metformin when eGFR falls below 60 mL/min/1.73 m^2 and stopping it completely below 30 [20].

Metformin has been used for decades and the caution about lactic acidosis is deeply rooted in medical teaching. However, a recent metanalysis of over 200 studies involving 100,000 people suggests that the risk may have been exaggerated [21]. Lactic acidosis is more likely to be due to the underlying condition than the metformin [22].

Because metformin is stopped in patients with a low GFR it is sometimes mistakenly thought to be nephrotoxic. Rather than metformin being a villain that damages kidneys, it is actually a victim of kidney failure.

Kidney Diseases Due to Toxins

Cocaine and Heroin

Use of cocaine and heroin has been associated with the nephrotic syndrome, acute glomerulonephritis, amyloidosis, interstitial nephritis, and rhabdomyolysis [23]. The kidney damage may be mediated by chronic viral infections such as Hepatitis B, C and HIV, and the existence of a specific 'heroin nephropathy' is now questioned. Cocaine is a potent vasoconstrictor and so leads to reduced renal blood flow and GFR. It accelerates atherosclerosis and platelet aggregation and can lead to malignant hypertension.

Mushroom Poisoning

Mushroom poisoning has been blamed for the death of many notable people, including The Buddha and the Roman Emperor Claudius, and has caused outbreaks of kidney failure throughout history.

Mushrooms of the *Cortinarius* species (the Deadly Webcap) can be confused with edible Chanterelle mushrooms. They cause severe acute kidney injury and permanent kidney failure. The toxic effect is due to orellanine, which causes tubular necrosis and interstitial nephritis. Clinical symptoms occur from 3 days to 3 weeks after ingestion. Identifying the spores and detecting the orellanine toxin in leftover mushrooms confirms the diagnosis. Orellanine is detectable by thin-layer chromatography technique in biopsy tissue for up to 6 months. There is no effective antidote [24].

Chemical Poisoning

The following are some of the more common chemicals known to be nephrotoxic:

- Heavy metals—cadmium, lead, mercury
- Melamine—added to baby milk formula
- Ethylene glycol antifreeze
- Glyphosate weed killer

As one of roles of the kidneys is the excretion of toxins, they are especially vulnerable to damage from these chemicals [25].

Chinese Herbal Medicines

Herbs used in Chinese medicines may contain nephrotoxic aristolochic acids and other plant alkaloids, anthraquinones, flavonoids, and glycosides. As well as the herbs being intrinsically nephrotoxic, the medicines may be adulterated with other compounds or heavy metals. They may also interact with other drugs.

These compounds have been linked to acute kidney injury, chronic kidney disease, kidney stones, rhabdomyolysis, Fanconi syndrome, and urothelial carcinoma [26].

References

1. Bundy JD, Bazzano LA, Xie D, Cohan J, Dolata J, Fink JC, Hsu CY, Jamerson K, Lash J, Makos G, Steigerwalt S, Wang X, Mills KT, Chen J, He J, CRIC Study Investigators. Self-reported tobacco, alcohol, and illicit drug use and progression of chronic kidney disease. Clin J Am Soc Nephrol. 2018;13(7):993–1001. https://doi.org/10.2215/CJN.11121017. https://cjasn.asnjournals.org/content/early/2018/06/06/CJN.11121017.long.

2. Jha V, Rathi M. Natural medicines causing acute kidney injury. Semin Nephrol. 2008;28(4):416–28. https://doi.org/10.1016/j.semnephrol.2008.04.010. http://www.seminarsinnephrology.org/article/S0270-9295(08)00088-0/abstract.

3. Lea-Henry TN, Carland JE, Stocker SL, Sevastos J, Roberts DM. Clinical pharmacokinetics in kidney disease: fundamental principles. Clin J Am Soc Nephrol. 2018;13(7):1085–95. https://doi.org/10.2215/CJN.00340118. Epub 2018 Jun 22. https://cjasn.asnjournals.org/content/13/7/1085.

4. Perazella MA. Pharmacology behind common drug nephrotoxicities. Clin J Am Soc Nephrol. 2018;13(12):1897–908. https://doi.org/10.2215/CJN.00150118. Epub 2018 Apr 5. https://cjasn.asnjournals.org/content/clinjasn/13/12/1897.full.pdf.

5. Markowitz GS, Bomback AS, Perazella MA. Drug-induced glomerular disease: direct cellular injury. Clin J Am Soc Nephrol. 2015;10(7):1291–9. https://doi.org/10.2215/CJN.00860115. http://cjasn.asnjournals.org/cgi/pmidlookup?view=long&pmid=25862776.

6. Hogan JJ, Markowitz GS, Radhakrishnan J. Drug-induced glomerular disease: immune-mediated injury. Clin J Am Soc Nephrol. 2015;10(7):1300–10. https://doi.org/10.2215/CJN.01910215. https://cjasn.asnjournals.org/content/10/7/1300.long.

7. Clark AL, Kalra PR, Petrie MC, Mark PB, Tomlinson LA, Tomson CRV. Change in renal function associated with drug treatment in heart failure: national guidance. Heart. 2019;105:904–10. https://heart.bmj.com/content/105/12/904.full.

8. O'Sullivan ED, Hughes J, Ferenbach DA. Renal aging: causes and consequences. J Am Soc Nephrol. 2017;28(2):407–20. https://doi.org/10.1681/ASN.2015121308. https://www.ncbi.nlm.nih.gov/pmc/articles/PMC5280008/.

9. Brodsky S, Eikelboom J, Hebert LA. Anticoagulant-related nephropathy. JASN. 2018;29(12):2787–93. https://doi.org/10.1681/ASN.201807074.

10. Alsady M, Baumgarten R, Deen PM, de Groot T. Lithium in the kidney: friend and foe? JASN. 2016;27(6):1587–95. https://doi.org/10.1681/ASN.2015080907. https://jasn.asnjournals.org/content/27/6/1587.long.

11. Lopez-Novoa JM, Quiros Y, Vicente L, Morales AI, Lopez-Hernandez FJ. New insights into the mechanism of aminoglycoside nephrotoxicity: an integrative point of view. Kidney Int. 2011;79:33–45. https://doi.org/10.1038/ki.2010.337. http://www.nature.com/ki/journal/v79/n1/full/ki2010337a.html.

12. Bell S, Davey P, Nathwani D, Marwick C, Vadiveloo T, Sneddon J, Patton A, Bennie M, Fleming S, Donnan PT. Risk of AKI with gentamicin as surgical prophylaxis. JASN. 2014;25(11):2625–32. https://doi.org/10.1681/ASN.2014010035. http://www.ncbi.nlm.nih.gov/pmc/articles/PMC4214537/.

13. Moledina DG, Perazella MA. Proton pump inhibitors and CKD. J Am Soc Nephrol. 2016;27(10):2926–8. https://www.ncbi.nlm.nih.gov/pmc/articles/PMC5042680/.

14. Kantor ED, Rehm CD, Haas JS, Chan AT, Giovannucci EL. Trends in prescription drug use among adults in the United States from 1999-2012. JAMA. 2015;314:1818–31. https://jamanetwork.com/journals/jama/fullarticle/10.1001/jama.2015.13766.

15. Lazarus B, Chen Y, Wilson FP, Sang Y, Chang AR, Coresh J, Grams ME. Proton pump inhibitor use and the risk of chronic kidney disease. JAMA Intern Med. 2016;176(2):238–46. https://doi.org/10.1001/jamainternmed.2015.7193. https://jamanetwork.com/journals/jamainternalmedicine/fullarticle/2481157.

16. Xie Y, Bowe B, Li T, Xian H, Balasubramanian S, Al-Aly Z. Proton pump inhibitors and risk of incident CKD and progression to ESRD. J Am Soc Nephrol. 2016;27(10):3153–63. https://doi.org/10.1681/ASN.2015121377. Epub 2016 Mar 14. PubMed PMID: 27080976; PubMed Central PMCID: PMC5042677. https://www.ncbi.nlm.nih.gov/pmc/articles/PMC5042677/.

17. Xie Y, Bowe B, Li T, Xian H, Yan Y, Al-Aly Z. Long-term kidney outcomes among users of proton pump inhibitors without intervening acute kidney injury. Kidney Int. 2017;91(6):1482–94. https://doi.org/10.1016/j.kint.2016.12.021. Epub 2017 Feb 22. https://www.kidney-international.org/article/S0085-2538(17)30005-4/fulltext.

18. Yepuri G, Sukhovershin R, Nazari-Shafti TZ, Petrascheck M, Ghebre YT, Cooke JP. Proton pump inhibitors accelerate endothelial senescence. Circ Res. 2016;118(12):e36–42. https://

doi.org/10.1161/CIRCRESAHA.116.308807.   https://www.ncbi.nlm.nih.gov/pmc/articles/PMC4902745.

19. Crowley MJ, Diamantidis CJ, McDuffie JR, Cameron CB, Stanifer JW, Mock CK, Wang X, Tang S, Nagi A, Kosinski AS, Williams JW. Clinical outcomes of metformin use in populations with chronic kidney disease, congestive heart failure, or chronic liver disease: a systematic review. Ann Intern Med. 2017;166:191–200. https://doi.org/10.7326/M16-1901.   http://annals.org/aim/article/2595889/clinical-outcomes-metformin-use-populations-chronic-kidney-disease-congestive-heart.

20. Lalau J-D, Kajbaf F, Bennis Y, Hurtel-Lemaire A-S, Belpaire F, De Broe ME. Metformin treatment in patients with type 2 diabetes and chronic kidney disease stages 3A, 3B, or 4. Diabetes Care. 2018;41(3):547–53. https://doi.org/10.2337/dc17-2231. https://care.diabetesjournals.org/content/41/3/547.long.

21. Salpeter SR, Greyber E, Pasternak GA, Salpeter EE. Risk of fatal and nonfatal lactic acidosis with metformin use in type 2 diabetes mellitus. Cochrane Database Syst Rev. 2006;1:CD002967. http://onlinelibrary.wiley.com/doi/10.1002/14651858.CD002967.pub4/full.

22. Fitzgerald E, Mathieu S, Ball A. Metformin associated lactic acidosis. BMJ. 2009;339:b3660. https://doi.org/10.1136/bmj.b3660. Published 16 September 2009. http://www.bmj.com/content/339/bmj.b3660.

23. Jaffe JA, Kimmel PL. Chronic nephropathies of cocaine and heroin abuse: a critical review. CJASN. 2006;1(4):655–67. https://doi.org/10.2215/CJN.00300106. http://cjasn.asnjournals.org/content/1/4/655.full.

24. Frank H, Zilker T, Kirchmair M, Eyer F, Haberl B, Tuerkoglu-Raach G, Wessely M, Gröne HJ, Heemann U. Acute renal failure by ingestion of Cortinarius species confounded with psychoactive mushrooms: a case series and literature survey. Clin Nephrol. 2009;71(5):557–62. http://www.dustri.com/nc/journals-in-english/mag/clinical-nephrology/vol/volume-71/issue/may-15.html.

25. Perazella MA. Renal vulnerability to drug toxicity. CJASN. 2009;4(7):1275–83. https://doi.org/10.2215/CJN.02050309. Published ahead of print June 11, 2009. http://cjasn.asnjournals.org/content/4/7/1275.full.

26. Bo Yang B, Xie Y, Guo M, Rosner MH, Yang H, Ronco C. Nephrotoxicity and Chinese herbal medicine. CJASN. 2018;13(10):1605–11. https://doi.org/10.2215/CJN.11571017. https://cjasn.asnjournals.org/content/13/10/1605.

Height and Weight: The Effects of Kidney Disease on Development; Links Between Obesity and Kidney Disease

10

Growing Up with Kidney Disease

Chronic kidney disease has a major impact on children's development and quality of life, particularly through its effects on growth. The lower a child's kidney function, the slower will be their rate of growth. As a result, about a third of children with chronic kidney disease fall below the third percentile for their age and gender. The effect is even greater when kidney function is reduced in infancy.

Head circumference and brain volume normally increase rapidly during the first year of life. Poor growth is associated with intellectual impairment and learning difficulties. In older children, reduced growth and delayed puberty are associated with worse physical functioning and increased mortality. Short stature may lead to low self-esteem and emotional difficulties as children grow up to be adults.

An essential part of the care of any child, especially one with kidney disease, is the charting of height, weight and, for infants, head circumference (Patient 10.1).

Patient 10.1 Congenital Nephrotic Syndrome

Rayaan was born to consanguineous parents at term. An ultrasound scan at 20 weeks gestation had shown increased echogenicity of the kidneys. A repeat scan after birth confirmed them to be slightly large and echogenic. Kidney function was normal but serum albumin was low, 17 g/L (1.7 g/dL). A urine dipstick test showed heavy proteinuria confirming congenital nephrotic syndrome.

Over the next few days he became progressively more oedematous. He was given the ACE inhibitor captopril and NSAID indomethacin to reduce renal blood flow and urinary protein loss, and was supplemented with daily intravenous infusions of 20% albumin.

Despite nasogastric feeding, his weight gain over the next 3 months was very slow and his head circumference barely increased (Fig. 10.1).

© Springer Nature Switzerland AG 2020
H. C. Rayner et al., *Understanding Kidney Diseases*,
https://doi.org/10.1007/978-3-030-43027-6_10

To further reduce urinary protein loss, one of his kidneys was removed surgically.

Over the next 4 months his head circumference and then body weight increased rapidly. By 12 months of age, his weight and head circumference were between the 9th and 25th centile and his length was on the 0.4th centile.

Fig. 10.1 Chart from a boy with congenital nephrotic syndrome showing delayed growth in head circumference, body length and body weight

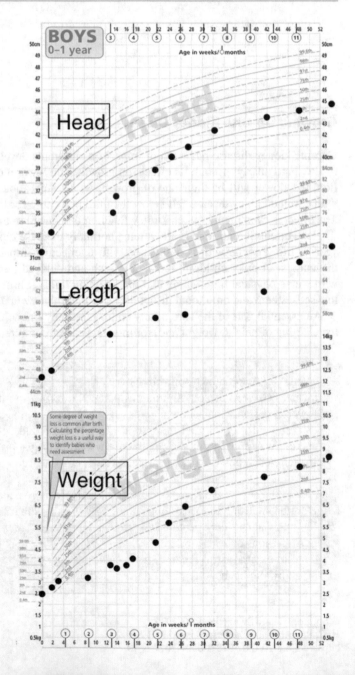

Growth failure in kidney disease is mainly due to a functional deficiency of Insulin-like Growth Factor 1 (IGF-1) [1]. Although the serum level of growth hormone is disproportionally high, its stimulatory effect on IGF-1 production by the liver is reduced. Bioactive IGF-1 is reduced and inhibitory IGF binding proteins are increased. The severity of these abnormalities is proportional to the reduction in GFR. Treatment with pharmacological doses of recombinant growth hormone can overcome some of the functional deficiency of IGF-1 (Patient 10.2) [2].

Children with CKD stage 3–5 or on dialysis can be given growth hormone if they have persistent growth failure, defined as a height below the third percentile for age and sex and a height velocity below the 25th percentile, once other potentially treatable risk factors for growth failure have been adequately addressed and provided the child has growth potential. In children who have received a kidney transplant and fulfil the above growth criteria, growth hormone can be started 1 year after transplantation if spontaneous catch-up growth does not occur and steroid-free immunosuppression is not possible [3].

Patient 10.2 Growth Retardation Due to Chronic Kidney Disease

Peter was born with dysplastic kidneys and reduced GFR. Despite nutritional supplements, calcium and vitamin D, his height remained below the 0.4th centile. Recombinant growth hormone injections were started and over the following 3 years his height velocity increased so that his height crossed the 0.4th centile (Fig. 10.2).

His renal function continued to decline and at 8.5 years of age he received a live-related kidney transplant. Over the next 18 months his height velocity accelerated so that he crossed the 25th centile for height, consistent with the height of his father.

Sadly, his family life became very difficult and at age 11.5 years he was taken into foster care. He was much happier in this environment; his height velocity increased and he entered puberty just below the 75th centile for height.

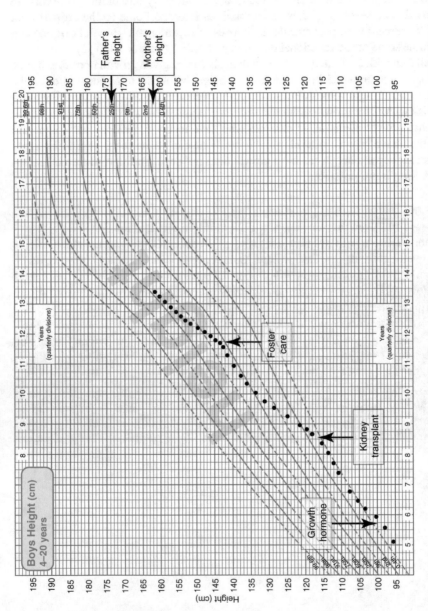

Fig. 10.2 Growth chart from a boy with chronic kidney disease showing the effects of growth hormone, kidney transplantation and improved social circumstances

As well as these hormonal abnormalities, growth can be affected by poor nutrition, metabolic acidosis, fluid and electrolyte abnormalities, renal bone disease and steroid therapy (Patient 10.3). Disadvantaged social circumstances may compound the medical problems. The most effective treatment is the restoration of normal kidney function with a successful transplant.

Patient 10.3 Growth Retardation and Obesity Due to Steroids

Aneesh attended the paediatric clinic for supervision of his asthma treatment. His height and weight were charted to monitor the effect of inhaled steroids on his growth. Until the age of seven both were increasing along the 50th centile (Fig. 10.3).

He then developed nephrotic syndrome, which is associated with atopy and asthma [4]. Glucocorticoid treatment led to remission of the proteinuria but stimulated his appetite. His weight accelerated and crossed the 75th centile.

During the following 2 years his nephrotic syndrome relapsed three times, requiring high doses of prednisolone on each occasion. His weight progressively increased, crossing the 91st centile, but his height velocity slowed to below the 50th centile.

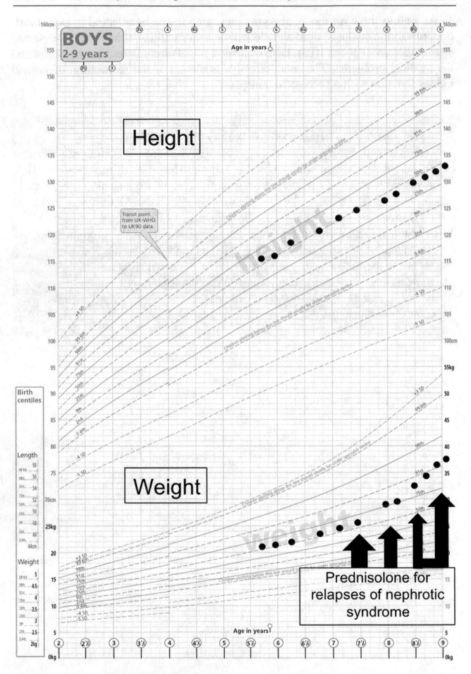

Fig. 10.3 Growth chart showing the effects of steroids on height and weight

Chronic kidney disease leads to a delay in puberty, on average by 2.5 years. When puberty does begin, the pubertal growth spurt may be shortened and less rapid. Bone maturation occurs at the end of puberty. If this is before growth has been completed the child will remain below the predicted height (Patient 10.4).

Patient 10.4 Growth and Puberty

Dominic's kidney disease was not apparent until the age of 15 when he presented acutely unwell with severely impaired kidney function and small shrunken kidneys. He was extremely short for his age and had delayed puberty, his radiological bone age being 4 years less than his chronological age (Fig. 10.4).

He was given recombinant growth hormone with some response in his height. Six months later he received a kidney transplant donated by his mother. Minimal doses of corticosteroid were used to allow maximum growth.

Because his bones were immature he was able to grow at a very rapid rate. By the time he completed his pubertal growth spurt he had reached a height between that of his parents.

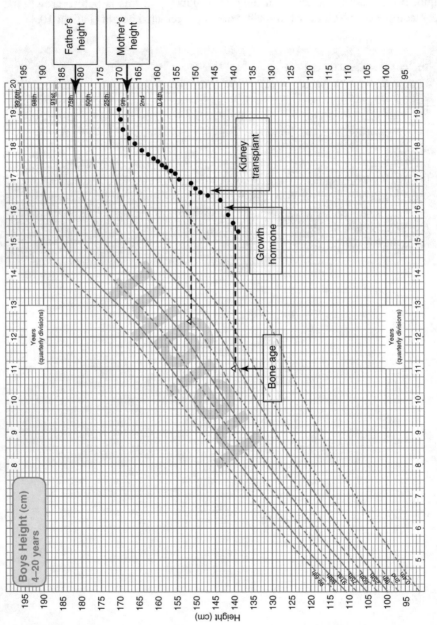

Fig. 10.4 Growth chart showing a delayed pubertal growth spurt in a boy with chronic kidney disease treated with growth hormone and a kidney transplant

Some children with chronic kidney disease may appear younger than their age because of their reduced growth and delayed puberty. In their teenage years others may treat them as children rather than young adults, delaying their emotional development.

Adolescent Care

Having kidney disease in childhood carries a lifelong legacy. The risk of developing end-stage kidney disease as an adult in increased fourfold, even if kidney function in adolescence is normal [5].

For adolescents with more advanced kidney disease, there comes a time when medical care needs to be transferred from the paediatric team to an adult kidney service. This can be a stressful experience for the young adult and his parents, especially if the support network built up over many years is lost. The break in continuity combined with the challenges of adolescence can precipitate a deterioration in health, for example an increased risk of kidney transplant rejection.

The age when the transfer should occur is best determined by the emotional maturity of the child and the readiness of the family. Ideally, the transition is made through a joint clinic provided by both paediatric and adult teams in an environment designed around the needs of adolescents [6].

Obesity and Risk

As an adult, being overweight or obese is associated with proteinuria due to focal segmental glomerulosclerosis [7] and increases the risk of kidney failure [8]. The effect appears to be mostly due to the metabolic syndrome, including high serum triglycerides, which is associated with a faster decline in GFR [9]. Obesity also increases the risk of kidney disease indirectly through high blood pressure, diabetes and cancer. In people with diabetes, long-term weight loss achieved through reduced food intake and increased exercise reduces the risk of a decline in GFR and an increase in albuminuria [10].

Weight loss or 'bariatric' surgery is the most effective treatment for extreme obesity as regards weight reduction, control of diabetes and cardiovascular disease. It also reduces the risk of developing chronic kidney disease [11] and halves the risk of a decline in kidney function [12]. Kidney stones become more common after surgery due to the increased absorption of oxalate.

In patients on dialysis, the usual association between obesity and mortality is not found; instead, increased body mass index (BMI) is associated with lower mortality. This is likely due to the benefit of a nutritional reserve in overweight dialysis patients during episodes of acute illness [13].

Obesity is associated with an increased risk of complications after transplant surgery. Many transplant centres apply a maximum acceptable BMI for transplantation to minimise the risks associated with the transplant procedure and maximise the survival chances of the graft. However, the 'obesity paradox' poses a dilemma for overweight dialysis patients. Losing weight may improve the outcomes after the transplant but worsen them while they remain on dialysis, especially if they have episodes of infection or inflammation [14].

References

1. Tönshoff B, Kiepe D, Ciarmatori S. Growth hormone/insulin-like growth factor system in children with chronic renal failure. Pediatr Nephrol. 2005;20(3):279. http://link.springer.com/article/10.1007%2Fs00467-005-1821-0.
2. Stonebrook E, Mahan JD. Treatment of growth retardation in a child with CKD. Clin J Am Soc Nephrol. 2019;14(11):1658–60. https://doi.org/10.2215/CJN.03960319. pii: CJN.03960319. https://cjasn.asnjournals.org/content/early/2019/07/25/CJN.03960319.
3. Drube J, Wan M, Bonthuis M, Wühl E, Bacchetta J, Santos F, Grenda R, Edefonti A, Harambat J, Shroff R, Tönshoff B, Haffner D, European Society for Paediatric Nephrology Chronic Kidney Disease Mineral and Bone Disorders, Dialysis, and Transplantation Working Groups. Clinical practice recommendations for growth hormone treatment in children with chronic kidney disease. Nat Rev Nephrol. 2019;15(9):577–89. https://doi.org/10.1038/s41581-019-0161-4. Epub 2019 Jun 13. https://www.nature.com/articles/s41581-019-0161-4.
4. Abdel-Hafez M, Shimada M, Lee PY, Johnson RJ, Garin EH. Idiopathic nephrotic syndrome and atopy: is there a common link? Am J Kidney Dis. 2009;54(5):945–53. https://doi.org/10.1053/j.ajkd.2009.03.019. http://www.ncbi.nlm.nih.gov/pmc/articles/PMC2895907.
5. Calderon-Margalit R, Golan E, Twig G, Leiba A, Tzur D, Afek A, Skorecki K, Vivante A. History of childhood kidney disease and risk of adult end-stage renal disease. N Engl J Med. 2018;378(5):428–38. https://doi.org/10.1056/NEJMoa1700993. https://www.nejm.org/doi/10.1056/NEJMoa1700993?url_ver=Z39.88-2003&rfr_id=ori:rid:crossref.org&rfr_dat=cr_pub%3dwww.ncbi.nlm.nih.gov.
6. Watson AR, Warady BA. Transition from pediatric to adult-centered care. Dial Transplant. 2011;40(4):156–8. http://onlinelibrary.wiley.com/enhanced/doi/10.1002/dat.20557/.
7. Mallamaci F, Tripepi G. Obesity and CKD progression: hard facts on fat CKD patients. Nephrol Dial Transplant. 2013;28(Suppl 4):iv105–8. https://doi.org/10.1093/ndt/gft391. http://ndt.oxfordjournals.org/content/28/suppl_4/iv105.full.pdf.
8. Herrington WG, Smith M, Bankhead C, Matsushita K, Stevens S, Holt T, Hobbs FD, Coresh J, Woodward M. Body-mass index and risk of advanced chronic kidney disease: prospective analyses from a primary care cohort of 1.4 million adults in England. PLoS One. 2017;12(3):e0173515. https://doi.org/10.1371/journal.pone.0173515. http://dx.plos.org/10.1371/journal.pone.0173515.
9. Stefansson VTN, Schei J, Solbu MD, Jenssen TG, Melsom T, Eriksen BO. Metabolic syndrome but not obesity measures are risk factors for accelerated age-related glomerular filtration rate decline in the general population. Kidney Int. 2018;93(5):1183–90. https://doi.org/10.1016/j.kint.2017.11.012. Epub 2018 Feb 1. https://www.kidney-international.org/article/S0085-2538(17)30828-1/fulltext.
10. The Look AHEAD Research Group. Effect of a long-term behavioural weight loss intervention on nephropathy in overweight or obese adults with type 2 diabetes: a secondary analysis of the Look AHEAD randomised clinical trial. Lancet Diabetes Endocrinol. 2014;2(10):801–9. http://www.thelancet.com/journals/landia/article/PIIS2213-8587(14)70156-1/abstract.
11. Friedman AN, Wahed AS, Wang J, Courcoulas AP, Dakin G, Hinojosa MW, Kimmel PL, Mitchell JE, Pomp A, Pories WJ, Purnell JQ, le Roux C, Spaniolas K, Steffen KJ, Thirlby R, Wolfe B. Effect of bariatric surgery on CKD risk. J Am Soc Nephrol. 2018;29(4):1289–300. https://doi.org/10.1681/ASN.2017060707. https://jasn.asnjournals.org/content/29/4/1289.long.

12. Chang AR, Chen Y, Still C, Wood GC, Kirchner HL, Lewis M, Kramer H, Hartle JE, Carey D, Appel LJ, Grams ME. Bariatric surgery is associated with improvement in kidney outcomes. Kidney Int. 2016;90(1):164–71. https://doi.org/10.1016/j.kint.2016.02.039. Epub 2016 May 12. https://www.ncbi.nlm.nih.gov/pmc/articles/PMC4912457.
13. Pifer TB, Mccullough KP, Port FK, Goodkin DA, Maroni BJ, Held PJ, Young EW. Mortality risk in hemodialysis patients and changes in nutritional indicators: DOPPS. Kidney Int. 2002;62:2238–45. https://doi.org/10.1046/j.1523-1755.2002.00658.x. http://www.nature.com/ki/journal/v62/n6/full/4493347a.html.
14. Stenvinkel P, Gillespie IA, Tunks J, Addison J, Kronenberg F, Drueke TB, Marcelli D, Schernthaner G, Eckardt KU, Floege J, Froissart M, Anker SD, ARO Steering Committee. Inflammation modifies the paradoxical association between body mass index and mortality in hemodialysis patients. J Am Soc Nephrol. 2016;27(5):1479–86. https://doi.org/10.1681/ASN.2015030252. Epub 2015 Nov 13. http://jasn.asnjournals.org/cgi/pmidlookup?view=long&pmid=26567245.

Blood Pressure: The Interactions Between Hypertension and Kidney Disease

11

High blood pressure is an important and treatable cardiovascular risk factor. Every 10 mmHg reduction in systolic blood pressure reduces the risk of coronary heart disease by 17%, stroke by 27%, heart failure by 28%, and all-cause mortality by 13% [1].

Blood pressure measured in the surgery or clinic may be raised by the 'white coat' effect, which affects over half of treated hypertensive patients. It can increase the systolic blood pressure by 30 mmHg or more, even in patients who are not overtly anxious. The size of the effect increases with the underlying blood pressure, making clinic readings of limited value for monitoring blood pressure control.

Taking regular home blood pressure readings leads to significantly better control than using infrequent clinic readings [2]. Validated automated arm cuff meters are available in chemist shops and on-line for about £20 (about US $30). The correct size of cuff for the arm circumference should be used—if it is too small the readings may be falsely high. If the pulse is irregular the meter may not give an accurate or any reading. Blood pressure should be measured on a bare arm; putting the cuff over the sleeve may increase the systolic pressure. Wrist blood pressure meters are not validated.

You should instruct patients in how to adjust their blood pressure treatment in response to their home readings. In a randomised trial comparing self-monitoring and self-titration of antihypertensive medication versus usual primary care, systolic blood pressure was on average 9 mmHg lower in the self-managing group after 12 months, without any increase in side effects [3]. A smartphone app for checking medications, recording blood pressure readings, symptoms and results, and receiving automated feedback helps patients gain confidence and feel more in control of their condition [4].

© Springer Nature Switzerland AG 2020
H. C. Rayner et al., *Understanding Kidney Diseases*,
https://doi.org/10.1007/978-3-030-43027-6_11

There is often a difference in blood pressure between the two arms [5]. This is more common in people with hypertension, diabetes and chronic kidney disease and is associated with an increased risk of cardiovascular and all-cause mortality. Patients should use the higher reading to guide treatment decisions if the difference is more than 15 mmHg.

A difference in blood pressure between the two arms of more than 35 mmHg may indicate an atherosclerotic stenosis of one subclavian artery. Smaller inequalities are more likely to be due to differences in the stiffness of the arteries in the arm than a localised stenosis.

Diurnal Variation in Blood Pressure

Blood pressure normally follows a pattern across the 24-h cycle—the diurnal rhythm. It dips before sleep then rises before wakening (Fig. 11.1).

In people with chronic kidney disease, this nocturnal dipping pattern is often lost; a non-dipping pattern is increasingly common as GFR decreases (Fig. 11.2). This pattern is associated with lower GFR, proteinuria, target organ damage [6] and a higher risk of developing chronic kidney disease [7].

In some patients, particularly when chronic kidney disease is more severe, the blood pressure may rise during sleep (Fig. 11.3).

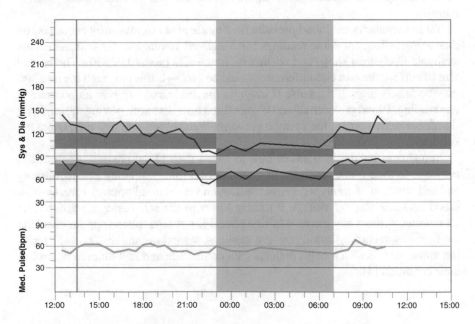

Fig. 11.1 A normal 24-h blood pressure recording showing the diurnal rhythm

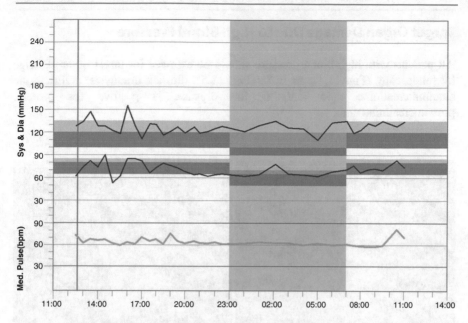

Fig. 11.2 24-h blood pressure recording in someone with chronic kidney disease. Daytime readings are normal but there is no dip during the night

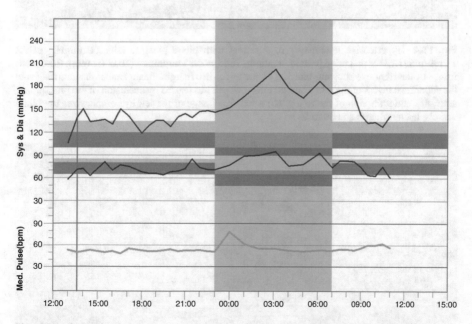

Fig. 11.3 24-h blood pressure recording in someone with chronic kidney disease stage 5, eGFR = 14 mL/min/1.73 m². Readings during the day are nearly normal but during the night they rise dramatically

Target Organ Damage Due to High Blood Pressure

All patients with high blood pressure should be assessed for target organ damage by fundoscopy (Fig. 11.4), an ECG (Fig. 11.5), dipstick urinalysis, eGFR, urine albumin:creatinine ratio and, if the dipstick is positive for protein, protein:creatinine ratio.

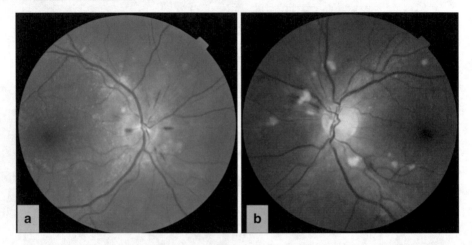

Fig. 11.4 Hypertensive retinopathy in a patient with blood pressure 240/160 mmHg, eGFR 11 mL/min/1.73 m² and urine protein:creatinine ratio = 2083 mg/mmol (20,000 mg/g). (**a**) Colour image of the right eye showing blurring of the optic disc margin, flame-shaped haemorrhages in the superficial layers of the retina and cotton-wool patches caused by occlusion of the precapillary arterioles and infarction of the retina; (**b**) a red-free image of the left eye emphasizes the blood vessels, haemorrhages and infarcts

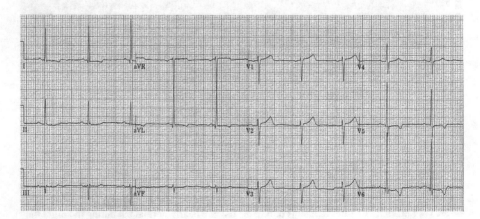

Fig. 11.5 ECG showing voltage criteria for left ventricular hypertrophy: S in V1 + R in V5 or V6 (whichever is larger) ≥35 mm, R in aVL ≥11 mm; T wave inversion in V5 and V6 indicates a strain pattern

Principles for Treating High Blood Pressure

Diet and Lifestyle

Lifestyle interventions should be part of the management of high blood pressure regardless of its severity or cause [8]. These include stopping smoking, eating a healthy diet and taking regular exercise, using relaxation techniques, and reducing intake of alcohol and caffeine if this is excessive. Being part of a group can help people stay motivated.

A moderate salt intake is ideal. Sodium intake of ≥ 7 g per day is associated with an increased risk of cardiovascular events and death in patients with hypertension, although interestingly not in people with normal blood pressure. A sodium intake of <3 g per day is also associated with an increased risk of cardiovascular events and death in people with and without hypertension [9].

In patients with chronic kidney disease, high salt intake is associated with an increased risk of cardiovascular disease [10]. In a randomized trial in patients an eGFR between 15 and 60 mL/min/1.73 m², a lower salt intake reduced blood pressure and extracellular fluid volume [11].

When to Use Antihypertensive Drugs

Patients with mild hypertension (defined as three consecutive blood pressure readings of 140/90–159/99 mmHg within 12 months), no target organ damage, and no history of cardiovascular disease or cardiovascular risk factors gain no benefit from antihypertensive drugs. Indeed, their risk of low blood pressure is increased by 69% and fainting by 28% [12].

Patients with mild, stage 1, hypertension and either cardiovascular disease, kidney disease, diabetes or a 10-year cardiovascular risk of $\geq 10\%$ should be offered antihypertensive drug treatment.

Patients with stage 2 hypertension (defined as $\geq 160/100$ mmHg and subsequent ambulatory 24-h daytime or home average blood pressure $\geq 150/95$ mmHg) should be offered antihypertensive drug treatment.

Patients with severe hypertension (defined as clinic systolic blood pressure ≥ 180 mmHg or clinic diastolic blood pressure ≥ 110 mmHg) or accelerated hypertension (defined as $>180/110$ mmHg with signs of papilloedema and/or retinal haemorrhage or suspected phaeochromocytoma with labile or postural hypotension, headache, palpitations, pallor and sweating) require urgent assessment and treatment.

Monitoring the Effect of Antihypertensive Drugs

The aim of treatment is to achieve normal diurnal blood pressure levels (Fig. 11.6). The dose of tablets should be adjusted according to the systolic readings.

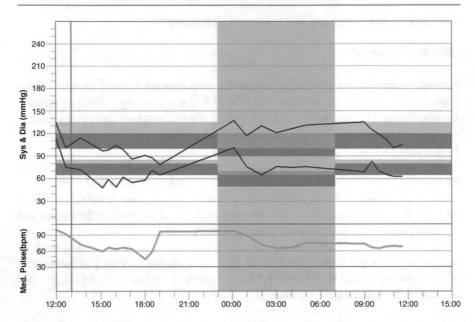

Fig. 11.6 24-h blood pressure recording in someone who took all their blood pressure treatment in the morning. Readings during the day are low after taking the tablets, which included a beta blocker—note the fall in pulse rate. The effect of the medication had worn off by the night, leaving the pressure high

Antihypertensive medication taken at night is more likely to produce a nocturnal dip (Fig. 11.7). Cardiovascular events such as death, myocardial infarction and stroke are reduced in patients taking all their medication at night compared with patients taking them all in the morning [13]. It can also reduce side effects, such as ankle swelling caused by calcium channel blockers.

Choice of Antihypertensive Drugs

A stepwise approach to introducing antihypertensives is recommended. Try to use once daily medications.
Step 1:

- Start with an angiotensin converting enzyme (ACE) inhibitor or angiotensin-II receptor blocker (ARB) for patients <55 years of age, and a calcium-channel blocker (CCB) for people aged >55 years and of African or Caribbean origin at any age.
- If a CCB is not suitable, use a thiazide diuretic.
- Beta-blockers may be used for younger people, particularly if they cannot tolerate other drugs

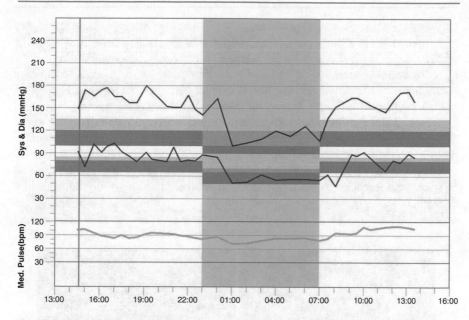

Fig. 11.7 24-h blood pressure recording in someone who took their blood pressure treatment before bedtime. Readings during the night are low after taking the tablets. The daytime pressure was high showing the need for more daytime medication

Step 2:

- Add a CCB in combination with either an ACE inhibitor or an ARB or add a thiazide diuretic

Step 3:

- If three drugs are needed, combine an ACE inhibitor or ARB, CCB and thiazide diuretic

Step 4:

- Consider low-dose spironolactone (25 mg once daily), watching serum potassium and eGFR, or an alpha- or beta-blocker.

Blood pressure that remains high despite a prescription of three or more drugs, so called resistant hypertension, is found in up to 20% of hypertensive patients [14]. Only about a half are truly drug resistant; the others are not fully adherent with their medication. If there is doubt whether the patient is taking the tablets, the levels of the drugs in urine can be checked. The effects of the medication can then be studied in a supervised setting (Patient 11.1) [15].

Patient 11.1 Non-adherence to Antihypertensive Drugs Due to Drug Intolerance
Mr. Cooper, a 70-year-old retired engineer, was referred to a specialist hypertension clinic because of high blood pressure despite being prescribed three antihypertensive drugs. His daytime ambulatory BP was 201/108 mmHg.

He had suffered angio-oedema of the mouth when taking the angiotensin receptor blocker candesartan and calcium channel blocker nifedipine (Fig. 11.8).

A urine antihypertensive drug screen was negative for all drugs. On further questioning he admitted to not taking his medications for fear of a further adverse reaction. He agreed to come to the day unit to be given the vasodilator hydralazine under supervision. His blood pressure was controlled with this agent (Fig. 11.9).

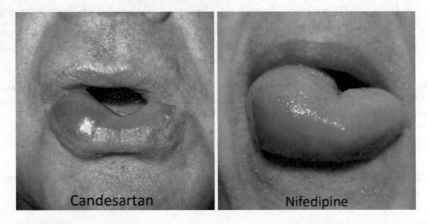

Fig. 11.8 Angio-oedema of the lip due to candesartan and tongue due to nifedipine

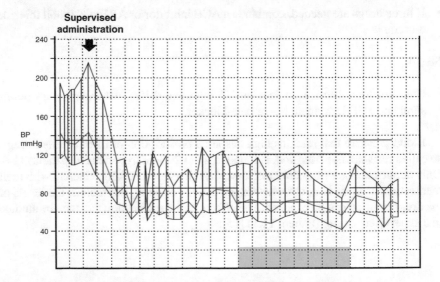

Fig. 11.9 The effect of hydralazine on Mr. Cooper's blood pressure over 24 h

Blood Pressure in Kidney Disease

Not all kidney diseases are associated with high blood pressure. Conditions in which the medullary region is damaged, for example ureteric obstruction, can result in the kidneys being unable to conserve sodium. The body is depleted of sodium, leading to reduced blood pressure, kidney blood flow and glomerular filtration rate.

In patients with chronic glomerular disease and high blood pressure, control is crucial for slowing the rate of decline in GFR. Having a systolic blood pressure >140 mmHg, compared with <120 mmHg, more than trebles the risk of reaching end-stage kidney disease or halving the eGFR [16].

The ideal is to lower the systolic pressure below 120 mmHg [17]. Strict blood pressure control is most beneficial in certain populations such as black people with the APOL1 genetic variant, which increases the risk of progressive kidney disease [18].

Intensive control of blood pressure can come at a price. Acute kidney injury and faints, but not injuries from falls, are more common with intensive treatment in the general population, although these problems are less prominent in patients with chronic kidney disease [19].

Older patients may be more likely to develop kidney failure with intensive blood pressure control [20]. Blood pressure that is slightly low in a young person can cause acute kidney injury in an elderly person who has lost the ability to dilate the kidney arterioles and preserve blood flow when systemic pressure is low—autoregulation.

Lowering the intraglomerular pressure reduces hydrostatic damage to the filtration barrier and slows down glomerulosclerosis (Patient 11.2). The first sign of this may be a reduction in proteinuria. Inhibitors of the renin-angiotensin-aldosterone system, such as ACE inhibitors and angiotensin receptor blockers (ARBs), are especially effective.

Patient 11.2 Slowing the Decline in Kidney Function by Controlling Blood Pressure

Mr. Boss had type 2 diabetes treated with insulin. He had cerebrovascular disease and had undergone coronary artery bypass grafting. He also had ischaemic optic neuropathy and was registered blind.

His blood pressure was poorly controlled; when seen in the diabetes-kidney clinic for the first time in 2013 it was 184/90 mmHg. eGFR had been falling at a rate of 4.5 mL/min/1.73 m^2 per year (Fig. 11.10).

His blood pressure treatment was intensified, in particular changing from a thiazide diuretic (indapamide) to a loop diuretic (furosemide) to remove excess salt and water. He learned to measure his blood pressure at home and achieved clinic systolic readings of 125/68 mmHg.

The decline in eGFR slowed to a rate of 1.5 mL/min/1.73 m^2 per year (Fig. 11.11).

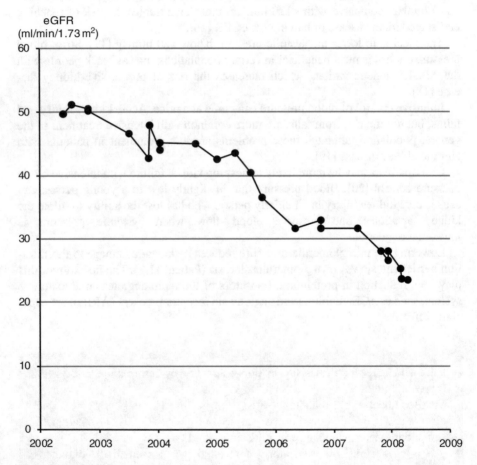

Fig. 11.10 Decline in eGFR due to diabetic nephropathy

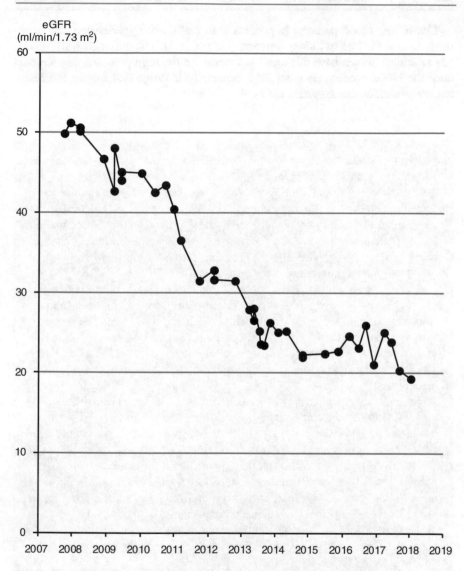

Fig. 11.11 Slowing of the rate of decline in eGFR following control of blood pressure

Starting treatment with an ACE or ARB often leads to an acute drop in eGFR due to the reduction in intraglomerular pressure. This is a reversible effect and not a sign of toxicity. There is no need to stop the treatment if the drop is not excessive, the serum potassium is less than 6.0 mmol/L, and the patient does not have symptomatic low blood pressure. It was thought that those patients who had a drop in eGFR gained more benefit from the treatment but recent studies do not support this [21, 22].

Controlling blood pressure in patients with malignant hypertension can sometimes reverse the loss of kidney function (Patient 11.3). The muscular walls of kidney arterioles, which have thickened in reaction to the high pressure, can remodel once the blood pressure is controlled, especially if drugs that inhibit the renin-angiotensin-aldosterone system are used.

Patient 11.3 Malignant Hypertension, Acute Kidney Injury, Haemolytic Anaemia and a Complicated Kidney Biopsy

Miss Korotkoff presented to hospital with headache, weakness and uncontrolled hypertension. Blood pressure in the left arm was 227/151 mmHg, in the right 207/144. She had been treated in the past for high blood pressure but had not taken any medication for over a year. Dipstick urinalysis showed heavy proteinuria, confirmed by a protein:creatinine ratio of 415 mg/mmol (4000 mg/g). Immunological screen was negative.

The eGFR on admission was 24 mL/min/1.73 m^2 and it continued to fall over the following days (Fig. 11.12). Haemoglobin concentration on admission was normal, 125 g/L (12.5 g/dL) but dropped to 84 g/L. The reticulocyte was raised at 181 × 10^9/L (normal range 33–102), haptoglobin was undetectable and lactate dehydrogenase raised at 1072 U/L (normal range 125–220). These abnormalities confirmed that the anaemia was due to haemolysis.

Both kidneys were of normal size on ultrasound but showed diffuse echogenicity with loss of cortico-medullary differentiation. Following control of her blood pressure she underwent a kidney biopsy on 25th June. This confirmed changes of malignant hypertension (Fig. 11.13).

On 5th July she developed left flank pain. Blood pressure and pulse were normal. The Hb had dropped further to 69 g/L (6.9 g/dL) (Fig. 11.12). Platelets and clotting screen were normal. Ultrasound scanning of the left kidney showed a 24 mm thick peri-renal haematoma caused by the biopsy.

Thereafter, kidney function continued to improve as blood pressure was controlled, initially with a calcium channel blocker and beta blocker and later with an ACE inhibitor.

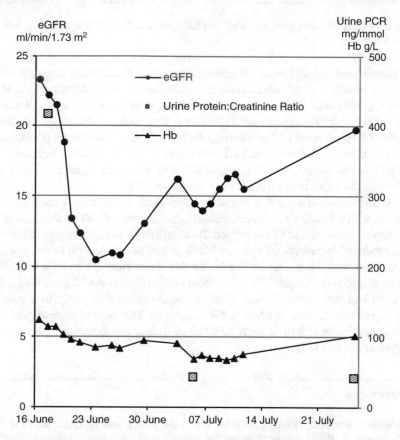

Fig. 11.12 Decline in eGFR and Hb due to malignant hypertension and haemolytic anaemia. The amount of proteinuria reduced as the blood pressure was controlled

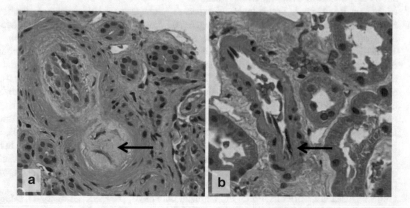

Fig. 11.13 Renal biopsy showing arterial changes due to malignant hypertension. Haemolytic anaemia results from damage to red cells as they are forced through the narrowed small artery lumens. (a) Small muscular artery showing expansion of the intima by myxoid material (arrow). Haematoxylin and eosin ×250. (b) Normal artery of similar calibre (arrow) for comparison. Haematoxylin and eosin ×400

The Effect of Kidney Function on Other Cardiovascular Risk Factors

The roles of diabetes and obesity in kidney disease are discussed in Chaps. 6 and 10. The other readily treatable cardiovascular risk factor is serum cholesterol. As eGFR decreases, treatment with statins to lower low-density lipoprotein (LDL) levels becomes less effective at preventing vascular events such as heart attack and stroke. For eGFR ≥ 60 mL/min/1.73 m^2 the risk of a first major vascular event is reduced by 21% per mmol/L reduction in LDL cholesterol. For eGFR <45 and >30 mL/min/1.73 m^2 the reduction is 15%. For eGFR <30 mL/min/1.73 m^2 and for patients on dialysis the effect is not statistically significant [23].

The high-sensitivity cardiac troponin I (hs-cTnI) blood test is used to assess someone with a possible myocardial infarction. The level of kidney function affects how the test result should be interpreted. Its sensitivity and negative predictive value are not reduced in patients with reduced GFR, so it can still be used to rule out myocardial infarction. However, its specificity decreases from 93 to 95% in patients with an eGFR >90 mL/min/1.73 m^2 to about 60% with eGFR <30 mL/min/1.73 m^2, and to 40% in patients on dialysis. Hence a positive result is less helpful in confirming a myocardial infarction when eGFR is reduced. The level of increse in hs-cTnI helps to predict the risk of dying at all levels of kidney function, the higher the level the greater the risk [24].

References

1. Ettehad D, Emdin CA, Kiran A, Anderson SG, Callender T, Emberson J, Chalmers J, Rodgers A, Rahimi K. Blood pressure lowering for prevention of cardiovascular disease and death: a systematic review and meta-analysis. Lancet. 2016;387(10022):957–67. https://doi.org/10.1016/S0140-6736(15)01225-8. Epub 2015 Dec 24. https://www.thelancet.com/action/showPdf?pii=S0140-6736%2815%2901225-8.
2. McManus RJ, Mant J, Franssen M, Nickless A, Schwartz C, Hodgkinson J, Bradburn P, Farmer A, Grant S, Greenfield SM, Heneghan C, Jowett S, Martin U, Milner S, Monahan M, Mort S, Ogburn E, Perera-Salazar R, Shah SA, Yu LM, Tarassenko L, Hobbs FDR, TASMINH4 Investigators. Efficacy of self-monitored blood pressure, with or without telemonitoring, for titration of antihypertensive medication (TASMINH4): an unmasked randomised controlled trial. Lancet. 2018;391(10124):949–59. https://doi.org/10.1016/S0140-6736(18)30309-X. Epub 2018 Feb 27. https://www.thelancet.com/journals/lancet/article/PIIS0140-6736%2818%2930309-X/fulltext.
3. McManus RJ, Mant J, Haque MS, Bray EP, Bryan S, Greenfield SM, Jones MI, Jowett S, Little P, Penaloza C, Schwartz C, Shackleford H, Shovelton C, Varghese J, Williams B, Hobbs FD. Effect of self-monitoring and medication self-titration on systolic blood pressure in hypertensive patients at high risk of cardiovascular disease: the TASMIN-SR randomized clinical trial. JAMA. 2014;312(8):799–808. https://doi.org/10.1001/jama.2014.10057. http://jama.jamanetwork.com/article.aspx?articleid=1899205.
4. Ong SW, Jassal SV, Miller JA, Porter EC, Cafazzo JA, Seto E, Thorpe KE, Logan AG. Integrating a smartphone-based self-management system into usual care of advanced CKD. Clin J Am Soc Nephrol. 2016;11(6):1054–62. https://doi.org/10.2215/CJN.10681015. Epub 2016 May 12. https://cjasn.asnjournals.org/content/11/6/1054.long.

5. Clark CE, Aboyans V. Interarm blood pressure difference: more than an epiphenomenon. Nephrol Dial Transplant. 2015;30(5):695–7. https://doi.org/10.1093/ndt/gfv075. https://academic.oup.com/ndt/article/30/5/695/2332879.

6. Drawz PE, Alper AB, Anderson AH, Brecklin CS, Charleston J, Chen J, Deo R, Fischer MJ, He J, Hsu CY, Huan Y, Keane MG, Kusek JW, Makos GK, Miller ER 3rd, Soliman EZ, Steigerwalt SP, Taliercio JJ, Townsend RR, Weir MR, Wright JT Jr, Xie D, Rahman M, Chronic Renal Insufficiency Cohort Study Investigators. Masked hypertension and elevated nighttime blood pressure in CKD: prevalence and association with target organ damage. Clin J Am Soc Nephrol. 2016;11(4):642–52. https://doi.org/10.2215/CJN.08530815. Epub 2016 Feb 18. https://cjasn.asnjournals.org/content/11/4/642.long.

7. Hermida RC, Ayala DE, Mojón A, Fernández JR. Sleep-time ambulatory BP is an independent prognostic marker of CKD. J Am Soc Nephrol. 2017;28(9):2802–11. https://doi.org/10.1681/ASN.2016111186. https://jasn.asnjournals.org/content/28/9/2802.long.

8. National Institute for Health and Care Excellence. Hypertension in adults: diagnosis and management. 2019. https://www.nice.org.uk/guidance/ng136.

9. Mente A, O'Donnell M, Rangarajan S, Dagenais G, Lear S, McQueen M, Diaz R, Avezum A, Lopez-Jaramillo P, Lanas F, Li W, Lu Y, Yi S, Rensheng L, Iqbal R, Mony P, Yusuf R, Yusoff K, Szuba A, Oguz A, Rosengren A, Bahonar A, Yusufali A, Schutte AE, Chifamba J, Mann JF, Anand SS, Teo K, Yusuf S, PURE, EPIDREAM and ONTARGET/TRANSCEND Investigators. Associations of urinary sodium excretion with cardiovascular events in individuals with and without hypertension: a pooled analysis of data from four studies. Lancet. 2016;388(10043):465–75. https://doi.org/10.1016/S0140-6736(16)30467-6. Epub 2016 May 20. https://www.thelancet.com/pdfs/journals/lancet/PIIS0140-6736(16)30467-6.pdf.

10. Mills KT, Chen J, Yang W, Appel LJ, Kusek JW, Alper A, Delafontaine P, Keane MG, Mohler E, Ojo A, Rahman M, Ricardo AC, Soliman EZ, Steigerwalt S, Townsend R, He J, Chronic Renal Insufficiency Cohort (CRIC) Study Investigators. Sodium excretion and the risk of cardiovascular disease in patients with chronic kidney disease. JAMA. 2016;315(20):2200–10. https://doi.org/10.1001/jama.2016.4447. https://jamanetwork.com/journals/jama/fullarticle/2524189.

11. Saran R, Padilla RL, Gillespie BW, Heung M, Hummel SL, Derebail VK, Pitt B, Levin NW, Zhu F, Abbas SR, Liu L, Kotanko P, Klemmer P. A randomized crossover trial of dietary sodium restriction in stage 3-4 CKD. Clin J Am Soc Nephrol. 2017;12(3):399–407. https://doi.org/10.2215/CJN.01120216. Epub 2017 Feb 16. https://cjasn.asnjournals.org/content/12/3/399.long.

12. Sheppard JP, Stevens S, Stevens R, Martin U, Mant J, Hobbs R, McManus R. Benefits and harms of antihypertensive treatment in low-risk patients with mild hypertension. JAMA Intern Med. 2018;178:1626–34. https://jamanetwork.com/journals/jamainternalmedicine/article-abstract/2708195.

13. Hermida RC, Crespo JJ, Domínguez-Sardiña M, Otero A, Moyá A, Ríos MT, Sineiro E, Castiñeira MC, Callejas PA, Pousa L, Salgado JL, Durán C, Sánchez JJ, Fernández JR, Mojón A, Ayala DE, Hygia Project Investigators. Bedtime hypertension treatment improves cardiovascular risk reduction: the Hygia Chronotherapy Trial. Eur Heart J. 2020;41(16):Page 1600. https://doi.org/10.1093/eurheartj/ehaa339.

14. Myat A, Redwood SR, Qureshi AC, Spertus JA, Williams B. Resistant hypertension. BMJ. 2012;345:e7473. https://www.bmj.com/content/bmj/345/bmj.e7473.full.pdf.

15. Hameed MA, Dasgupta I. Medication adherence and treatment-resistant hypertension: a review. Drugs Context. 2019;8:212560. https://doi.org/10.7573/dic.212560. https://www.drugsincontext.com/medication-adherence-and-treatment-resistant-hypertension-a-review/.

16. Anderson AH, Yang W, Townsend RR, Pan Q, Chertow GM, Kusek JW, Charleston J, He J, Kallem R, Lash JP, Miller ER 3rd, Rahman M, Steigerwalt S, Weir M, Wright JT Jr, Feldman HI. Chronic Renal Insufficiency Cohort Study Investigators: time-updated systolic blood pressure and the progression of chronic kidney disease: a cohort study. Ann Intern Med. 2015;162:258–65. https://doi.org/10.7326/M14-0488. https://www.ncbi.nlm.nih.gov/pmc/articles/PMC4404622/.

17. Cheung AK, Rahman M, Reboussin DM, Craven TE, Greene T, Kimmel PL, Cushman WC, Hawfield AT, Johnson KC, Lewis CE, Oparil S, Rocco MV, Sink KM, Whelton PK, Wright JT Jr, Basile J, Beddhu S, Bhatt U, Chang TI, Chertow GM, Chonchol M, Freedman BI, Haley W, Ix JH, Katz LA, Killeen AA, Papademetriou V, Ricardo AC, Servilla K, Wall B, Wolfgram D, Yee J, SPRINT Research Group. Effects of intensive BP control in CKD. J Am Soc Nephrol. 2017;28(9):2812–23. https://doi.org/10.1681/ASN.2017020148. https://jasn.asnjournals.org/content/28/9/2812.long.
18. Ku E, Lipkowitz MS, Appel LJ, Parsa A, Gassman J, Glidden DV, Smogorzewski M, Hsu CY. Strict blood pressure control associates with decreased mortality risk by APOL1 genotype. Kidney Int. 2017;91(2):443–50. https://doi.org/10.1016/j.kint.2016.09.033. Epub 2016 Dec 4. https://www.ncbi.nlm.nih.gov/pmc/articles/PMC5237400/.
19. SPRINT Research Group, Wright JT Jr, Williamson JD, Whelton PK, Snyder JK, Sink KM, Rocco MV, Reboussin DM, Rahman M, Oparil S, Lewis CE, Kimmel PL, Johnson KC, Goff DC Jr, Fine LJ, Cutler JA, Cushman WC, Cheung AK, Ambrosius WT. A randomized trial of intensive versus standard blood-pressure control. N Engl J Med. 2015;373(22):2103–16. https://doi.org/10.1056/NEJMoa1511939. Epub 2015 Nov 9. https://www.nejm.org/doi/10.1056/NEJMoa1511939?url_ver=Z39.88-2003&rfr_id=ori:rid:crossref.org&rfr_dat=cr_pub%3dwww.ncbi.nlm.nih.gov.
20. Bavishi C, Bangalore S, Messerli FH. Outcomes of intensive blood pressure lowering in older hypertensive patients. J Am Coll Cardiol. 2016;69(5):486–93. https://doi.org/10.1016/j.jacc.2016.10.077. http://www.onlinejacc.org/content/69/5/486.
21. Clase CM, Barzilay J, Gao P, Smyth A, Schmieder RE, Tobe S, Teo KK, Yusuf S, Mann JFE. Acute change in glomerular filtration rate with inhibition of the renin-angiotensin system does not predict subsequent renal and cardiovascular outcomes. Kidney Int. 2017;91(3):683–90. https://doi.org/10.1016/j.kint.2016.09.038.
22. Beddhu S, Shen J, Cheung AK, Kimmel PL, Chertow GM, Wei G, Boucher RE, Chonchol M, Arman F, Campbell RC, Contreras G, Dwyer JP, Freedman BI, Ix JH, Kirchner K, Papademetriou V, Pisoni R, Rocco MV, Whelton PK, Greene T. Implications of early decline in eGFR due to intensive BP control for cardiovascular outcomes in SPRINT. J Am Soc Nephrol. 2019;30(8):1523–33. https://doi.org/10.1681/ASN.2018121261. https://jasn.asnjournals.org/content/30/8/1523.
23. Cholesterol Treatment Trialists' (CTT) Collaboration, Herrington WG, Emberson J, Mihaylova B, Blackwell L, Reith C, Solbu MD, Mark PB, Fellström B, Jardine AG, Wanner C, Holdaas H, Fulcher J, Haynes R, Landray MJ, Keech A, Simes J, Collins R, Baigent C. Impact of renal function on the effects of LDL cholesterol lowering with statin-based regimens: a meta-analysis of individual participant data from 28 randomised trials. Lancet Diabetes Endocrinol. 2016;4(10):829–39. https://doi.org/10.1016/S2213-8587(16)30156-5. Epub 2016 Jul 29. https://www.thelancet.com/action/showPdf?pii=S2213-8587%2816%2930156-5.
24. Gunsolus I, Sandoval Y, Smith SW, Sexter A, Schulz K, Herzog CA, Apple FS. Renal dysfunction influences the diagnostic and prognostic performance of high-sensitivity cardiac troponin I. J Am Soc Nephrol. 2018;29(2):636–43. https://doi.org/10.1681/ASN.2017030341. Epub 2017 Oct 27. https://jasn.asnjournals.org/content/jnephrol/29/2/636.full.pdf.

Test the Urine: Understanding Haematuria, Proteinuria and Urinary Infection

12

Urine testing strips are simple and informative tools for investigating kidney diseases (Fig. 12.1). The assessment of a patient with possible kidney disease is incomplete without urinalysis.

Haematuria

Seeing blood in your urine is alarming. As little as 1 mL of blood makes a litre of urine look blood-stained, so the colour exaggerates the amount of blood being lost.

It is important to take a precise history of the appearance of the urine.

- Is it bright red? (= fresh bleeding) or brick red? (= altered blood, Fig. 12.2)
- Are there clots? (= urothelial rather than glomerular bleeding)
- Is the whole stream red from start to finish? (= blood entered the urine above the bladder outlet)
- Does the urine start red and then clear? (= blood from the prostate or urethra washed out by urine from the bladder)

All men with visible haematuria should have a digital rectal examination and serum prostate specific antigen level measured as a basic check for prostate cancer.

Adults aged ≥45 years with unexplained visible haematuria without urinary tract infection or with haematuria that persists or recurs after successful treatment of urinary tract infection should be investigated for bladder and kidney cancer.

Adults aged ≥60 years with unexplained non-visible haematuria and either dysuria or a raised white cell count on a blood test should also be investigated for bladder and kidney cancer [1].

Anticoagulant treatment alone is not an adequate explanation for haematuria. However, if a patient is over-anticoagulated and has an underlying glomerular disease, glomerular bleeding can cause haematuria and acute kidney injury (Patient 9.4).

© Springer Nature Switzerland AG 2020
H. C. Rayner et al., *Understanding Kidney Diseases*,
https://doi.org/10.1007/978-3-030-43027-6_12

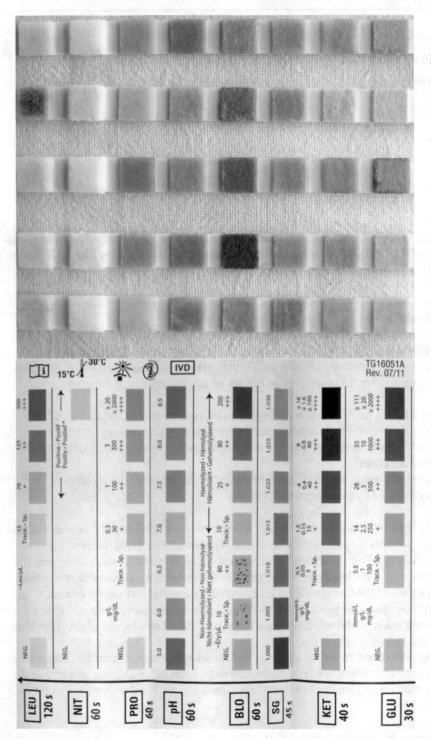

Fig. 12.1 Colour patterns from urine testing strips or 'dipsticks'. The chart on the left is used to interpret the colour changes on the strips on the right

Fig. 12.2 Brick-red urine from a patient with severe acute nephritis. It is opaque due to cells and casts, which form a sediment at the bottom

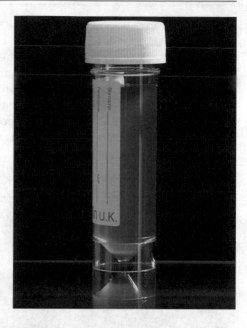

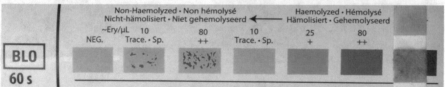

Fig. 12.3 Non-haemolysed microscopic haematuria detected on a urine dipstick test (*right*)

Asymptomatic microscopic haematuria is found in up to 8% of healthy women and 3% of healthy men (Fig. 12.3). The challenge is to identify the small number of people in whom it is clinically important.

The dipstick test distinguishes between free haemoglobin and non-haemolysed red cells. Free haemoglobin can come from intravascular haemolysis or lysis of red cells in the urine. The test strip also reacts to myoglobin.

Dark urine with a negative dipstick test for blood can be caused by food dyes, laxatives containing phenolphthalein, rifampicin and, rarely, porphyria and alkaptonuria.

How Red Cells Cross the Glomerular Filtration Barrier

If the glomerular filtration barrier is broken, blood and protein can appear in the urine. When combined with reduced GFR and high blood pressure, this constitutes the nephritic syndrome. If the barrier is weakened but otherwise intact, red cells can appear in the urine without protein and with a normal GFR. This is called isolated microscopic haematuria.

Red cells squeeze through the fenestrations in the endothelial cells and cross into Bowman's space. They are often damaged as they are forced through the glomerular filtration barrier and so have irregular shapes in the urine. Rarely, they have been caught in the act of traversing the barrier on electron microscopy (Patient 12.1) [2]. As they pass down the tubule they may become embedded in uromodulin (Tamm-Horsfall protein) and appear in the urine as red cell casts (Patient 12.2).

> **Patient 12.1 A Red Cell Caught in the Act**
> A 22-year-old woman underwent a kidney biopsy to investigate persistent microscopic hematuria. There was no macroscopic hematuria, no proteinuria and serum creatinine was normal. There was no family history of kidney disease and no hearing loss.
>
> The glomeruli were normal under light microscopy and immunostaining for immunoglobulins and complement was negative. Electron microscopy showed the capillary walls to be thinner than normal. In one capillary loop, a red blood cell was found almost bisected by the glomerular capillary basement membrane (Fig. 12.4).
>
> Similar pictures of the extravasation of red cells through gaps in endothelial cells have been produced experimentally in frog capillaries exposed to increasing amounts of pressure until they burst [3].

The Clinical Significance of Haematuria

Although seeing blood in your urine is alarming, haematuria is a less ominous sign than proteinuria in the context of glomerular diseases. For example, thin glomerular basement membrane disease (Patient 12.1) causes haematuria but is a benign condition that does not lead to kidney failure.

The risk of a fit young person with only microscopic haematuria going on to develop end-stage kidney failure is increased but still very low—34 per 100,000 person years compared to a normal rate of 2 per 100,000 person years [4].

The commonest type of glomerular disease causing haematuria in adults is immunoglobulin A (IgA) nephropathy [5]. Patients with this condition have IgA1 in their serum that contains abnormally small amounts of galactose [6]. Specific IgG autoantibodies against galactose-deficient IgA1 and complement C3 bind to the IgA1 in the serum to form immune complexes that are deposited in glomeruli [7].

IgA nephropathy is primarily a kidney disease. Sometimes, especially in children and adolescents, it is accompanied by involvement of the skin, joints and bowel, when it is called Henoch-Schönlein Purpura. Patients with IgA nephropathy often describe generalised symptoms: 81% of those using the website patientslikeme.com report feeling fatigued, and 50% report having pain.

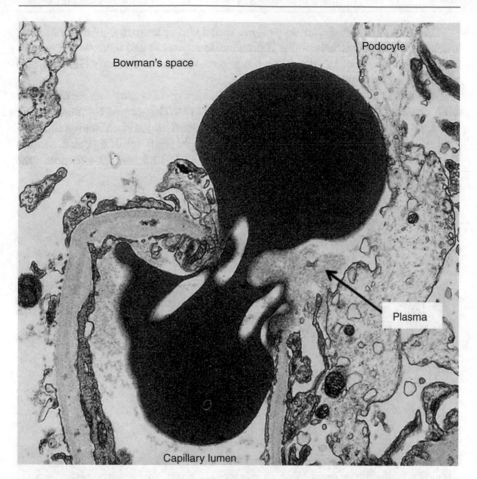

Fig. 12.4 A red cell passing upwards from the capillary lumen at the bottom of the picture through gaps in the cytoplasm of an endothelial cell. The podocyte foot processes have lost contact with the basement membrane and the cell body has been displaced by the red cell. Material similar in density to plasma (arrow) is present on the epithelial side of the membrane. This small amount of plasma would have been reabsorbed by the tubule, leaving the red cell alone to appear in the urine. (Reproduced with permission from [2])

Several diseases, including cirrhosis, inflammatory bowel disease, infections, and autoimmune diseases, can cause deposition of IgA in the glomerular mesangium [8]. Immunostaining for galactose-deficient IgA is weaker than in typical IgA nephropathy [9].

Some patients present with visible (macroscopic) haematuria at the time of a sore throat—synpharyngitic haematuria. This is in contrast to the haematuria in post-streptococcal glomerulonephritis that occurs about 2 weeks after the sore throat. Although appearing more serious, this presentation of IgA nephropathy has a more benign long-term prognosis, especially when there are repeated episodes of macroscopic haematuria [10].

The risk of kidney failure in patients with IgA nephropathy, as in glomerular diseases more generally, is higher if proteinuria is present and increases in proportion to the amount of protein. High blood pressure and a reduced eGFR are also signs of a worse prognosis.

The abnormalities on the kidney biopsy in IgA nephropathy can be combined with clinical features to give a prognostic score [11]. This can be calculated using an app: https://qxmd.com/calculate/calculator_499/international-igan-prediction-tool. Fibrosis in the kidney interstitium is a stronger predictor of a poor prognosis than many of the glomerular changes. Patients 12.2, 12.3 and 12.4 illustrate the range of outcomes.

Patient 12.2 IgA Nephropathy: Recovery After a Worrying Presentation
Mr. Austin, aged 30 years, presented to hospital with abdominal pain and visible haematuria that had developed after an episode of diarrhoea and vomiting. Urine dipstick showed blood +++ and protein +++. Urine microscopy showed >500 red blood cells/mm^3 but <5 white blood cells/mm^3 and no malignant cells. Urine culture was negative.

Full blood count was normal and serum creatinine = 86 micromol/L (1 mg/dL). The kidneys looked normal on an ultrasound scan. Plasma immunoglobulins were:

Immunoglobulin IgG	9.98 g/L	(Normal 6.00–16.00)
Immunoglobulin IgA	3.96 g/L	(0.80–2.80)
Immunoglobulin IgM	1.01 g/L	(0.50–1.90)

Two days after admission, his eGFR dropped to 56 mL/min/1.73 m^2.

A renal biopsy specimen showed 13 largely normal glomeruli but an increase in cells in part of one glomerulus—a focal segmental glomerulonephritis. Immunofluorescent staining showed many granular deposits of IgA and complement C3 in the mesangial cells of all glomeruli (Fig. 12.5). The mesangial cells lie between the glomerular capillaries and are attached to their basement membrane. They are phagocytic and take up deposits containing IgA and C3 that are trapped by the filtration barrier. These appearances are typical of IgA nephropathy.

Occasional tubules contained red blood cell casts (Fig. 12.6).

The acute kidney injury was attributed to the red cell casts obstructing the tubules [12]. Over the following 3 months the eGFR recovered to its previous normal level (Fig. 12.7).

Three years later Mr. Austin was reviewed in clinic. His urine had been intermittently blood-stained, each time associated with vomiting and joint pain. His serum creatinine was the same as when he first presented—86 micromol/L (1.0 mg/dL).

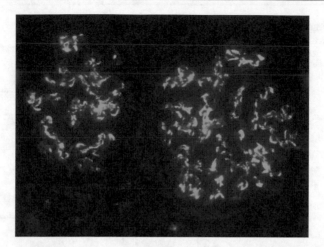

Fig. 12.5 Immunofluorescence microscopy showing positive staining for IgA in the glomerular mesangium. ×400

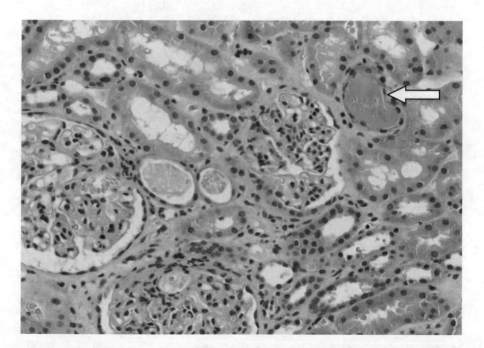

Fig. 12.6 Section through kidney cortex showing glomerular changes of IgA nephropathy, including mesangial hypercellularity and thickening. A number of tubules contain red cell casts, one of which is occluding the lumen (*arrow*). Haematoxylin and eosin ×200

Fig. 12.7 Transient drop in eGFR due to red cell casts in IgA nephropathy

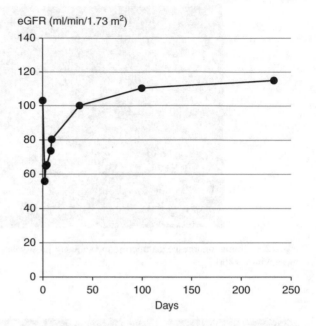

Patient 12.3 IgA Nephropathy: From Haematuria to CKD Stage G5 in 43 Years
Paul first presented in 1971 at the age of 22 years with fever, sore throat, frank haematuria and four episodes of loin pain. His blood pressure was high, ranging from 160/102 to 195/120 mmHg. The urine protein:creatinine ratio was 43.1 mg/mmol (380 mg/g) and a 24-h urine collection contained 0.68 g of protein.

A renal biopsy specimen showed some sclerosed glomeruli and others with segmental proliferation consistent with IgA nephropathy. There were some fibrotic scars in the interstitium.

His blood pressure was difficult to control due to drug side effects. However, he remained very fit and twice ran the London marathon in under 4 h.

His kidney function declined over the following 43 years, charted over the last 18 years in Fig. 12.8.

Myoglobinuria

Myoglobinuria results from the breakdown of large amounts of muscle tissue. Physical damage can be due to: compression from prolonged immobility or crush injury; ischaemia from embolism; electric shock; or severe exercise (Patient 12.5). Prescribed drugs, notably statins, and infectious or inflammatory diseases can cause myositis and muscle breakdown. Metabolic conditions such as McArdle disease,

Fig. 12.8 Decline in eGFR at a rate of approximately 2 mL/min/1.73 m² per year due to IgA nephropathy

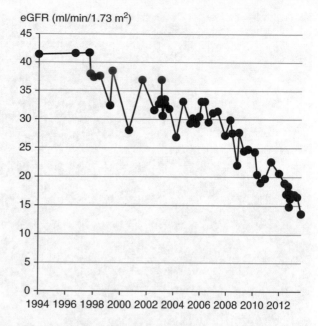

eGFR (ml/min/1.73 m²)

Patient 12.4 IgA Nephropathy: No Visible Haematuria But End-Stage Kidney Failure in 2 Years

Mr. Mitchell presented for an insurance medical examination at the age of 47. He was a heavy smoker. His urine was found to contain microscopic haematuria and heavy proteinuria; urine protein:creatinine ratio = 565 mg/mmol (4972 mg/g). His eGFR was 69 mL/min/1.73 m².

A renal biopsy specimen showed expansion and increased cellularity of the mesangial region with interstitial and periglomerular fibrosis (Fig. 12.9).

Immunofluorescent staining showed the typical features of IgA nephropathy (Fig. 12.5).

His eGFR rapidly declined over the following 2 years (Fig. 12.10). Smoking may have accelerated the decline; smokers with IgA nephropathy are twice as likely to lose kidney function [13].

He later had a successful kidney transplant.

hypokalaemia or an enzyme deficiency make the muscles more vulnerable to damage [14].

Myoglobinuria causes acute kidney injury though a number of mechanisms. Necrotic muscle swells up leading to hypovolaemia and shock. Myoglobin is filtered and then concentrated in the tubules, where it precipitates with uromodulin to form casts that obstruct the tubule. Increased uric acid production from muscle protein leads to uric acid casts, which are more likely to precipitate in the low urine pH

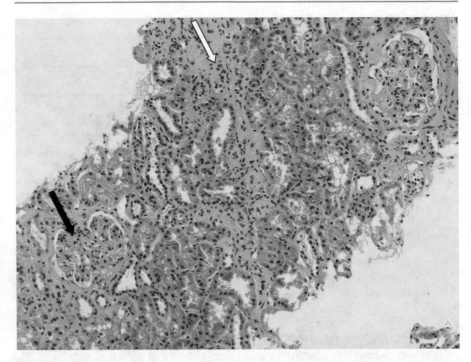

Fig. 12.9 Light micrograph showing expansion and hypercellularity of the mesangial region with glomerulosclerosis (*black arrow*). There is interstitial fibrosis and tubular atrophy, best seen as a vertical band of pale cellular tissue between the tubules in the middle of the section (*white arrow*) and around the glomerulus in the upper right corner. Haematoxylin and eosin ×100

Fig. 12.10 Decline in eGFR at a rate of 30 mL/min/1.73 m^2 per year due to IgA nephropathy

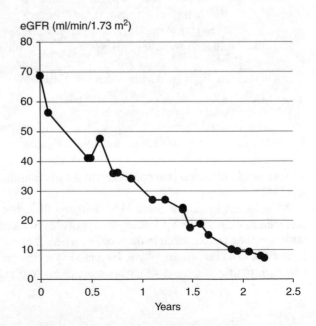

caused by metabolic acidosis. And finally, the tubular cells that reabsorb the myoglobin are damaged by the haem centre of the myoglobin molecule.

The exposed sarcoplasm and myofibrils in damaged muscle release potassium and phosphate into the circulation and bind calcium, causing hypocalcaemia and cardiac arrhythmias. The damaged muscles can take up so much calcium that they become calcified. During the recovery phase as the muscles heal, the bound calcium is released causing hypercalcaemia.

Patient 12.5 Rhabdomyolysis, Myoglobinuria and Acute Kidney Injury

Ryan, a 23-year-old unemployed man, was admitted as an emergency having been found unconscious on the floor. He had lain there for at least 12 h. He had a history of epilepsy and alcohol dependency, and used intravenous heroin.

On arrival at the casualty department, the skin over his legs had already begun to blister from pressure damage, and his muscles were tense. He was oliguric and his urine was like cola (Fig. 12.11).

His serum creatinine had increased from 78 micromols/L (0.9 mg/dL) 7 months previously to 172 (1.9) on arrival and 297 (3.4) 13 h later (AKI Stage 3). Serum creatine phosphokinase was >50,000 IU/L.

On arrival, his serum potassium was high (8.6 mmol/L, mEq/L) and calcium was low (corrected for serum albumin = 1.78 mmol/L, 7.1 mg/dL) due to the release of potassium and binding of calcium by damaged muscle fibres.

Because the pressure within all the muscle compartments of his legs was extremely high (100–125 mmHg) multiple fasciotomies were performed. The muscles were swollen and some visibly necrotic (Fig. 12.12).

Fig. 12.11 Cola-coloured urine due to myoglobinuria

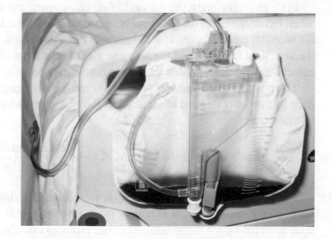

Fig. 12.12 Multiple fasciotomies revealing necrotic muscle. There is blistering of the skin by the right knee caused by prolonged pressure and oedema

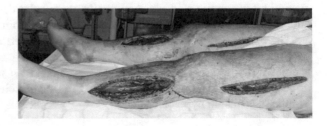

Proteinuria

Testing for albuminuria or proteinuria is an essential part of the assessment of someone with suspected kidney disease. The simplest method to use is the urine dipstick. The protein test pad uses a reagent that reacts more strongly to albumin than to other proteins (Fig. 12.13) and is not able to detect proteins such as free light chains.

Normal glomerular filtration allows an estimated 3.3–5.7 g of albumin to pass into the proximal tubules per day. Almost all of this is reabsorbed and very little appears in the urine. If the filtration barrier is damaged, the amount of albumin and other proteins that pass into the tubules can overwhelm their absorptive capacity so that more appears in the urine.

Large amounts of albumin make the urine foamy. Normal urine can make froth if it is concentrated and rapidly urinated. This is caused mainly by metabolites of bile salts. Only about a third of patients who complain of foamy urine are found to have proteinuria and if the protein:creatinine ratio is normal no further investigation is needed [15].

Urine that contains large amounts of semen due to retrograde ejaculation can be foamy. Bubbly urine can be passed by patients with a vesico-colic fistula or with urine infected by gas-forming organisms.

Perhaps surprisingly, the passage of albumin across the filtration barrier is easier when the thickness of the glomerular basement membrane is increased (Fig. 12.14). Conversely, patients with thin basement membranes do not have proteinuria. It is the structural integrity and the size and electrical charge of pores in the membrane rather than its thickness that determine how easily proteins can pass through.

The amount of albumin lost per day is most easily measured by calculating the ratio of the concentration of albumin to the concentration of creatinine in a sample of urine:

$$\text{Albumin : creatinine ratio} \left(\text{ACR} \right) = \frac{\text{Urine albumin concentration}}{\text{Urine creatinine concentration}}$$

The protein:creatinine ratio (PCR) is calculated in a similar way. The difference between the ACR and PCR is mainly made up of uromodulin (Tamm-Horsfall protein) secreted by the distal tubules. Other proteins that are not detected by the dipstick reagent but are measured by the laboratory assay, such as free light chains and myoglobin, will increase the difference between ACR and PCR.

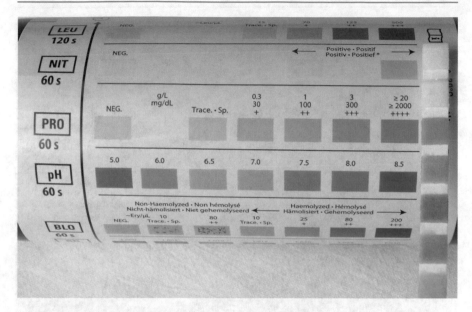

Fig. 12.13 Heavy proteinuria on a urine dipstick test (*PRO* +++)

Using the ratio between the albumin and creatinine concentrations removes the effect of changes in the dilution of urine from hour to hour and day to day. If the urine is more dilute, the concentrations of albumin and creatinine are both reduced and so the ratio remains the same. As the rate of production of creatinine remains fairly constant from day to day, sequential ACR results show the trend in the rate of albuminuria.

In UK laboratories, ACR and PCR are reported as mg protein per mmol creatinine. Although the daily excretion rate of creatinine varies according to muscle mass, a convenient average figure is 10 mmol creatinine per day. Multiplying the ACR or PCR in mg/mmol by 10 gives an estimate of the number of grams of protein lost per day.

In the United States, ACR and PCR are expressed as mg/g. This is 8.8 times the value in mg/mmol and is similar to the amount in milligrams per day in a 24 h urine collection.

Table 12.1 shows the conventional stages of albuminuria in mg/mmol, with their equivalents in mg/g.

Chronic kidney disease is staged according to the eGFR and the ACR. For example, a man with CKD stage G4A2 would have an eGFR between 15 and 29 mL/min/1.73 m^2 and an albumin:creatinine ratio between 2.5 and 30 mg/mmol (20 and 300 mg/g).

Figure 12.15 compares albuminuria and proteinuria in a patient with diabetes. 30 mg/mmol (250 mg/g) of albuminuria, the threshold between microalbuminuria and proteinuria, is equivalent to 45 mg/mmol (approx. 400 mg/g) of proteinuria.

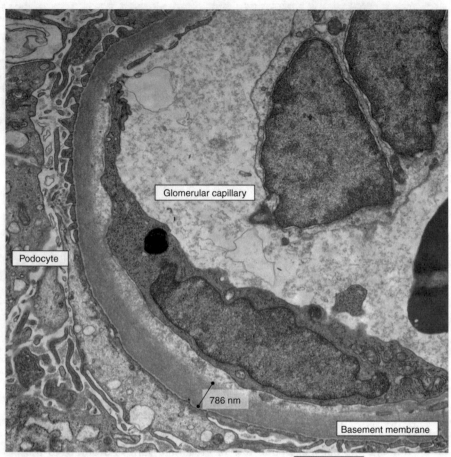

2 µm
HV=100.0kV
Direct Mag: 9300x

Fig. 12.14 Electron micrograph showing thickening of the glomerular basement membrane up to 786 nm in a patient with diabetes and nephrotic range proteinuria. The average width of a normal glomerular basement membrane is 280 nm. Magnification ×9300

Table 12.1 Stages of albuminuria

A1: normal—Male	ACR <2.5 mg/mmol	<20 mg/g
A1: normal—Female	ACR <3.5 mg/mmol	<30 mg/g
A2: microalbuminuria—Male	ACR 2.5–30 mg/mmol	20 to <300 mg/g
A2: microalbuminuria—Female	ACR 3.5–30 mg/mmol	30 to <300 mg/g
A3: macroalbuminuria	ACR >30 mg/mmol	>300 mg/g
Nephrotic-range proteinuria [16]	ACR >220 mg/mmol	>2200 mg/g
	PCR >350 mg/mmol	>3500 mg/g

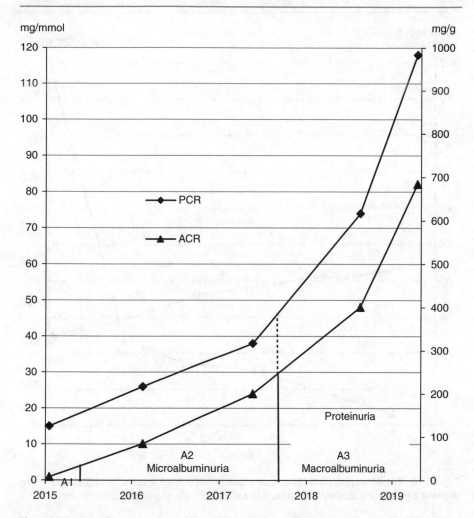

Fig. 12.15 Simultaneous measurements of urinary protein:creatinine ratio (*upper line*) and albumin:creatinine ratio (*lower line*) in a patient with increasing proteinuria due to diabetic nephropathy

It is best to use the first sample of urine passed in the day to measure the ACR. Losses of albumin increase with exercise, blood pressure and salt intake, and so are higher and more variable during the day than during the night. There is considerable variation from day to day in ACR on a morning sample. In someone with an ACR >30 mg/mmol, a difference of more than 83% between two samples is needed to be confident that there has been a real change in the underlying disease [17].

The long-term trend in ACR or PCR is a useful guide to changes in kidney disease. A progressive and sustained reduction in proteinuria is an encouraging sign

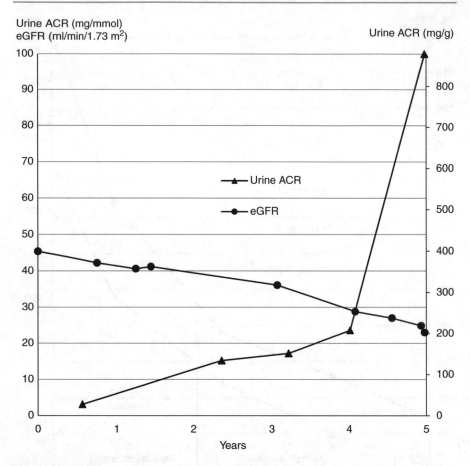

Fig. 12.16 Trends in urine albumin:creatinine ratio and eGFR in a man with diabetic nephropathy showing a progressive increase in albuminuria and reduction in glomerular filtration rate

that treatment, such as improved control of blood pressure, is working. The opposite trend highlights the need for better control (Fig. 12.16).

Whether proteinuria actually damages nephrons and so contributes directly to the progression of disease has been the subject of much debate. If it does, reducing proteinuria would in itself be a worthy aim. Proteinuria has been used as a surrogate endpoint for many trials investigating whether drugs slow the progression of CKD. Changes in proteinuria can be measured over a shorter timescale than changes in mortality, so we get a quicker answer [18].

However, changes in proteinuria may not be a reliable guide to hard endpoints. For example, giving patients with diabetic nephropathy a combination of two drugs that inhibit the renin-angiotensin-aldosterone system may lead to a reduction in proteinuria and a slowing of the rate of decline in eGFR over the short term. Unfortunately, with longer follow-up the combination may also cause acute kidney injury and does not reduce mortality or cardiovascular events [19].

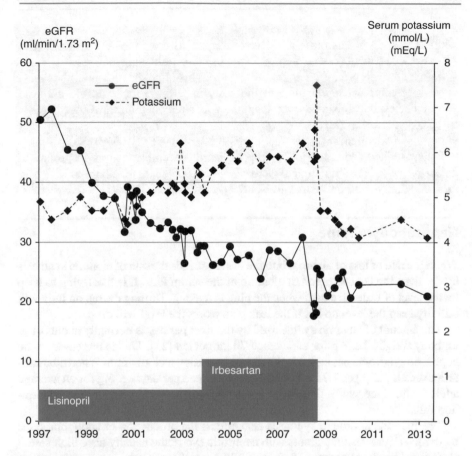

Fig. 12.17 Trends in eGFR and serum potassium concentration with combined ACE inhibitor and angiotensin receptor blocker treatment

Patient 12.6 The Effect of a Combination of ACE Inhibitor and ARB

Robert was treated for his diabetic nephropathy with the ACE inhibitor lisinopril for many years. Because his blood pressure remained too high and eGFR was falling, the angiotensin receptor blocker (ARB) irbesartan was added in 2003 (Fig. 12.17).

In 2006 a systematic review of this combination [20] concluded "the combination of ACE inhibitor and ARB therapy … is safe, without clinically meaningful changes in serum potassium levels or glomerular filtration rates (and) a significant decrease in proteinuria … in the short term".

Over the next 4 years his eGFR remained stable and his serum potassium was elevated but safe. Then in 2008, without any warning, there was a sudden drop in eGFR and rises in urea to 22 mmol/L (BUN = 62 mg/dL) and potassium to 7.5 mmol/L (mEq/L).

Both lisinopril and irbesartan were stopped, serum potassium returned to normal and there was an improvement in eGFR, although not back to the previous level. From showing no proteinuria, his urine dipstick now showed +++ protein. Thereafter, despite the recurrence of proteinuria, the eGFR remained stable, raising doubts about the apparent benefit of the drug combination seen from 2004.

This patient encapsulates the results of the VA-NEPHRON D study and other studies, which led to a European Union recommendation not to prescribe an ACE inhibitor and angiotensin receptor blocker together.

Nephrotic Syndrome

When the rate of loss of albumin into the urine exceeds the rate of albumin synthesis by the liver, the concentration of albumin in the serum falls. It is like trying to keep up the level of water in a bath when the plug is leaking. Turning the tap on fully will initially keep the level up but if the leak gets worse the level will drop.

The amount of albumin synthesized by the liver per day is normally about 0.1 g/kg body weight, i.e. 7 g for an average 70 kg person [21]. This is increased in the nephrotic syndrome but so too is the rate of breakdown of albumin. When albuminuria exceeds 3.5 g per 1.73 m^2 of body-surface area per day, i.e. 5 g for an average adult male, liver synthesis cannot keep up and the serum albumin concentration falls.

The increase in protein synthesis also affects the production of apolipoproteins by the liver. As a result, patients with nephrotic syndrome usually have high serum cholesterol levels, often over 10 mmol/L (400 mg/dL).

Nephrotic syndrome is a triad of urine albumin excretion >3.5 g per 1.73 m^2 per day, low serum albumin concentration, usually ≤25 g/L (≤2.5 g/dL), and oedema (Fig. 12.18). Rather than analysing a full 24-h collection, the albuminuria is more easily estimated from the urine protein:creatinine ratio, the nephrotic range being above 350 mg/mmol (3500 mg/g) in adults and 200 mg/mmol (2000 mg/g) in children.

All three criteria must be met to make a diagnosis of nephrotic syndrome. A low serum albumin concentration and oedema without heavy proteinuria can be found in many conditions. For example, in chronic liver disease there is reduced synthesis of albumin and oedema due to salt retention. Systemic inflammation lowers the serum albumin concentration by reducing its rate of synthesis and increasing its breakdown. For this reason, serum albumin is described as a negative acute-phase reactant.

Oedema in nephrotic syndrome is commonly put down to reduced oncotic pressure from the low serum albumin allowing salt and water to leak into the tissues. However, this traditional explanation is not the full story. For example, adults with congenital analbuminaemia, an autosomal recessive disorder where serum albumin is absent, have a low plasma oncotic pressure but little or no oedema. Also, children

Fig. 12.18 This man has chronic nephrotic syndrome due to severe diabetic nephropathy. The urine protein:creatinine ratio was 549 mg/mmol (4831 mg/g) and the serum albumin was 19 g/L (1.9 g/dL). The oedema in his legs has caused pigmented thickening (lichenification) of the skin and ulceration. The ulcers have healed leaving white scars

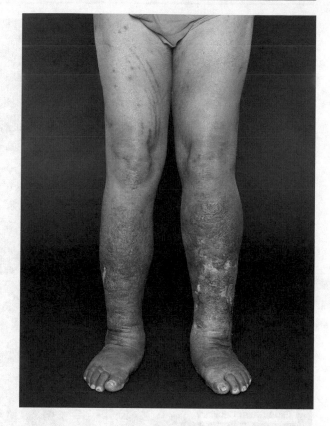

with nephrotic syndrome that responds to steroid treatment excrete the excess sodium as soon as the proteinuria stops and before the serum albumin recovers.

The oedema is actually caused by retention of sodium by the kidneys. The retained sodium then leaks into the tissues more easily than normal due to increased permeability of the capillary walls. The increased retention of sodium by the kidney tubules is caused by enzymes that leak through the glomeruli into the tubules, where they activate the sodium channels [22]. This is explained in more detail in Chap. 13.

Diuretics given at usual doses are often ineffective in nephrotic syndrome. Much higher doses of loop diuretics, sometimes in combination with a thiazide diuretic, are needed to block sodium reabsorption sufficiently to achieve a diuresis. The diuretic amiloride blocks the sodium channel in the distal tubule and so is very effective for treating oedema in nephrotic syndrome. However, it can cause dangerous potassium retention and is not routinely used [23].

A histological abnormality in all patients with nephrotic syndrome is fusion of the podocyte foot processes (Fig. 12.19). The digits of the podocyte merge across the slit diaphragm to form a continuous layer over the surface of the glomerular basement membrane. The width of the basement membrane is increased, suggesting that the collagen protein molecules are packed less tightly together, allowing protein molecules to pass between them. These changes are only visible under the electron

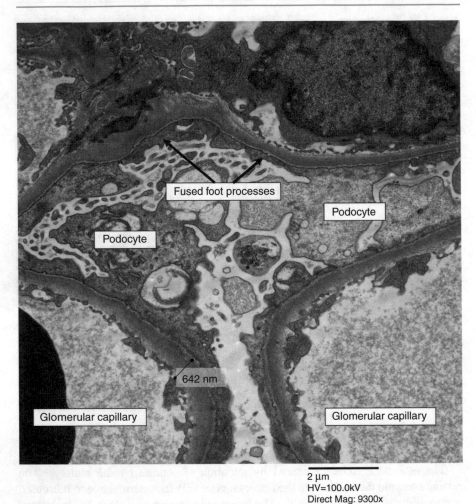

Fig. 12.19 Electron micrograph showing complete fusion of the podocyte foot processes and thickening of the glomerular basement membrane in a patient with minimal change nephrotic syndrome. The average width of a normal membrane is 280 nm. Magnification ×9300

microscope. Under light microscopy the specimen may show no definite abnormalities, in which case it is called minimal change nephrotic syndrome [24]. This is the commonest appearance in children over the age of 1 year, found in up to 90%, whereas only about 15% of adults have this finding.

Nephrotic syndrome may be caused by a primary kidney disease such as congenital disease, minimal change disease, focal segmental glomerulosclerosis or membranous nephropathy, or may be secondary to another condition, most commonly diabetes mellitus and amyloidosis [25]. Which cause is the commonest changes with age, congenital disease being most common in infancy, minimal change disease in childhood, and diabetes in middle and older age. In adults, causes vary with race, focal segmental glomerulosclerosis being more common in black populations and membranous nephropathy in white populations.

Acute kidney injury may accompany the onset of nephrotic syndrome. This may be due to changes in the glomerular filtration barrier and podocyte foot process fusion or to vasoconstriction within the kidney [26].

Patients with nephrotic syndrome are at risk of venous thrombosis due to the loss of antithrombin III in the urine. Antithrombin III is an anticoagulant protein that has a molecular weight lower than serum albumin (58.2 kDa compared to 66.5 kDa). Clotting can occur in unusual venous territories such as the renal, cerebral or mesenteric veins [27]. Swelling from pelvic and leg vein thrombosis may be hard to distinguish from oedema due to the nephrotic syndrome and the thrombosis may only be evident later when pulmonary embolism occurs.

The lower the serum albumin, the greater is the risk of thrombosis. Prophylactic anticoagulation is often given when the serum albumin concentration is <20 g/L (<2 g/dL), especially in patients with membranous nephropathy. Tools have been developed to estimate the risks and benefits of anticoagulation [28].

Immunoglobulins and complement are also lost into the urine, increasing the risk of infections, particularly in children and in developing countries [29].

Urine Infection

Infection in the urinary tract presents with a range of symptoms and signs (Fig. 12.20). This section explains how to approach the diagnosis and treatment of infection.

Figure 12.21 shows a dipstick urine test from Adele, a 23-year-old woman with bilateral vesico-ureteric reflux and scarring of both kidneys. She has had recurrent attacks of burning dysuria and loin pain. Does she have a urine infection?

In a woman, the best guide to whether a urine infection is present are her symptoms—frequency, dysuria, haematuria, fever, loin pain—and the absence of vaginal irritation or discharge. If the symptoms are present when the urine is tested, the dipstick test does not add much; whatever the stick test shows, a urine culture is needed.

The stick tests for nitrites and leucocytes are best used as 'rule-out' tests. A negative urine dipstick test for both nitrites and leucocytes makes a urinary tract infection unlikely, but a mid-stream urine (MSU) culture should still be done in patients with symptoms. If someone has only loin pain and a negative urine dipstick test for nitrites and leucocytes, urinary infection is unlikely to be the cause of the pain [30].

Although Adele's urine is ++ for leucocytes and positive for nitrites, she had no symptoms at the time of the sample and her urine culture was negative. She did not have sufficient evidence to warrant antibiotic treatment at that time but is at high risk of future infection because of her reflux nephropathy.

Urine infection most definitely cannot be diagnosed from a positive urine dipstick test for blood and/or protein. Despite this, a high proportion of acutely unwell older people with blood and protein on a urine dipstick test are given a diagnosis of

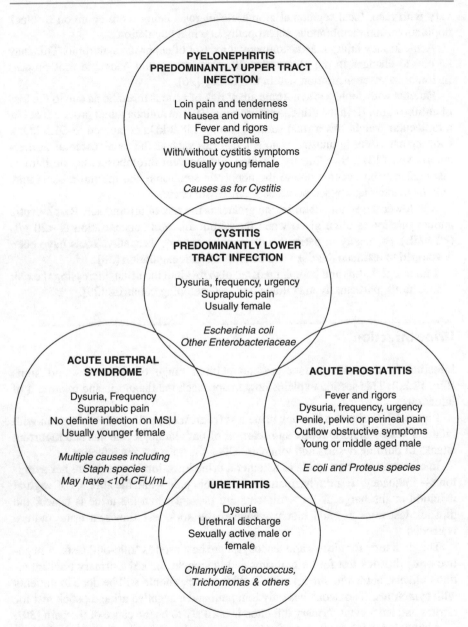

Fig. 12.20 Acute urinary tract infection syndromes in adults. Although shown as discrete syndromes, they may overlap. The commoner causative organisms are in italics

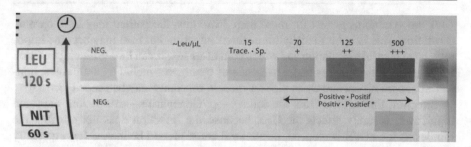

Fig. 12.21 Leucocytes and nitrites detected on a urine dipstick test

'?UTI' and inappropriately started on antibiotics. A small number of them actually have glomerulonephritis, as discussed earlier in this chapter.

As urine flows out of the urethra is can be contaminated by organisms from the skin surface. The threshold number of organisms (Colony Forming Units) grown from a correctly collected MSU specimen that distinguishes between contaminants and an infection is $>10^5$ CFU/mL. A diagnosis of urinary tract infection can be made in a patient with a colony count above this threshold *and* symptoms suggestive of infection.

Dipstick tests on urine specimens taken from a urinary catheter (CSU) are even less meaningful than an MSU. A culture should only be done if there are symptoms. The result can be interpreted as for an MSU. A positive culture without systemic symptoms does not warrant treatment with antibiotics because the catheter is likely to be coated with a biofilm containing the micro-organisms. The risk of colonisation of a urinary catheter increases by about 5% per day after insertion.

Specimens from a nephrostomy should be highlighted to the laboratory. The sample is less likely to be contaminated so any organisms grown, whatever the CFU count, will be identified to guide antimicrobial treatment.

People aged 60 years and over with recurrent or persistent unexplained urinary tract infection should be considered for investigation for bladder cancer [1].

It is important to take a sexual history in all women with a urinary tract infection. The likelihood of urine infection in both pre- and post-menopausal women correlates with the frequency of sexual intercourse [31, 32].

In men, urine infection is much less common and should always prompt a search for an underlying cause. The species of organism grown may give a clue. For example, *Proteus mirabilis* produces urease, which breaks down urea and reduces the acidity of urine, leading to the formation of kidney or bladder stones. The bacteria then stick to the stone, where they are protected from antibiotics.

Men can develop inflammation and infection of the prostate gland. Acute symptoms may include aches, pains and a fever with pain in or around the penis, testes, anus, lower abdomen or lower back, which is worse when passing urine. There may be nocturnal frequency and urgency with difficulty starting urination that can lead to acute retention of urine. Haematuria and a small amount of thick discharge blood may be produced. Acute symptoms are usually caused by infection and are treated with antibiotics and pain relief.

If the symptoms persist for more than 3 months, the patient may have chronic prostatitis. This is not a sexually transmitted infection but men may become impotent, have painful ejaculation and worse pain after sex. It can be a difficult condition to diagnose with certainty and a sequence of treatments including antibiotics, nonsteroidal pain killers and alpha blocker muscle relaxants may be needed [33].

Infection that ascends into the kidney—pyelonephritis—causes loin pain and high fever. It rarely affects the GFR because the infection does not obstruct the tubules. If the eGFR is reduced, a structural cause should be looked for, especially if a more unusual organism is grown (Patient 12.7).

Patient 12.7 Urine Infection by an Unusual Bacterium Suggests an Underlying Pathology

Angie, aged 36, presented to her GP with symptoms of a urine infection. She had had urinary frequency and pain on and off over the previous 10 months. A mid-stream urine sample subsequently yielded a heavy growth of *Enterococcus faecalis* and she was treated with antibiotics according to the organism's sensitivities. The GP also measured her renal function and the eGFR was only 17 mL/min/1.73 m². She was sent urgently to hospital.

In the emergency assessment unit, she described having left lower back pain for the previous 2 days. She had intense urinary frequency, having to go to the toilet halfway through the conversation.

An ultrasound scan of the kidneys and bladder showed bilateral hydronephrosis, with marked thinning of the renal cortex on the right indicating chronic damage. The left kidney cortex was thicker suggesting more recent obstruction, consistent with her symptoms (Fig. 12.22).

In the pelvis there was a central solid mass adherent to the bladder. When asked about any previous gynaecological problems, she said she had had a hysterectomy for cervical carcinoma 5 years previously.

By this time, her eGFR had dropped to 7 mL/min/1.73 m². Bilateral nephrostomies were inserted (Fig. 12.23) and her kidney function improved over the next 10 days (Fig. 12.24).

An MRI scan confirmed the ultrasound scan findings (Fig. 12.25).

A nuclear medicine whole body fluoro-deoxyglucose Positron Emission Tomography scan (FDG PET scan) (Fig. 12.26) combined with CT (Fig. 12.27) showed marked activity in the mass adjacent to the bladder, consistent with recurrent cervical carcinoma.

The nephrostomies were replaced by bilateral ureteric stents and she was transferred to the oncology unit for a course of chemotherapy and radiotherapy.

Treatment of Urinary Tract Infection in Adults

Personal hygiene and micturition after intercourse may reduce the risk of urine infection. Sadly, cranberry juice is not effective [34].

In deciding whether to prescribe antibiotics, the presence or absence of symptoms is crucial. Many older women, especially with diabetes, yield a significant growth of organisms on an MSU culture but have no symptoms. They are colonised with organisms and treatment with antibiotics does not lead to improved kidney

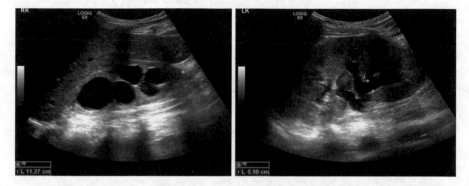

Fig. 12.22 Ultrasound scan showing bilateral hydronephrosis, with marked thinning of the right renal cortex. *RK* right kidney, *LK* left kidney

Fig. 12.23 Nephrostogram showing hydronephrosis and a dilated upper ureter

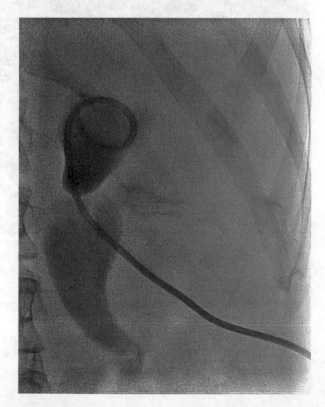

Fig. 12.24 Relief of obstruction by nephrostomies led to recovery in kidney function

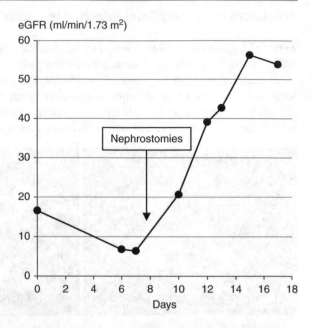

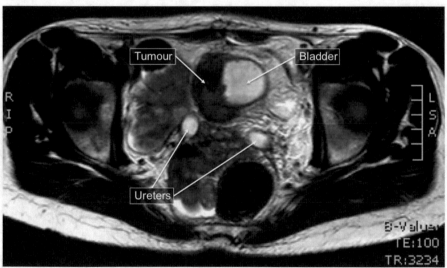

Fig. 12.25 MRI scan on the pelvis showing a tumour adjacent to the bladder and dilated ureters

function or a lower risk of future symptomatic urine infections. It is recommended that such asymptomatic bacteriuria is only treated in pregnant women or before urological surgery [35].

On the other hand, a patient with painful lower urinary tract symptoms, increased urinary white blood cells but a negative urine culture can benefit from long-term antibiotic treatment [36].

Fig. 12.26 FDG PET scan showing high level of activity in the pelvis

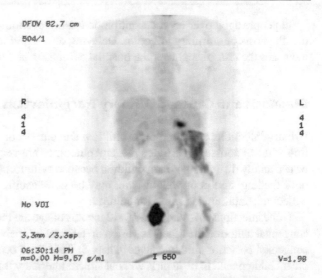

Fig. 12.27 PET CT scan showing that the high level of radioactivity is located in the tumour mass

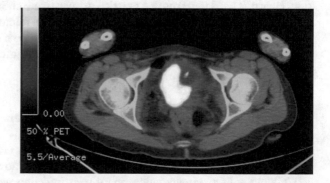

For patients with recurrent symptomatic urinary infections, antibiotics can be used at three levels of intensity:

Low: Instruct the patient to attend their general practitioner or primary care doctor when symptoms start and then treat accordingly. This risks a delay in starting treatment and a prolongation of the symptoms.

Medium: Provide the patient with a course of appropriate antibiotics to keep at home and instruct them to take them when symptoms start. This reduces the delay in treatment and the impact that the infections have on the patient's life.

High: Use a regular nocturnal prophylactic antibiotic. This is appropriate for patients with very frequent infections or symptoms that are having a significant impact on their education, work or social life. For patients with normal kidney function, a nightly dose of nitrofurantoin is a good choice. Otherwise the choice should be based upon the level of kidney function and the antibiotic sensitivities of the organisms grown.

In people aged over 65 years antibiotic treatment should be given promptly after the diagnosis of a urinary infection. Delaying or not giving antibiotics substantially increases the risk of septicaemia, hospital admission and death [37].

Diagnosis and Causes of Urinary Tract Infection in Children

Urinary infections are common in children and can occur at any age. The presentation, clinical course, recurrence risk and outcomes are very variable. Diagnosis can be especially difficult in young children because symptoms, such as vomiting, fever, poor feeding, and poor weight gain, may be non-specific and it can be difficult to collect uncontaminated urine for culture.

Urine infections that start under 6–12 months of age are more likely to be linked with congenital abnormalities such as vesico-ureteric reflux, pelvi-ureteric obstruction, and congenital posterior urethral valves (Chap. 8). Infections occurring for the first time in older children tend to be in girls without structural urinary tract abnormalities.

Urine infections associated with vesico-ureteric reflux may cause kidney scarring. Hence, it used to be routine practice to investigate children with urine infection using ultrasound to exclude urinary obstruction and a micturating cystourethrogram to exclude vesico-ureteric reflux. More recently, practice has changed to only investigating infants and children with atypical or recurrent infections who are at higher risk (Table 12.2) [38].

Treatment of Urinary Tract Infection in Children

Asymptomatic bacteriuria is commonly found in girls aged 5–15 years. While there is no need to treat this, children should be treated if they go on to develop symptoms.

Children with a symptomatic urinary tract infection who are systemically well should be treated with between 3 and 7 days of oral antibiotics, the choice of antibiotic being based on the local pattern of antibiotic resistance [39]. Children who are systemically unwell should be treated for up to 14 days and if oral antibiotics are not tolerated or the child is severely unwell, intravenous antibiotics should be used for the first 2–4 days.

Prevention of Recurrent Urinary Tract Infection in Children

Children with a structurally normal urinary tract should be encouraged to maintain a normal fluid intake of about 1.5 L/m^2 per day and to pass urine regularly throughout the day and before bedtime. Girls should be taught how to maintain good perineal hygiene.

Table 12.2 Recommendations for investigating a child with urinary tract infection stratified by age and type of urine infection (from [38])

Test	Responds well to treatment	Severe or atypical urinary tract infection[a]	Recurrent urinary tract infection
Infants aged 0–6 months			
Early ultrasound	No	Yes	Yes
Late ultrasound	Yes (within 6 weeks)	No	No
Early DMSA scan	No	No	No
Late DMSA scan	No	Yes	Yes
Micturating cystourethrogram	No	Yes	Yes
Children from 6 months of age to toilet-trained			
Early ultrasound	No	Yes	No
Late ultrasound	No	No	Yes
Early DMSA scan	No	No	No
Late DMSA scan	No	Yes	Yes
Micturating cystourethrogram	No	No	No
Children toilet-trained and older			
Early ultrasound	No	Yes	No
Late ultrasound	No	No	Yes
Early DMSA scan	No	No	No
Late DMSA scan	No	No	Yes
Micturating cystourethrogram	No	No	No

[a]Atypical urinary tract infection: Still febrile after 48 h of appropriate treatment, poor urine flow or infection with organism other than E. coli

Constipation is often associated with bladder dysfunction and should also be treated. A history of bladder dysfunction, such as bed wetting, daytime wetting, urgency, poor stream, staccato voiding and incomplete bladder emptying, warrants further investigation and treatment by bladder training with or without medication.

The use of prophylactic antibiotics and surgical correction of vesico-ureteric reflux to prevent kidney scarring has changed over the years. The Birmingham Reflux Study showed that there was no reduction in the rate of new scarring with prophylactic antibiotics [40]. The RIVUR trial found that the risk of urinary tract infection was reduced by half in children with vesico-ureteric reflux who were treated with prophylactic antibiotics [41]. A re-analysis of the data showed that the greatest benefit was in children at high risk (Table 12.3) [42], leading to a more targeted approach to treatment [39].

Table 12.3 Classification system for the risk of urinary tract infection in children (from [42])

| **Low risk of urinary tract infection:** |
| Circumcised males with grade 1–3 vesico-ureteric reflux |
| Females with grade 1–3 vesico-ureteric reflux |
| AND no constipation or evidence of disordered bowel or bladder function |
| **High risk of urinary tract infection:** |
| Uncircumcised males with grade 1–3 vesico-ureteric reflux with or without bladder or bowel dysfunction |
| All males with grade 4 vesico-ureteric reflux |
| Females with grade 1–3 vesico-ureteric reflux with or without bladder or bowel dysfunction |
| All females and males with grade 4 vesico-ureteric reflux |

During childhood, vesico-ureteric reflux can reduce in severity or resolve completely [43] and surgery to reduce the reflux does not prevent kidney scarring [40]

References

1. National Collaborating Centre for Cancer. Suspected cancer: recognition and referral. NICE Guideline [NG12]. https://www.nice.org.uk/guidance/ng12/chapter/1-Recommendations-organised-by-site-of-cancer#urological-cancers.
2. Collar JE, Ladva S, Cairns TDH, Cattell V. Red cell traverse through thin glomerular basement membranes. Kidney Int. 2001;59:2069–72. https://doi.org/10.1046/j.1523-1755.2001.00721.x. http://www.nature.com/ki/journal/v59/n6/full/4492253a.html#bib7.
3. Neal CR, Michel CC. Openings in frog microvascular endothelium induced by high intravascular pressures. J Physiol. 1996;492(1):39–52. http://www.ncbi.nlm.nih.gov/pmc/articles/PMC1158859/.
4. Vivante A, Afek A, Frenkel-Nir Y, Tzur D, Farfel A, Golan E, Chaiter Y, Shohat T, Skorecki K, Calderon-Margalit R. Persistent asymptomatic isolated microscopic hematuria in Israeli adolescents and young adults and risk for end-stage renal disease. JAMA. 2011;306(7):729–36. https://doi.org/10.1001/jama.2011.1141. http://jama.jamanetwork.com/article.aspx?articleid=1104231.
5. Rodrigues JC, Haas M, Reich HN. IgA nephropathy. Clin J Am Soc Nephrol. 2017;12(4):677–86. https://doi.org/10.2215/CJN.07420716. https://cjasn.asnjournals.org/content/12/4/677.long.
6. Suzuki H, Yasutake J, Makita Y, Tanbo Y, Yamasaki K, Sofue T, Kano T, Suzuki Y. IgA nephropathy and IgA vasculitis with nephritis have a shared feature involving galactose-deficient IgA1-oriented pathogenesis. Kidney Int. 2018;93(3):700–5. https://doi.org/10.1016/j.kint.2017.10.019. Epub 2018 Jan 10. https://www.kidney-international.org/article/S0085-2538(17)30799-8/fulltext.
7. Rizk DV, Saha MK, Hall S, Novak L, Brown R, Huang Z-O, Fatima H, Julian BA, Novak J. Glomerular immunodeposits of patients with IgA nephropathy are enriched for IgG autoantibodies specific for galactose-deficient IgA1. JASN. 2019;30(10):2017–26. https://doi.org/10.1681/ASN.2018111156. Published ahead of print August 23, 2019. https://jasn.asnjournals.org/content/early/2019/08/22/ASN.2018111156.abstract.
8. Saha MK, Julian BA, Novak J, Rizk DV. Secondary IgA nephropathy. Kidney Int. 2018;94(4):674–81. https://doi.org/10.1016/j.kint.2018.02.030. Epub 2018 May 24. https://www.kidney-international.org/article/S0085-2538(18)30245-X/fulltext.
9. Cassol CA, Bott C, Nadasdy GM, Alberton V, Malvar A, Nagaraja HN, Nadasdy T, Rovin BH, Satoskar AA. Immunostaining for galactose-deficient immunoglobulin A is not specific for primary immunoglobulin A nephropathy. Nephrol Dial Transplant. 2019; pii: gfz152. https://doi.org/10.1093/ndt/gfz152. https://www.academic.oup.com/ndt/advance-article-abstract/doi/10.1093/ndt/gfz152/5542608?redirectedFrom=fulltext.

10. Le W, Liang S, Chen H, Wang S, Zhang W, Wang X, Wang J, Zeng C-H, Liu Z-H. Long-term outcome of IgA nephropathy patients with recurrent macroscopic hematuria. Am J Nephrol. 2014;40:43–50. http://www.karger.com/Article/Abstract/364954.

11. Roberts IS. Oxford classification of immunoglobulin A nephropathy: an update. Curr Opin Nephrol Hypertens. 2013;22(3):281–6. https://doi.org/10.1097/MNH.0b013e32835fe65c. http://journals.lww.com/co-nephrolhypertens/Abstract/2013/05000/Oxford_classification_of_immunoglobulin_A.6.aspx.

12. Gutiérrez E, González E, Hernández E, Morales E, Martínez MA, Usera G, Praga M. Factors that determine an incomplete recovery of renal function in macrohematuria-induced acute renal failure of IgA nephropathy. Clin J Am Soc Nephrol. 2007;2(1):51. http://cjasn.asnjournals.org/content/2/1/51.long.

13. Yamamoto R, Nagasawa Y, Shoji T, Iwatani H, Hamano T, Kawada N, Inoue K, Uehata T, Kaneko T, Okada N, Moriyama T, Horio M, Yamauchi A, Tsubakihara Y, Imai E, Rakugi H, Isaka Y. Cigarette smoking and progression of IgA nephropathy. Am J Kidney Dis. 2010;56(2):313. http://www.ajkd.org/article/S0272-6386(10)00682-7/abstract.

14. Vanholder R, Sever MS, Erek E, Lameire N. Rhabdomyolysis. JASN. 2000;11:1553–61. http://jasn.asnjournals.org/content/11/8/1553.full.

15. Khitan ZJ, Glassock RJ. Foamy urine. CJASN. 2019;14(11):1664–6. https://doi.org/10.2215/CJN.06840619. https://cjasn.asnjournals.org/content/early/2019/09/30/CJN.06840619.

16. Stoycheff N, Stevens LA, Schmid CH, Tighiouart H, Lewis J, Atkins RC, Levey AS. Nephrotic syndrome in diabetic kidney disease: an evaluation and update of the definition. Am J Kidney Dis. 2009;54(5):840–9. https://doi.org/10.1053/j.ajkd.2009.04.016. Epub 2009 Jun 25. http://www.ncbi.nlm.nih.gov/pmc/articles/PMC4036614/.

17. Naresh CN, Hayen A, Weening A, Craig JC, Chadban SJ. Day-to-day variability in spot urine albumin-creatinine ratio. Am J Kidney Dis. 2013;62(6):1095–101. http://www.ajkd.org/article/S0272-6386(13)01007-X/abstract.

18. Lambers Heerspink HJ, Kröpelin TF, Hoekman J, Zeeuw D, Reducing Albuminuria as Surrogate Endpoint (REASSURE) Consortium. Drug-induced reduction in albuminuria is associated with subsequent renoprotection: a meta-analysis. J Am Soc Nephrol. 2015;26(8):2055–64. https://doi.org/10.1681/ASN.2014070688. https://jasn.asnjournals.org/content/26/8/2055.long.

19. Fried LF, Emanuele N, Zhang JH, Brophy M, Conner TA, Duckworth W, Leehey DJ, McCullough PA, O'Connor T, Palevsky PM, Reilly RF, Seliger SL, Warren SR, Watnick S, Peduzzi P, Guarino P, VA NEPHRON-D Investigators. Combined angiotensin inhibition for the treatment of diabetic nephropathy. N Engl J Med. 2013;369(20):1892–903. https://doi.org/10.1056/NEJMoa1303154. Epub 2013 Nov 9. http://www.nejm.org/doi/full/10.1056/NEJMoa1303154#t=articleTop.

20. MacKinnon M, Shurraw S, Akbari A, Knoll GA, Jaffey J, Clark HD. Combination therapy with an angiotensin receptor blocker and an ACE inhibitor in proteinuric renal disease: a systematic review of the efficacy and safety data. Am J Kidney Dis. 2006;48(1):8–20. http://www.ajkd.org/article/S0272-6386(06)00769-4/abstract.

21. Barle H, Nyberg B, Essén P, Andersson K, McNurlan MA, Wernerman J, Garlick PJ. The synthesis rates of total liver protein and plasma albumin determined simultaneously in vivo in humans. Hepatology. 1997;25(1):154–8. http://onlinelibrary.wiley.com/doi/10.1002/hep.510250128/epdf.

22. Bohnert BN, Menacher M, Janessa A, Wörn M, Schork A, Daiminger S, Kalbacher H, Häring HU, Daniel C, Amann K, Sure F, Bertog M, Haerteis S, Korbmacher C, Artunc F. Aprotinin prevents proteolytic epithelial sodium channel (ENaC) activation and volume retention in nephrotic syndrome. Kidney Int. 2018;93(1):159–72. https://doi.org/10.1016/j.kint.2017.07.023. https://www.sciencedirect.com/science/article/abs/pii/S008525381730569016.

23. Hinrichs GR, Mortensen LA, Jensen BL, Bistrup C. Amiloride resolves resistant edema and hypertension in a patient with nephrotic syndrome; a case report. Physiol Rep. 2018;6(12):e13743. https://doi.org/10.14814/phy2.13743. https://physoc.onlinelibrary.wiley.com/doi/full/10.14814/phy2.13743.

24. Vivarelli M, Massella L, Ruggiero B, Emma F. Minimal change disease. Clin J Am Soc Nephrol. 2017;12(2):332–45. https://doi.org/10.2215/CJN.05000516. https://cjasn.asnjournals.org/content/12/2/332.long.
25. Hull RP, Goldsmith DJA. Nephrotic syndrome in adults. BMJ. 2008;336(7654):1185–9. www.ncbi.nlm.nih.gov/pmc/articles/PMC2394708/.
26. Meyrier A, Niaudet P. Acute kidney injury complicating nephrotic syndrome of minimal change disease. Kidney Int. 2018;94(5):861–9. https://doi.org/10.1016/j.kint.2018.04.024. Epub 2018 Jul 3. https://www.kidney-international.org/article/S0085-2538(18)30352-1/fulltext.
27. Loscalzo J. Venous thrombosis in the nephrotic syndrome. N Engl J Med. 2013;368:956–8. https://doi.org/10.1056/NEJMcibr1209459.   http://www.nejm.org/doi/full/10.1056/NEJMcibr1209459.
28. Lee T, Biddle AK, Lionaki S, Derebail VK, Barbour SJ, Tannous S, Hladunewich MA, Hu Y, Poulton CJ, Mahoney SL, Jennette JC, Hogan SL, Falk RL, Cattran DC, Reich HN, Nachman PH. Personalized prophylactic anticoagulation decision analysis in patients with membranous nephropathy. Kidney Int. 2014;85(6):1412–20. https://doi.org/10.1038/ki.2013.476. http://www.nature.com/ki/journal/v85/n6/full/ki2013476a.html.
29. Alwadhi RK, Mathew JL, Rath B. Clinical profile of children with nephrotic syndrome not on glucocorticoid therapy, but presenting with infection. J Paediatr Child Health. 2004;40(1–2):28–32. http://onlinelibrary.wiley.com/doi/10.1111/j.1440-1754.2004.00285.x/abstract.
30. St John A, Boyd JC, Lowes AJ, Price CP. The use of urinary dipstick tests to exclude urinary tract infection: a systematic review of the literature. Am J Clin Pathol. 2006;126(3):428–36. http://ajcp.ascpjournals.org/content/126/3/428.full.pdf.
31. Hooton TM, Scholes D, Hughes JP, Winter C, Roberts PL, Stapleton AE, Stergachis A, Stamm WE. A prospective study of risk factors for symptomatic urinary tract infection in young women. N Engl J Med. 1996;335(7):468–74. http://www.nejm.org/doi/full/10.1056/NEJM199608153350703#t=articleTop.
32. Moore EE, Hawes SE, Scholes D, Boyko EJ, Hughes JP, Fihn SD. Sexual intercourse and risk of symptomatic urinary tract infection in post-menopausal women. J Gen Intern Med. 2008;23(5):595–9. https://doi.org/10.1007/s11606-008-0535-y. Epub 2008 Feb 12. http://link.springer.com/article/10.1007%2Fs11606-008-0535-y.
33. National Institute for Health and Care Excellence. Prostatitis—chronic. https://cks.nice.org.uk/prostatitis-chronic#!topicSummary.
34. Jepson RG, Williams G, Craig JC. Cranberries for preventing urinary tract infections. Cochrane Database Syst Rev. 2012;10:CD001321. https://doi.org/10.1002/14651858.CD001321.pub5. https://www.cochranelibrary.com/cdsr/doi/10.1002/14651858.CD001321.pub5/full.
35. Nicolle LE, Bradley S, Colgan R, Rice JC, Schaeffer A, Hooton TM, Infectious Diseases Society of America; American Society of Nephrology; American Geriatric Society. Infectious Diseases Society of America guidelines for the diagnosis and treatment of asymptomatic bacteriuria in adult. Clin Infect Dis. 2005;40(5):643–54. Epub 2005 Feb 4. http://www.idsociety.org/uploadedFiles/IDSA/Guidelines-Patient_Care/PDF_Library/Asymptomatic%20Bacteriuria.pdf.
36. Swamy S, Kupelian AS, Khasriya R, Dharmasena D, Toteva H, Dehpour T, Collins L, Rohn JL, Malone-Lee J. Cross-over data supporting long-term antibiotic treatment in patients with painful lower urinary tract symptoms, pyuria and negative urinalysis. Int Urogynecol J. 2019;30(3):409–14. https://doi.org/10.1007/s00192-018-3846-5. Epub 2018 Dec 18. https://www.ncbi.nlm.nih.gov/pmc/articles/PMC6394536/.
37. Gharbi M, Drysdale JH, Lishman H, Goudie R, Molokhia M, Johnson AP, et al. Antibiotic management of urinary tract infection in elderly patients in primary care and its association with bloodstream infections and all cause mortality: population based cohort study. BMJ. 2019;364:l525. https://doi.org/10.1136/bmj.l525.
38. National Institute for Health and Care Excellence. Clinical guideline [CG54]. Urinary tract infection in under 16s: diagnosis and management. https://www.nice.org.uk/guidance/cg54.

39. National Institute for Health and Care Excellence. NICE guideline [NG109]. Urinary tract infection (lower): antimicrobial prescribing. https://www.nice.org.uk/guidance/ng109.

40. Birmingham Reflux Study Group. Prospective trial of operative versus non-operative treatment of severe vesicoureteric reflux in children: five years' observation. Br Med J (Clin Res Ed). 1987;295:237–41. http://www.bmj.com/content/295/6592/237.

41. Hoberman A, Greenfield SP, Mattoo TK, et al. The RIVUR Trial Investigators. Antimicrobial prophylaxis for children with vesicoureteral reflux. N Engl J Med. 2014;370:2367–76. http://www.nejm.org/doi/full/10.1056/NEJMoa1401811#t=articleTop.

42. Wang ZT, Wehbi E, Alam Y, Khoury A. A reanalysis of the RIVUR trial using a risk classification system. J Urol. 2018;199:1608–14. https://www.auajournals.org/doi/10.1016/j.juro.2017.11.080.

43. Edwards D, Normand ICS, Prescod N, Smellie JM. Disappearance of vesicoureteric reflux during long-term prophylaxis of urinary tract infection in children. Br Med J. 1977;2:285–8. http://www.bmj.com/content/2/6082/285.

Examine the Patient: Physical Signs Related to Kidney Diseases

13

Fluid Balance

How Salt and Water Is Distributed in the Body

Salt and water are distributed in three functionally separate compartments in the body—inside the cells (intracellular fluid), around the cells (interstitial fluid) and in blood vessels (plasma).

Before trying to judge a patient's salt and water balance from the physical examination, first take a history. For example, if someone has had diarrhoea and vomiting for a week and has lost weight, they will be salt and water depleted. The examination is then used to judge the severity of the salt and water depletion and whether it is affecting plasma volume as well as the interstitial fluid.

In children, an estimate of the percentage change in body weight is used to guide the route and volume of fluid replacement. Weight loss of more than 10% of body weight indicates reduced plasma volume and requires intravenous fluid replacement. In adults, low blood pressure and a rise in pulse rate of >20 beats per minute from sitting to standing or >30 bpm from supine to standing indicate reduced plasma volume.

The traditional signs of reduced interstitial fluid volume, such as reduced skin turgor, are not reliable in the elderly [1].

Oedema indicates excess interstitial fluid. Interstitial fluid is formed at the arterial end of the capillary bed by hydrostatic pressure forcing fluid across the capillary wall. It is removed at the venous end by osmotic force drawing it back into the capillary lumen, and also by the lymphatic system (Fig. 13.1).

Salt and water overload lead to increased hydrostatic pressure and oedema. A little puffiness at the ankles indicates a kilogram or two of excess fluid. Oedema to the knees may indicate 5 kg; oedema up to the abdomen may mean more than 20 kg of fluid overload. Fluid may also accumulate in spaces that are normally dry, for example pleural effusions and ascites.

© Springer Nature Switzerland AG 2020
H. C. Rayner et al., *Understanding Kidney Diseases*,
https://doi.org/10.1007/978-3-030-43027-6_13

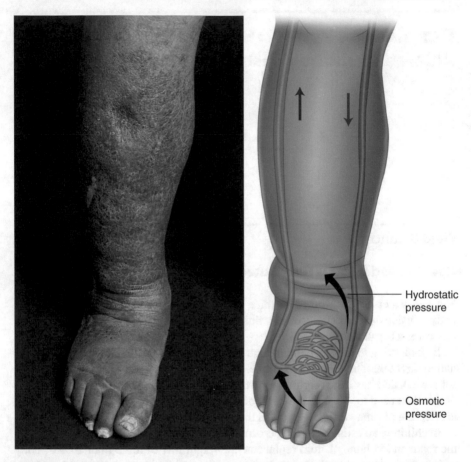

Fig 13.1 The formation of oedema. Fluid is forced from the capillary bed at the arterial end by hydrostatic pressure and returns at the venous end by osmotic pressure

Older people develop oedema more readily than younger people. It can be hard to detect fluid overload in younger patients because they become hypertensive but do not show oedema. Patients with low serum albumin tend to form oedema more easily due to the reduced capillary osmotic pressure.

Interstitial fluid can flow within subcutaneous tissue. This allows oedema to form a pit when your thumb compresses it over the tibia (Fig. 13.2). Lymphoedema is non-pitting because the fluid is in lymphatic vessels and cannot move easily.

Fluid Retention in Chronic Kidney Disease

Patients with chronic kidney disease commonly have an increased total body sodium content. This is more common if the patient has proteinuria and is characteristic of the nephrotic syndrome. The mechanism of sodium retention in patients with

Fig. 13.2 This man has had nephrotic syndrome for a few weeks. The oedema is soft and pits easily with gentle pressure. An imprint left by fingers pressing on the tibia is seen above the gloved hand

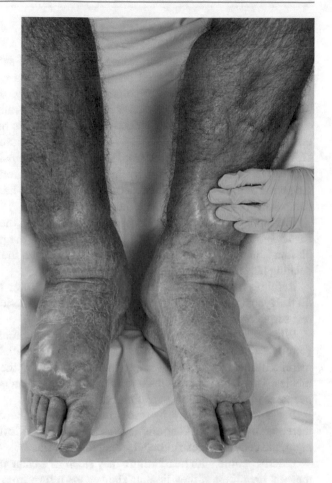

proteinuria has been revealed through studies of the effects of urine on oocytes from the African clawed frog *Xenopus laevis*. These large cells express the same epithelial sodium channels (ENaC) that reabsorb sodium in tubular epithelial cells. Electrodes can be inserted into the oocyte to measure the flow of current across the membrane via the sodium channel [2]. When urine from patients with proteinuria is applied to the oocytes, the sodium channels are activated.

Activation of the sodium channel is mediated by plasmin. Plasmin is derived from plasminogen, which is produced by vascular endothelial cells and binds to fibrin clots in the circulation. Plasmin is a protease, an enzyme that breaks down proteins, and it clears away clots by a process called fibrinolysis.

In patients with proteinuria, plasminogen is filtered and converted into plasmin in the tubules by urokinase-like plasminogen activator. The plasmin activates the epithelial sodium channels and sodium is reabsorbed. The greater the proteinuria, the greater the amounts of plasminogen and plasmin in the urine, and these correlate well with how much excess extracellular volume is found in the body [3].

Management of Excess Salt and Water

For oedema to be removed, salt excretion must exceed salt intake. As most drinks are hypotonic, imposing a limit on fluid intake—fluid restriction—is effectively water deprivation. This is either pointless, as the kidneys will counteract it by concentrating the urine, or dangerous, as it will eventually cause hypernatraemia.

Restricting salt intake may reduce oedema in chronic heart failure [4], although this is controversial [5], and helps to lower blood pressure and slow the decline in GFR in chronic kidney disease [6]. However, the principal treatment of fluid overload is to increase salt excretion by the kidneys with diuretic drugs. Avoiding salt in the period of the day after the effect of a dose of diuretic has worn off can reduce the compensatory salt retention that otherwise occurs [7].

The kidneys can only excrete salt and water that is in the plasma; interstitial fluid has to re-enter the plasma before it can be excreted. If the rate of excretion from the plasma is in equilibrium with the rate of refilling from the interstitial fluid, the circulating plasma volume is maintained.

Refilling from pleural effusions and ascites is slower than from the interstitial fluid. Hypoalbuminaemia lowers the low plasma osmotic pressure and slows the reabsorption of interstitial fluid.

When salt and water are excreted faster than the circulation is refilled, plasma volume is reduced and glomerular filtration rate may fall. The reabsorption of glomerular filtrate by the tubules is then increased, slowing the flow of filtrate along the tubules. This allows more urea to diffuse out of the tubules into the plasma, which increases the serum urea-to-creatinine ratio.

Leg swelling typically increases during the day because venous pressure is increased by gravity. When the legs are raised to the level of the heart in bed at night, the oedema is reabsorbed, leading to nocturia.

Elderly people with heart failure may sleep in a chair rather than a bed because they get breathless if they lie flat. The venous return from their legs is continually exposed to gravity and fluid cannot leave the tissues. This can lead to chronic oedema and venous ulceration.

Similarly, refilling of the circulation from leg oedema is slow in patients with high venous pressure due to right heart failure—cor pulmonale—and diuretic treatment is more likely to affect kidney function.

How to Use Diuretics

There are three main classes of diuretic drugs: thiazides, e.g. bendroflumethiazide, mainly used to treat hypertension; potassium sparing diuretics, e.g. spironolactone, mainly used to treat heart failure and hypertension resistant to other drugs; and loop diuretics, e.g. furosemide, used to treat fluid overload [8].

Amiloride is a diuretic that specifically blocks the epithelial sodium channel (ENaC). It would therefore seem a logical choice in the treatment of patients with proteinuria and fluid overload. Unfortunately, trials of amiloride have shown a high risk of hyperkalaemia and acute kidney injury and so it is not routinely used [9].

Loop diuretics are secreted into the tubule and block sodium reabsorption in the ascending limb of the loop of Henle. The concentration of the drug within the tubule needs to go above a therapeutic threshold to increase the volume of urine. The dose required to achieve this varies greatly between patients. To find the correct dose, ask the patient, "Does the tablet make you go to the toilet and how much urine do you pass?" If there is no increase in urine volume after one dose, giving the same dose again later in the day will not help. You need to give the kidneys a bigger 'kick' with a higher dose that goes above the threshold.

The effect of a loop diuretic lasts about 5 h. If the patient has polyuria throughout the day and night this is more likely to be the effect of being fluid overloaded rather than the diuretic.

As the GFR decreases and proteinuria increases, larger doses of diuretic are needed to achieve the same volume of urine from the smaller number of nephrons. At very low levels of GFR, a combination of diuretics that work in different places on the nephron may be needed, e.g. the thiazide diuretic metolazone with furosemide. The combined effect can be very powerful and needs careful monitoring of fluid balance and biochemistry.

In oedematous patients, absorption of an oral diuretic from the gut may be slower but the overall dose absorbed and the diuretic effect is essentially the same as in someone without intestinal oedema, so giving it intravenously is not necessary. There is also no evidence that an intravenous infusion is more effective than giving intravenous boluses [8].

The patient should weigh themselves each morning to guide the dose and frequency needed that day. Some increase in serum urea and creatinine is not a good reason to reduce the dose. An effective diuresis in someone with oedema is likely to reduce intravascular volume and the resulting drop in eGFR is not a sign of nephrotoxicity. The patient's symptoms and signs are more important guides for adjusting the dose than the blood results.

Physical Signs of Kidney Disease

Traditional physical signs of advanced kidney disease, such as uraemic frost and pigmentation, are rarely seen now that the detection and treatment of kidney disease has improved.

Skin signs are usually related to systemic diseases that affect the kidneys. Vasculitis is the commonest and can have a range of appearances depending upon the size and location of the vessels affected (Figs. 13.3, 13.4, 13.5, 13.6, and 13.7).

Fig. 13.3 Purpuric
vasculitic rash in a patient
with Henoch-
Schönlein Purpura

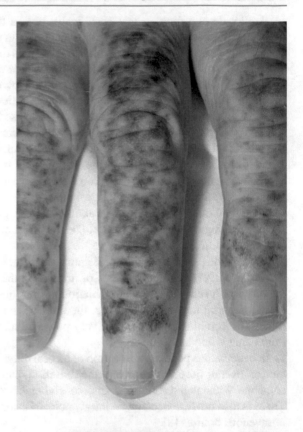

Fig. 13.4 Splinter
haemorrhages in a patient
with ANCA-positive
systemic necrotising
vasculitis

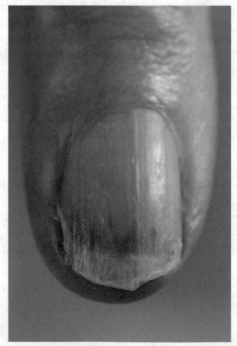

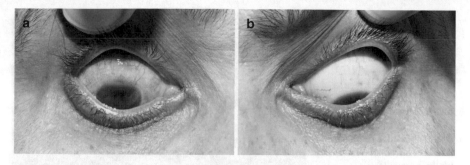

Fig. 13.5 Vasculitis of the sclerae of the right (**a**) and left (**b**) eyes in a patient with granulomatosis with polyangiitis

Fig. 13.6 Vasculitic and purpuric rash affecting the legs of a patient with Henoch-Schönlein purpura. Skin biopsy showed a leucocytoclastic vasculitis

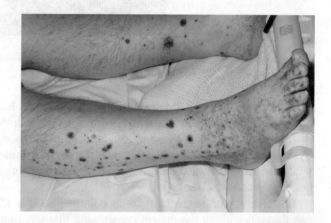

Fig. 13.7 Oedema and vasculitic lesions with skin necrosis in a man with ulcerative colitis and antiphospholipid syndrome. He also suffered a bowel infarction requiring total colectomy. The dressing covers the wound from a skin biopsy that showed a vasculitic process with fibrin thrombi affecting all the vessels

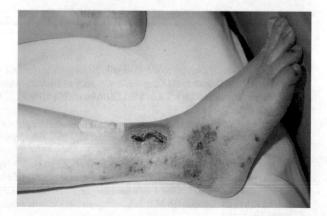

Fig. 13.8 Ultrasound scan of a patient with chronic bladder outflow obstruction. The bladder is distended and the wall is thickened with an irregular trabeculated surface. In a man, obstruction is usually caused by prostatic enlargement. These images are from a woman with a urethral stricture

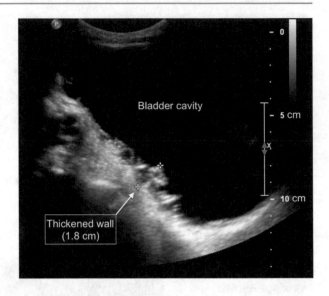

Examine the Abdomen

If you are able to feel a kidney by bimanual palpation, it is enlarged. This may be due to a tumour, gross hydronephrosis or polycystic kidney disease.

In patients with hypertension, it is traditional to listen for an abdominal bruit. Systolic bruits are frequently heard over the aorta or femoral arteries. In someone with atherosclerotic vascular disease, a bruit heard in both systole and diastole suggests renovascular disease [10].

It is always worth examining for an enlarged bladder. Chronic retention of urine can develop without the patient recognising that anything is wrong. The bladder may not be tense but is stony dull to percussion. It is easy to measure the volume using an ultrasound bladder scanner (Fig. 13.8).

References

1. Fortes MB, Owen JA, Raymond-Barker P, Bishop C, Elghenzai S, Oliver SJ, Walsh NP. Is this elderly patient dehydrated? Diagnostic accuracy of hydration assessment using physical signs, urine, and saliva markers. J Am Med Dir Assoc. 2015;16(3):221–8. http://www.ncbi.nlm.nih. gov/pubmed/25444573.
2. Papke RL, Smith-Maxwell C. High throughput electrophysiology with Xenopus oocytes. Comb Chem High Throughput Screen. 2009;12(1):38–50. https://www.ncbi.nlm.nih.gov/pmc/ articles/PMC3005249/.
3. Schork A, Woern M, Kalbacher H, Voelter W, Nacken R, Bertog M, Haerteis S, Korbmacher C, Heyne N, Peter A, Häring HU, Artunc F. Association of plasminuria with overhydration in patients with CKD. Clin J Am Soc Nephrol. 2016;11(5):761–9. https://doi.org/10.2215/ CJN.12261115. Epub 2016 Mar 1. http://cjasn.asnjournals.org/cgi/pmidlookup?view=long&p mid=26933188.

4. Philipson H, Ekman I, Forslund HB, Swedberg K, Schaufelberger M. Salt and fluid restriction is effective in patients with chronic heart failure. Eur J Heart Fail. 2013;15(11):1304–10. https://doi.org/10.1093/eurjhf/hft097. Epub 2013 Jun 19. http://onlinelibrary.wiley.com/doi/10.1093/eurjhf/hft097/full.

5. Konerman MC, Hummel SL. Sodium restriction in heart failure: benefit or harm? Curr Treat Options Cardiovasc Med. 2014;16(2):286. https://doi.org/10.1007/s11936-013-0286-x. http://onlinelibrary.wiley.com/doi/10.1093/eurjhf/hft097/full.

6. Vegter S, Perna A, Postma MJ, Navis G, Remuzzi G, Ruggenenti P. Sodium intake, ACE inhibition, and progression to ESRD. J Am Soc Nephrol. 2012;23(1):165–73. https://doi.org/10.1681/ASN.2011040430. Epub 2011 Dec 1. http://jasn.asnjournals.org/content/23/1/165.long.

7. Ellison DH. Clinical pharmacology in diuretic use. Clin J Am Soc Nephrol. 2019;14:1248–57. https://doi.org/10.2215/CJN.09630818. https://cjasn.asnjournals.org/content/clin-jasn/14/8/1248.full.pdf.

8. Anisman SD, Stephen B, Erickson SB, Morden NE. How to prescribe loop diuretics in oedema. BMJ. 2019;364:l359. https://doi.org/10.1136/bmj.l359. https://www.bmj.com/content/bmj/364/bmj.l359.full.pdf.

9. Unruh ML, Pankratz S, Demko JE, Ray EC, Hughey RP, Kleyman TR. Trial of amiloride in type 2 diabetes with proteinuria. Kidney Int Rep. 2017;2(5):893–904. https://doi.org/10.1016/j.ekir.2017.05.008. https://www.sciencedirect.com/science/article/pii/S2468024917301262.

10. Krijnen P, van Jaarsveld BC, Steyerberg EW, Man in 't Veld AJ, Schalekamp MA, Habbema JD. A clinical prediction rule for renal artery stenosis. Ann Intern Med. 1998;129(9):705–11. http://annals.org/article.aspx?articleid=711773.

Full Blood Count: Haematological Changes in Kidney Diseases

14

Anaemia

As kidney function declines, haemoglobin concentration declines with it. Ten percent of patients with a GFR between 50 and 40 mL/min/1.73 m^2 have a haemoglobin concentration less than 110 g/L. By the time GFR has fallen below 20 mL/min/1.73 m^2 this has risen to 40% [1] (Patient 14.1). This is important because anaemia in chronic kidney disease is associated with a worse quality of life, admission to hospital, cardiovascular disease, cognitive impairment, and mortality.

> **Patient 14.1 The Development of Anaemia in Chronic Kidney Disease**
> Mr. Roberts was under regular follow up for chronic kidney disease and hypertension. Over the course of a year his eGFR dropped by half. An ultrasound scan showed a shrunken right kidney.
>
> As the right kidney atrophied, glomerular filtration rate and erythropoietin production declined, leading to a decline in both eGFR and haemoglobin concentration (Fig. 14.1).

The normal physiology of red blood cell production is shown in Fig. 14.2.

In chronic kidney disease, erythropoietin production is insufficient to maintain a normal haemoglobin concentration. In addition, red cell life span is shortened and iron metabolism is abnormal. The resulting anaemia is typically normocytic, normochromic and hypoproliferative [2].

If someone with kidney disease has abnormal red cells or changes in white cells or platelets, an alternative cause should be sought. Common causes include iron deficiency from gastrointestinal blood loss or coeliac disease, folate or vitamin B12 deficiency causing macrocytic anaemia, and bone marrow disorders such as myelodysplastic syndrome.

© Springer Nature Switzerland AG 2020
H. C. Rayner et al., *Understanding Kidney Diseases*,
https://doi.org/10.1007/978-3-030-43027-6_14

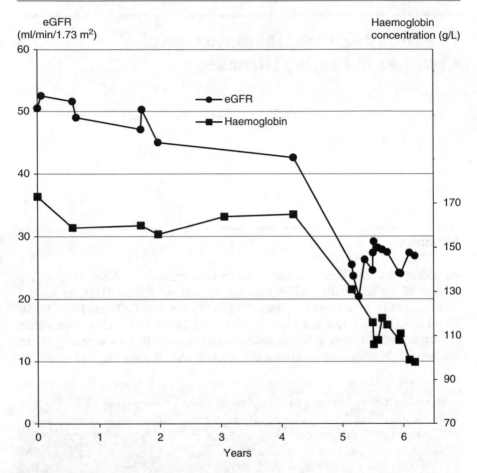

Fig. 14.1 Parallel reductions in eGFR and haemoglobin concentration due to atrophy of one kidney in a patient with pre-existing chronic kidney disease

Erythropoietin and the Regulation of Haemoglobin Concentration

Red cells are formed from erythroid progenitor cells in the bone marrow. Erythropoietin binds to receptors on the progenitor cells and triggers a cascade of phosphorylations of intracellular proteins. These activated proteins set the progenitor cells on a path to form mature red cells.

In the fetus and newborn baby, erythropoietin is produced mainly by the liver. In infancy, production shifts to the kidneys as their blood flow and function increase. In adults, 90% of erythropoietin comes from the kidneys.

Erythropoietin production is controlled by changes in the partial pressure of oxygen (pO₂) dissolved in tissue fluid. In 2019, the Nobel Prize in Physiology or

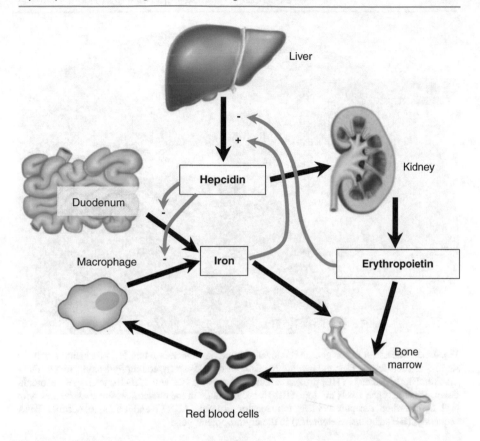

Fig. 14.2 The physiology of red cell production. Black arrows represent the movements of iron and the hormones hepcidin and erythropoietin around the body. Grey arrows represent their regulatory effects

Medicine was awarded jointly to Professors Kaelin, Ratcliffe (a British nephrologist) and Semenza for their discoveries of how cells sense and adapt to oxygen availability.

The regulation of erythropoietin production takes place inside interstitial fibroblast cells, located close to peritubular capillaries in the deep layer of the renal cortex [3]. It is mediated by hypoxia-inducible factors (HIFs) (Fig. 14.3). When pO_2 is normal, HIF-1α is hydroxylated by oxygen-dependent HIF prolyl-4-hydroxylase domain (PHD) enzymes. The hydroxylated HIF-1α then binds to von Hippel-Lindau (VHL) protein and a small peptide, ubiquitin, is added. Ubiquitin functions as a tag to mark proteins that go on to be broken down by enzyme complexes called proteasomes.

Under hypoxic conditions, the PHD enzymes are not hydroxylated and so HIF-1α levels increase. HIF-1α enters the cell nucleus, binds to specific DNA sequences (HIF-responsive elements) in the erythropoietin gene, and turns on erythropoietin production. Erythropoietin levels in blood may increase 1000-fold.

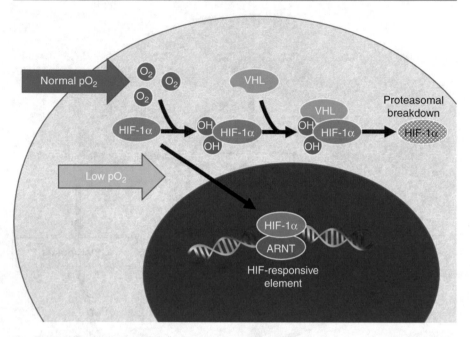

Fig. 14.3 The effect of oxygen on the level of hypoxia-inducible factor HIF-1α inside a cell. At normal oxygen levels, O₂ regulates the breakdown of HIF-1α by adding hydroxyl groups (OH). The von Hippel-Lindau (VHL) protein can then form a complex with HIF-1α, leading to its breakdown. When oxygen levels are low, HIF-1α accumulates in the nucleus, where it associates with aryl hydrocarbon receptor nuclear translocator protein (ARNT) and binds to specific DNA sequences (HIF-responsive elements) in the erythropoietin gene

HIF binds to HIF-responsive elements in a number of genes in a wide range of tissues. As well as regulating erythropoietin, it is involved in the adaptation of muscles to hypoxia during intense exercise, the immune system, the generation of new blood vessels in the fetus, and the development of the placenta. It also has an important role in the growth of tumours. In von Hippel-Lindau disease, faulty VHL protein is produced leading to a large rise in HIF-regulated gene activity. This is linked to the growth of cysts and tumours in a number of organs.

Erythropoietin production declines as kidney tissue is lost and GFR drops, due to the fall in the number of interstitial cells and reduced HIF activity within each cell. If HIF levels are increased by pharmacological inhibition of the PHD enzymes, erythropoietin production and haemoglobin concentration increase [4].

Why Is Haemoglobin Regulated by the Kidneys?

Why are the kidneys central to the regulation of red cell production by the bone marrow? The answer to this question becomes clear from thinking about the role of haemoglobin in survival and evolution.

The regulatory mechanism maintains a rate of red cell production that replaces red cells cleared from the circulation at the end of their life. If the loss of red cells increases, the haemoglobin concentration falls and the regulatory mechanism stimulates red cell production to restore it to its optimum level.

The optimal haemoglobin concentration is the one that delivers oxygen most efficiently to the tissues. Too high a concentration increases the risk of hyperviscosity and clotting; too low a concentration risks high-output cardiac failure.

A low haemoglobin concentration provides an inadequate supply of O_2 to the tissues. This may be compensated by an increase in blood flow; for example, in exercising muscles blood flow can increase by 20-fold. Tissues that are unable to compensate by increasing their blood flow are vulnerable to hypoxic damage.

If the blood flow to the kidneys increased in response to anaemia, GFR would also increase. This would increase the amount of sodium in the tubules and the amount of O_2 and energy required to reabsorb it. The increased O_2 consumption would eventually exceed the extra O_2 provided by the increased blood flow. Kidney blood flow is therefore tightly regulated.

Because hypoxia in the kidneys cannot be compensated by increased blood flow, they are at risk of hypoxic damage due to anaemia. Locating the haemoglobin regulatory mechanism in the region of the kidney most at risk—the deep cortex—guards against this and so provides the greatest survival advantage.

Iron Metabolism in Kidney Disease

Iron deficiency is common in patients with chronic kidney disease. It is due to decreased iron absorption from the gut and increased iron loss from gastrointestinal bleeding. In addition, iron metabolism is abnormal.

Iron is absorbed from the duodenum and distributed around the body bound to transferrin in the plasma. Liver cells and macrophages take up iron-transferrin complexes and store the iron in ferritin. When red cells are broken down, the iron that is released is taken up and stored by macrophages (Fig. 14.2).

Iron is released from duodenal cells, liver cells and macrophages by a protein called ferroportin located in their membranes. This process is controlled by hepcidin, a small peptide produced by the liver. A rise in plasma iron concentration increases the production of hepcidin, which binds to ferroportin in the cell membrane. The hepcidin-ferroportin complex is taken into the cell by endocytosis and broken down. The loss of ferroportin reduces the release of iron from the cell and the plasma iron concentration falls.

The production of hepcidin by the liver is inhibited by erythropoietin, and hepcidin is excreted by the kidneys. Hence, when kidney function is reduced, hepcidin levels rise due to impaired production of erythropoietin and reduced excretion of hepcidin. This is exacerbated by inflammation, which increases hepcidin production by the liver.

Increased hepcidin levels reduce the delivery of iron into plasma, so called functional iron deficiency [5]. Because iron absorption from the duodenum is impaired, iron supplements used to overcome this are often given intravenously rather than orally.

The Pros and Cons of Anaemia in Kidney Disease

The anaemia of chronic kidney disease provides some survival advantage against cardiovascular disease. Blood clots less readily due to anaemia and impaired platelet function. If the anaemia is corrected with recombinant erythropoietin, the risk of stroke increases [6].

The increased risk may be an effect of recombinant erythropoietin rather than the correction of anaemia. Patients on haemodialysis who have higher hemoglobin concentrations without transfusion or erythropoietin treatment, such as patients with polycystic kidney disease or respiratory disease, do not have an increased mortality risk [7]. Also, there is evidence that using longer acting erythropoietin is associated with a higher risk of mortality than shorter acting agents [8].

Anaemia has indirectly increased survival from kidney failure through haemodialysis. Long-term haemodialysis is made possible by the arterio-venous fistula that allows repeated safe access to the circulation. If one attempts to create a fistula in someone with normal kidney function, the vein clots almost immediately. Similarly, if a dialysis patient regains normal kidney function with a transplant, the fistula usually clots. The anaemia and bleeding tendency of kidney failure have permitted the evolution of haemodialysis by allowing arterio-venous fistulas to function.

Kidney Diseases Linked to Causes of Anaemia

Anaemia may sometimes be caused by the same condition that causes kidney disease. Sickle cell anaemia is common; paroxysmal nocturnal haemoglobinuria (PNH) and haemolytic uraemic syndrome (HUS) are rare [9]. In all three, anaemia is caused by intravascular haemolysis. If haemolysis is suspected, check for a raised serum lactate dehydrogenase (LDH), which is released from damaged red cells.

Patients with **sickle cell disease** may have a wide range of clinical presentations including haematuria, proteinuria, nephrotic syndrome, acute and chronic kidney disease. The pathological mechanisms underlying many of these complications remain unclear [10].

Kidney function declines more quickly in patients with more severe sickle cell disease and in patients with sickle cell disease compared to the trait [11]. Nonetheless, patients with sickle cell trait still have twice the normal risk of end-stage kidney failure [12]. In sickle cell trait, high hemoglobin S and haemoglobins F and A2 are associated with a slower decline in eGFR [11].

Sickle cell disease and trait both cause infarction of the renal medulla and papillae due to sickling of red cells in this hypoxic region. Necrotic papillae slough off into the renal pelvis and can cause haematuria, ureteric colic and obstruction. Chronic

Fig. 14.4 Blood film showing microangiopathic haemolytic anaemia. There are large numbers of fragmented and abnormally shaped red cells called schistocytes, indicating damage to red cell membranes, and low numbers of platelets

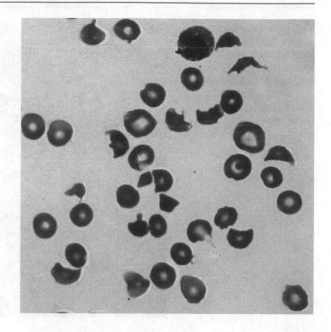

medullary ischaemia impairs the kidney's ability to concentrate urine and excrete acid and potassium. Patients with sickle cell disease and trait have double the usual risk of haematuria but should be investigated for other causes in the normal way before concluding that sickling is the cause [13].

Paroxysmal nocturnal haemoglobinuria (PNH) is caused by an acquired defect of protective proteins on the red cell membrane—a deficiency of glycophosphatidylinositol. It may occur in isolation or as part of a bone marrow disorder such as aplastic anemia. Only a quarter of patients have red urine (haemoglobinuria) in the morning. It may present with acute or chronic kidney disease, caused by haemoglobin occluding or damaging tubules and stimulating interstitial fibrosis [14]. It can be treated with eculizumab, a monoclonal antibody that inhibits the complement activation that attacks the red cell membranes.

Haemolytic uraemic syndrome (HUS) is divided into three forms: typical diarrhoea-positive (D+ HUS), atypical (aHUS), and HUS secondary to a range of other causes.

D+ HUS is the consequence of an infection, usually Escherichia coli subtype O157. The infection is typically contracted from undercooked beef, contaminated dairy products, or contact with the organism in the environment such as at petting farms. E. coli O157 produces a shiga-like toxin, also known as verocytotoxin, which damages endothelial cells, activates neutrophils and triggers the coagulation pathway. This consumes platelets and causes a microangiopathic haemolytic anaemia (MAHA) (Fig. 14.4).

Microthrombi occlude the glomerular capillaries, causing acute kidney injury (Fig. 14.5).

Fig. 14.5 Section of a
glomerulus from a patient
with HUS showing
glomerular capillaries
containing microthrombi
and red cells (arrow).
Haematoxylin and
eosin ×60

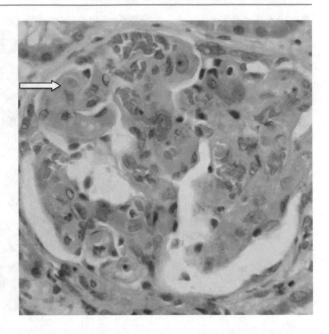

Once the acute illness is passed, the glomerular microthrombi resolve and the capillaries reopen. Hence treatment of the condition is supportive; about 50% of patients require dialysis, usually for up to 2 weeks (Patient 14.2).

Patient 14.2 Typical Diarrhoea-Positive (D+ HUS)
Ten-year-old Rosie was admitted to hospital with a 3-day history of diarrhoea, with blood for the last 24 h. She had drunk unpasteurised milk 4 days before the diarrhoea. Serum electrolytes and creatinine were normal for her age (creatinine 50 μmol/L = 0.6 mg/dL). Haemoglobin concentration was increased due to acute dehydration (174 g/L = 17.4 g/dL). Neutrophils were raised (17.7 × 10⁹/L) but platelets and clotting were normal. She was given oral rehydration mixture.

Two days later serum sodium had fallen to 130 mmol/L and creatinine increased to 345 μmol/L (3.9 mg/dL). Haemoglobin had fallen to 117 g/L (11.7 g/dL) and platelets to 76 × 10⁹/L. A faecal culture grew *Escherichia coli* O157.

Over the next 5 days her creatinine rose to 975 μmol/L (11.0 mg/dL) and she commenced peritoneal dialysis, which continued for 13 days. Her haemoglobin fell further to 74 g/L (7.4 g/dL) and the film showed fragmented red cells typical of microangiopathic haemolytic anaemia. She was given a blood transfusion.

Two months later her creatinine had returned to a normal level and she has since remained well.

Atypical HUS (aHUS) is atypical in that there is usually no or only mild diarrhoea and no E. coli infection. Hypertension is common and can be severe. Up to 70% of affected patients progress to end-stage kidney failure and there is a high risk of recurrence after a kidney transplant.

The condition can present at any age, with 60% of cases being in childhood. It may be familial and up to 80% have a genetic abnormality of complement regulation (Patient 14.3).

Patient 14.3 Atypical HUS (aHUS)

Peter, aged 5, was admitted with a 3-day history of vomiting, jaundice and abdominal cramps without diarrhoea. He was pale, jaundiced and had a petechial rash on his limbs and trunk. Blood count confirmed a low haemoglobin concentration with fragmented red blood cells on the film. Serum lactate dehydrogenase and creatinine were raised (Fig. 14.6).

His older brother had had an episode of low platelets and transient anaemia at the age of 5 years, diagnosed as thrombotic thrombocytopenic purpura, and had made a full recovery.

A diagnosis of atypical HUS was made and Peter was treated with daily plasma exchange. His kidney function and blood count recovered quickly. He was then maintained on eculizumab infusions every 2 weeks.

Genetic studies identified a mutation of the gene encoding CD46 membrane cofactor protein in both Peter and his brother. This cofactor degrades complement components C3b and C4b, interrupting the complement cascade. Loss of its function leads to unregulated formation of complement membrane attack complex that causes endothelial cell damage.

Eculizumab infusions were discontinued after 6 months but he was admitted 9 months later with a recurrence of HUS (Fig. 14.6). This responded rapidly to eculizumab alone and he remains on 3 weekly infusions.

When aHUS involves other organs, notably the nervous system causing seizures and coma, it is termed thrombotic thrombocytopenic purpura-hemolytic uremic syndrome (TTP-HUS). Patients with TTP classically have a severe deficiency of the protease enzyme ADAMTS13. ADAMTS13 normally suppresses blood clotting by breaking down multimers of von Willebrand factor [15].

Treatment of aHUS used to involve plasmapheresis and infusions of fresh-frozen plasma but had a 40% rate of dialysis or death. Because the condition, like PNH, is mediated by the complement cascade, the monoclonal antibody eculizumab is now used, with much better results.

Secondary HUS can be caused by drugs, autoimmune diseases, infections including invasive *Streptococcus pneumoniae* infection, malignancies, glomerular disease, organ transplantation, and pancreatitis. Up to half of patients require dialysis and about 1 in 5 have neurological symptoms of TTP-HUS. The condition is not caused by an abnormality of the complement pathway and does not relapse once the acute illness has resolved [16].

Haemoglobin (g/L)
Platelets (x10⁹/L)   Lactate
Creatinine (micromol/L)   dehydrogenase
(mg/dL)   (IU/L)

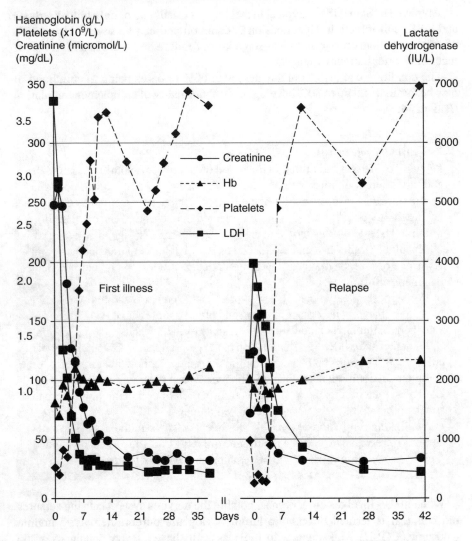

Fig. 14.6 Patterns of creatinine, blood count and lactate dehydrogenase (LDH) during two episodes of aHUS

References

1. Moranne O, Froissart M, Rossert J, et al. Timing of onset of CKD-related metabolic complications. J Am Soc Nephrol. 2009;20:164–71. https://doi.org/10.1681/ASN.2008020159. https://jasn.asnjournals.org/content/20/1/164.long.
2. Babitt JL, Lin HY. Mechanisms of Anemia in CKD. J Am Soc Nephrol. 2012;23(10):1631–4. https://doi.org/10.1681/ASN.2011111078. https://jasn.asnjournals.org/content/23/10/1631.
3. Zeisberg M, Kalluri R. Physiology of the renal interstitium. Clin J Am Soc Nephrol. 2015;10(10):1831–40. https://doi.org/10.2215/CJN.00640114. http://cjasn.asnjournals.org/cgi/pmidlookup?view=long&pmid=25813241.

4. Provenzano R, Besarab A, Sun CH, Diamond SA, Durham JH, Cangiano JL, Aiello JR, Novak JE, Lee T, Leong R, Roberts BK, Saikali KG, Hemmerich S, Szczech LA, Yu KH, Neff TB. Oral hypoxia-inducible factor prolyl hydroxylase inhibitor roxadustat (FG-4592) for the treatment of anemia in patients with CKD. Clin J Am Soc Nephrol. 2016;11(6):982–91. https://doi.org/10.2215/CJN.06890615. Epub 2016 Apr 19. https://www.ncbi.nlm.nih.gov/pmc/articles/PMC4891748/.

5. Ganz T, Nemeth E. Iron balance and the role of hepcidin in chronic kidney disease. Semin Nephrol. 2016;36(2):87–93. https://doi.org/10.1016/j.semnephrol.2016.02.001. https://www.ncbi.nlm.nih.gov/pmc/articles/PMC4884601/.

6. Mc Causland FR, Claggett B, Burdmann EA, Chertow GM, Cooper ME, Eckardt KU, Ivanovich P, Levey AS, Lewis EF, McGill JB, McMurray JJV, Parfrey P, Parving HH, Remuzzi G, Singh AK, Solomon SD, Toto RD, Pfeffer MA. Treatment of anemia with darbepoetin prior to dialysis initiation and clinical outcomes: analyses from the trial to reduce cardiovascular events with aranesp therapy (TREAT). Am J Kidney Dis. 2019;73(3):309–15. https://doi.org/10.1053/j.ajkd.2018.10.006. Epub 2018 Dec 19. https://www.ajkd.org/article/S0272-6386(18)31087-4/fulltext.

7. Goodkin DA, Fuller DS, Robinson BM, Combe C, Fluck R, Mendelssohn D, Akizawa T, Pisoni RL, Port FK. Naturally occurring higher hemoglobin concentration does not increase mortality among hemodialysis patients. J Am Soc Nephrol. 2011;22(2):358–65. https://doi.org/10.1681/ASN.2010020173. Epub 2010 Dec 16. https://www.ncbi.nlm.nih.gov/pmc/articles/PMC3029908.

8. Sakaguchi Y, Hamano T, Wada A, Masakane I. Types of erythropoietin-stimulating agents and mortality among patients undergoing hemodialysis. J Am Soc Nephrol. 2019;30(6):1037–48. https://doi.org/10.1681/ASN.2018101007. https://jasn.asnjournals.org/content/early/2019/04/22/ASN.2018101007.

9. Brocklebank V, Wood KM, Kavanagh D. Thrombotic microangiopathy and the kidney. Clin J Am Soc Nephrol. 2018;13(2):300–17. https://doi.org/10.2215/CJN.00620117. Epub 2017 Oct 17. https://cjasn.asnjournals.org/content/13/2/300.long.

10. Pham P-T T, Pham P-C T, Wilkinson AH, Lew SQ. Renal abnormalities in sickle cell disease. Kidney Int. 2000;57:1–8. https://doi.org/10.1046/j.1523-1755.2000.00806.x. http://www.nature.com/ki/journal/v57/n1/full/4491289a.html.

11. Olaniran KO, Allegretti AS, Zhao SH, Achebe MM, Eneanya ND, Thadhani RI, Nigwekar SU, Kalim S. Kidney function decline among black patients with sickle cell trait and sickle cell disease: an observational cohort study. J Am Soc Nephrol. 2020;31(2):393–404. https://doi.org/10.1681/ASN.2019050502. https://jasn.asnjournals.org/content/early/2019/12/05/ASN.2019050502.abstract?papetoc.

12. Naik RP, Irvin MR, Judd S, Gutiérrez OM, Zakai NA, Derebail VK, Peralta C, Lewis MR, Zhi D, Arnett D, McClellan W, Wilson JG, Reiner AP, Kopp JB, Winkler CA, Cushman M. Sickle cell trait and the risk of ESRD in blacks. J Am Soc Nephrol. 2017;28(7):2180–7. https://doi.org/10.1681/ASN.2016101086. Epub 2017 Mar 9. PubMed PMID: 28280138; PubMed Central PMCID: PMC5491293. https://www.ncbi.nlm.nih.gov/pmc/articles/PMC5491293/.

13. Kiryluk K, Jadoon A, Gupta M, Radhakrishnan J. Sickle cell trait and gross hematuria. Kidney Int. 2007;71(7):706–10. https://www.kidney-international.org/article/S0085-2538(15)52425-3/fulltext.

14. Nair RK, Khaira A, Sharma A, Mahajan S, Dinda AK. Spectrum of renal involvement in paroxysmal nocturnal hemoglobinuria: report of three cases and a brief review of the literature. Int Urol Nephrol. 2008;40(2):471–5. https://doi.org/10.1007/s11255-008-9356-5. http://link.springer.com/article/10.1007%2Fs11255-008-9356-5.

15. Noris M, Mescia F, Remuzzi G. STEC-HUS, atypical HUS and TTP are all diseases of complement activation. Nat Rev Nephrol. 2012;8:622–33. https://doi.org/10.1038/nrneph.2012.195. http://www.nature.com/nrneph/journal/v8/n11/full/nrneph.2012.195.html.

16. Le Clech A, Simon-Tillaux N, Provôt F, Delmas Y, Vieira-Martins P, Limou S, Halimi J, Le Quintrec M, Lebourg L, Grangé S, Karras A, Ribes D, Jourde-Chiche N, Rondeau E, Frémeaux-Bacchi V, Fakhouri F. Atypical and secondary hemolytic uremic syndromes have a distinct presentation and no common genetic risk factors. Kidney Int. 2019;95(6):1443–52. https://www.kidney-international.org/article/S0085-2538(19)30165-6/pdf.

Acid, Base and the Kidneys: The Role of the Kidneys in Acid-Base Disorders

15

A Brief Reminder of Acid-Base Chemistry and Homeostasis

An acid is a substance that can donate a hydrogen ion (H^+), the proton of a hydrogen atom. A base or alkali is a substance that can accept a hydrogen ion. A buffer is substance that resists changes in pH when small quantities of acid or alkali are added to it.

A strong acid donates its H^+ readily. It is harder to remove the H^+ from a weak acid, such as carbonic acid, so only a small fraction is in the ionised form.

	Acid		Base
Carbonic acid	H_2CO_3	$\leftrightarrow H^+ +$	HCO_3^-
Ammonium	NH_4^+	$\leftrightarrow H^+ +$	NH_3
Dihydrogen phosphate	$H_2PO_4^-$	$\leftrightarrow H^+ +$	HPO_4^{2-}

Free hydrogen ions are highly reactive and have powerful effects on the body's metabolism. Their concentration is tightly controlled at a nanomolar level (Table 15.1), about one-millionth of the concentration of bicarbonate.

For many patients who are not critically ill, a venous blood gas provides a sufficiently accurate measure of acid-base status that is easier and less painful to obtain than an arterial sample [1]. However, venous blood will not provide a good measure of arterial oxygenation.

Changes in pH are regulated by negatively charged buffers: bicarbonate anions (HCO_3^-) in the extracellular fluid; monohydrogen phosphate (HPO_4^{2-}) on cellular proteins; and carbonate (CO_3^{2-}) in bone.

CO_2 and bicarbonate are controlled independently in the extracellular fluid:

$$H_2O + CO_2 \overset{Slow*}{\leftrightarrow} H_2CO_3 \overset{Fast}{\leftrightarrow} H^+ + HCO_3^-$$

* catalysed by carbonic anhydrase

© Springer Nature Switzerland AG 2020
H. C. Rayner et al., *Understanding Kidney Diseases*,
https://doi.org/10.1007/978-3-030-43027-6_15

Table 15.1 · Typical normal ranges for arterial and venous blood gas variables, and the differences between venous and arterial values

	pO_2	pCO_2	pH	$[H^+]$ nmol/L	$[HCO_3^-]^a$ mmol/L	Standard base excess[b] mmol/L	Anion gap mEq/L
Arterial blood (SI units)	10.5–13.5 kPa	4.7–6.0 kPa	7.35–7.45	35–45	22–26	0 ± 2	8–16[c]
Arterial blood (conventional)	80–100 mmHg	35–45 mmHg					
Venous blood (SI units)[d]		5.5–6.8 kPa	7.32–7.41	38–48	23–27		
Difference between venous and arterial blood[d]		0.8 kPa (6 mmHg) higher	0.035 lower	3 nmol/L higher	1.4 mmol/L higher	0.1 mmol/L lower	

1 mmHg = 0.13 kiloPascals (kPa); mmHg = kPa × 7.5

[a]Measured as actual bicarbonate

[b]Amount of acid needed to be added to return the pH to 7.4 under standard conditions

[c]The normal range varies between analysers

[d]See [1] for details; all values are approximate

Acidosis, an excess of hydrogen ions in the body, can be caused by a rise in the level of pCO_2 or a fall in the level of HCO_3^- as demonstrated by this modification of the Henderson-Hasselbach equation, showing that hydrogen ion concentration is proportional to the CO_2 level divided by the bicarbonate level:

$$\left[H^+\right] \alpha \frac{pCO_2}{\left[HCO_3^-\right]}$$

The laboratory may measure the serum total CO_2 content instead of the serum bicarbonate concentration. Total CO_2 includes bicarbonate ions, dissolved CO_2 and carbonic acid. Bicarbonate comprises about 95% of total CO_2.

Normal metabolism on a Western diet produces 50–100 mmol of acid per day, such as sulphuric acid (H_2SO_4) from the metabolism of sulphur-containing amino acids. The body's buffers initially absorb the acid but it must be excreted to maintain acid-base balance. The lungs and kidneys play key roles in this. The lungs excrete acid as CO_2 in breath and regulate the blood pCO_2; the kidneys excrete H^+ in urine and regulate the blood HCO_3^- concentration [2].

Acid is excreted in the urine mainly as ammonium ions (NH_4^+). The smell of stale urine comes from the breakdown of ammonium chloride and urea to ammonia. In Roman times, stale urine was collected and used for whitening teeth and for cleaning.

How the Kidney Tubules Regulate Serum Bicarbonate and Acid Excretion

The regulation of serum bicarbonate involves two processes in the kidney tubules: the reabsorption of 80–90% of filtered HCO_3^- and the production of new HCO_3^- to make up for HCO_3^- bound by metabolic acid. These mechanisms are shown in diagrammatic form in Figs. 15.1, 15.2 and 15.3.

Carbonic anhydrase inside proximal tubular cells catalyses the conversion of CO_2 and H_2O into the charged ions H^+ and HCO_3^-. Charged ions cannot cross cell membranes and need a protein transporter or channel to move in and out of cells. The HCO_3^- is returned to blood in the peritubular capillaries by Sodium-Bicarbonate Co-transporter-1 (NBC1). The H^+ is secreted into the tubular filtrate by Sodium-Hydrogen Exchanger-3 (NHE-3), where it combines with HCO_3^- to form H_2CO_3. This is broken down into CO_2 and H_2O by carbonic anhydrase in the tubular cell brush border and the CO_2 diffuses into the cell. Overall, bicarbonate is removed from the tubular filtrate and added to the peritubular blood, and so effectively is reabsorbed (Fig. 15.1).

In the early proximal tubule, NH_4^+ and HCO_3^- are produced from glutamine (Fig. 15.1). The Sodium-Hydrogen Exchanger-3 (NHE3) secretes NH_4^+ instead of H^+ into the tubular lumen. In the thick ascending limb of the loop of Henle, NH_4^+ is reabsorbed from the lumen into the medullary interstitium by the Sodium-Potassium-2 Chloride Cotransporter (NKCC2), NH_4^+ replacing K^+. NH_4^+ and NH_3 are trapped in the medulla and NH_3 diffuses into the lumen of the collecting duct, where it binds with H^+ to form NH_4^+ and is excreted in urine.

The distal nephron is where the final composition and pH of urine is controlled. In the distal tubule, H^+ is secreted into the lumen by type A intercalated cells

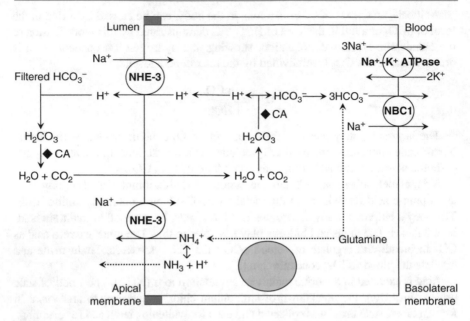

Fig. 15.1 Bicarbonate reabsorption and acid secretion by the proximal tubule. Ammonium (NH_4^+) is produced from glutamine and is secreted into the lumen; ammonia (NH_3) diffuses into the lumen. *NHE-3* sodium-hydrogen exchanger-3, *NBC1* sodium-bicarbonate co-transporter-1, *CA* carbonic anhydrase, located inside the cell and in the apical, brush border membrane

(Fig. 15.2), where it binds with monohydrogen phosphate (HPO_4^{2-}) to form dihydrogen phosphate ($H_2PO_4^-$). In the collecting duct, the type A cells have an apical H^+ ATPase that secretes H^+ into the urine. HCO_3^- generated from this process is pumped into the blood by the basolateral Cl^-/HCO_3^- exchanger (AE1). Type B intercalated cells (Fig. 15.3) have a Cl^-/HCO_3^- exchanger (Pendrin) in the apical membrane that secretes HCO_3^- into the lumen.

H^+ and K^+ secretion into the distal tubule is easier if the lumen is more negatively charged. Reabsorption of sodium (Na^+) makes the lumen more negative and so increases H^+ excretion (Fig. 15.2). Aldosterone stimulates the reabsorption of sodium via the epithelial sodium channel (ENaC) and so increases distal tubular acid excretion, as does angiotensin II.

The secretion of acid results in a progressive fall in the pH of filtrate along the nephron:

Nephron segment	pH	[H^+] nmol/L
Glomerular filtrate	7.4	40
End of proximal tubule	6.7	200
Distal tubule	5.5	3200
Distal collecting duct	4.5	32,000

The concentration of H^+ in the distal collecting duct is about 800-times higher than the surrounding extracellular fluid. This concentration gradient is maintained by the lipid cell membrane and tight junctions between cells that are impermeable to H^+.

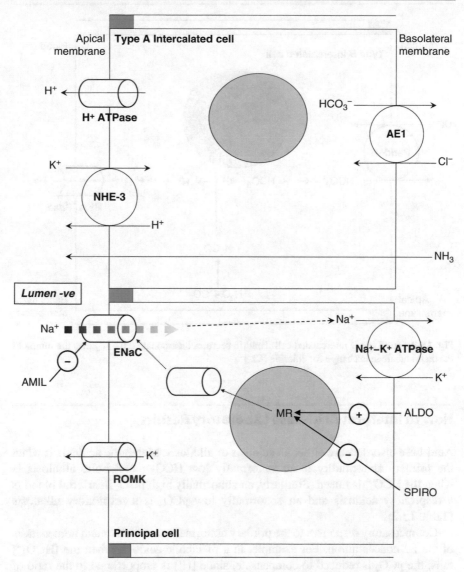

Fig. 15.2 The Type A acid-secreting intercalated cell and the principal cell in the collecting duct. Production of the epithelial sodium channel (ENaC) is stimulated the mineralocorticoid receptor (MR). MR is activated by aldosterone (ALDO). The action of aldosterone is competitively inhibited by spironolactone (SPIRO). ENaC is inhibited by amiloride (AMIL). Sodium ions (Na$^+$) flow down a concentration gradient into the principal cell through sodium channels (ENaC), leaving a negative charge in the lumen. This facilitates K$^+$ secretion into the lumen via the ROMK potassium channel. ROMK rat outer medullary potassium channel, *AE1* anion exchanger-1, *NHE3* sodium-hydrogen exchanger-3

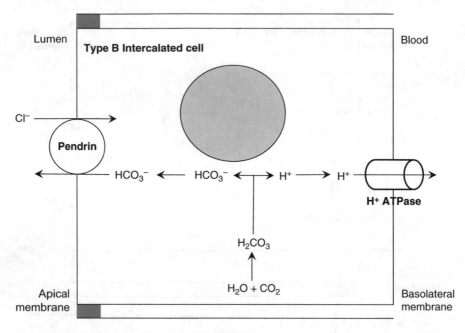

Fig. 15.3 The Type B intercalated cell. Pendrin secretes bicarbonate (HCO₃⁻) into the lumen of the distal tubule in exchange for chloride (Cl⁻)

How to Interpret Acid-Base Laboratory Results

Acid-base disorders are either an acidosis or alkalosis. Metabolic acidosis is when the primary abnormality is an abnormally low HCO_3^-; metabolic alkalosis is when the HCO_3^- is raised. Similarly, an abnormally high pCO_2 in arterial blood is a respiratory acidosis and an abnormally low pCO_2 is a respiratory alkalosis (Table 15.2).

Compensatory responses to the primary abnormality act to maintain homeostasis of the H⁺ concentration. For example, in a metabolic acidosis when the $[HCO_3^-]$ falls, the pCO_2 is reduced to compensate, since [H⁺] is proportional to the ratio of pCO_2 to $[HCO_3^-]$.

The respiratory system attempts to compensate for primarily metabolic disorders; the kidneys attempt to compensate for respiratory disorders. Changes in pH and pCO_2 differ between metabolic and respiratory disorders. They move in the same direction in metabolic disorders and in opposite directions in respiratory disorders (Table 15.2).

Answering the following questions will help you to interpret acid-base laboratory results.

Table 15.2 Acid-base disorders: their causes, consequences and compensatory changes

Condition	Initiating mechanism	Primary consequence	[H⁺]	pH	Compensation
Metabolic acidosis	Increased acid production or bicarbonate loss	Fall in [HCO₃⁻]	Increased	Reduced	Reduced pCO₂ by increased alveolar ventilation
Metabolic alkalosis	Gain of alkali or loss of acid	Rise in [HCO₃⁻]	Reduced	Increased	Increased pCO₂ by reduced alveolar ventilation
Respiratory acidosis	Decreased alveolar ventilation—respiratory failure	Rise in pCO₂	Increased	Reduced	Increased [HCO₃⁻] i. Acute—due to buffering ii. Chronic—due to kidney response
Respiratory alkalosis	Increased alveolar ventilation	Fall in pCO₂	Reduced	Increased	Reduced [HCO₃⁻] i. Acute—due to buffering ii. Chronic—due to kidney response

1. **What is the oxygenation?**
   An arterial pO_2 >10 kPa (75 mmHg) on room air is regarded as normal.
2. **What is the pH?**
   (a) pH <7.35   An acidaemia is present
   (b) pH >7.45   An alkalaemia is present
3. **What is the pCO_2?**
   (a) pCO_2 >6.0 kPa   Hypercapnia is present; alveolar ventilation is reduced
       (>45 mmHg)
   (b) pCO_2 <4.7 kPa   Hypocapnia is present; alveolar ventilation is increased
       (<35 mmHg)
4. **What is the bicarbonate concentration?**
   (a) [HCO₃⁻] >26 mmol/L   Increased bicarbonate concentration
   (b) [HCO₃⁻] <22 mmol/L   Reduced bicarbonate concentration
5. **What is the standard base excess (SBE)?**
   (a) SBE >2 mmol/L   Metabolic alkalosis
   (b) SBE <−2 mmol/L   Metabolic acidosis
       <−6 mmol/L indicates severe metabolic acidosis [3]
6. **What are the relative changes in pH and pCO_2?**
   (a) Opposite direction: there is a respiratory disorder
   (b) Same direction: there is a metabolic disorder
7. **What compensatory changes have happened?**
   (a) Respiratory compensation for metabolic disorders occurs in minutes to hours
   (b) Metabolic compensation for respiratory disorders occurs over several days

The Anion Gap

All body fluids, including urine, have to be electro-chemically neutral—the positively charged cations must equal the negatively charged anions. Not all the cations and anions in plasma are measured routinely and the measured cations (mainly sodium, potassium is usually ignored) exceed the measured anions (chloride and bicarbonate). Hence, there is an apparent 'anion gap' [4]:

$$Anion\,gap = Measured\,cations - Measured\,anions$$
$$= \left[Na^+\right] - \left(\left[Cl^-\right] + \left[HCO_3^-\right]\right)$$

A normal anion gap = 140 − (105 + 24) = 11 mmol/L (mEq/L). The normal range is typically 8–16 mmol/L (mEq/L) (Table 15.1).

In some types of metabolic acidosis, only the measured anions Cl^- and HCO_3^- are affected so the anion gap is unchanged (Fig. 15.4). This is called a normal anion

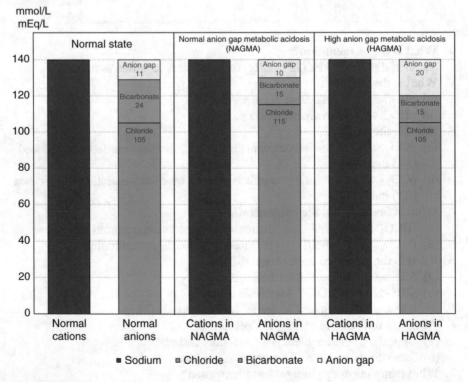

Fig. 15.4 Plasma cations, anions and the anion gap in different types of metabolic acidosis. In normal anion gap metabolic acidosis (NAGMA), bicarbonate (HCO_3^-) is lost and Cl^- is added. In high anion gap metabolic acidosis (HAGMA), unmeasured anions are added and the bicarbonate (HCO_3^-) concentration is reduced

gap metabolic acidosis (NAGMA). In other types, unmeasured anions are present so the anion gap increases. This is called a high anion gap metabolic acidosis (HAGMA).

The anion gap is made up organic acids, sulphate, monohydrogen phosphate, and proteins including albumin. In patients with a low serum albumin concentration, the anion gap should be corrected, otherwise it will be underestimated: corrected AG = AG + (0.25 × (40 − [albumin] g/L)).

In urine, the measured ions are sodium, potassium and chloride, so the urine anion gap = ([Na$^+$] + [K$^+$]) − [Cl$^-$]. Ammonium (NH$_4^+$) and bicarbonate (HCO$_3^-$) are not measured. The urine anion gap is normally positive, about +30 to +50 mmol/L (mEq/L) [5].

In acidosis, the normal kidney response is to acidify the urine with an increase in NH$_4^+$ excretion. Electro-chemical neutrality of the urine is maintained by an accompanying increase in Cl$^-$ excretion, making the urine anion gap negative, −20 to −50 mmol/L (mEq/L) or less.

Normal Anion Gap Metabolic Acidosis (NAGMA)

Normal anion gap metabolic acidosis (NAGMA) occurs when there is: excessive loss of bicarbonate from the gastrointestinal tract or the kidneys; inadequate excretion of acid by the kidneys; or, uncommmonly, an ingested toxin (Table 15.3).

The cause of a normal anion gap metabolic acidosis can be determined from the patient's history and the following three questions [6] (Fig. 15.5):

- What is the serum potassium?
- What is the urine pH?
- What is the urine anion gap?

Table 15.3 Causes of a Normal Anion Gap Metabolic Acidosis (NAGMA)

Bicarbonate loss	
Gastrointestinal bicarbonate loss	Diarrhoea, ileostomy, ureterosigmoidostomy
Renal bicarbonate loss	Type 2 proximal renal tubular acidosis
Acid accumulation	
Chronic kidney disease	Some cases can have a normal anion gap
Failed renal acid excretion	Type 1 distal renal tubular acidosis
Hypoaldosteronism	Type 4 renal tubular acidosis
Certain ingestions or poisonings	Ammonium chloride and others

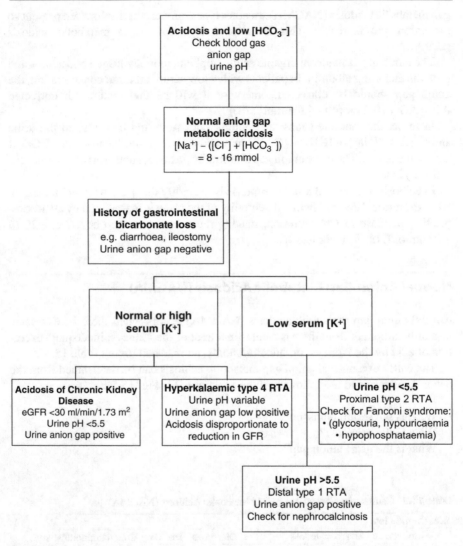

Fig. 15.5 A simplified approach to the diagnosis of a normal anion gap metabolic acidosis (NAGMA). [HCO_3^-] serum bicarbonate concentration, [Na^+] sodium concentration, [Cl^-] chloride concentration, [K^+] potassium concentration, *RTA* renal tubular acidosis. Urine dipstick tests of pH may be inaccurate at low and high values. Urine pH is best checked in the laboratory with a pH meter, using an early morning specimen

Patient 15.1 illustrates how to intepret laboratory results in a patient with acidosis.

Patient 15.1 How to Interpret Laboratory Results in a Patient with Acidosis
Mrs Distaff, aged 35 years, was brought to the emergency department by her family. Over the previous 2 weeks she had found it increasingly difficult to stand or walk. In the last few days she had become breathless and drowsy. Her family reported that she normally took ibuprofen 400 mg three times every day for headaches. In the last 4 days, she had increased the dose because of flu-like symptoms.

Test	Result SI units (*Conventional units*)	Normal range and units
Sodium	143	135–145 mmol/L
Potassium	1.0	3.5–5.5 mmol/L
Chloride	119	98–106 mmol/L
Urea (BUN)	13.2 (*37*)	3.0–7.0 mmol/L (*8–20 mg/dL*)
Creatinine	239 (*2.7*)	60–115 μmol/L (*0.7–1.3 mg/dL*)
eGFR	21	>60 mL/min/1.73 m²
Hydrogen ions	87	35–45 nmol/L
Arterial pH	7.06	7.35–7.45
Arterial pO$_2$	10.9 (*82*)	10.5–13.5 kPa (*80–100 mmHg*)
Arterial pCO$_2$	4.0 (*30*)	4.7–6.0 kPa (*35–45 mmHg*)
Lactate	0.7	Normal <2; intermediate 2.0–3.9; high ≥4.0 mmol/L
Bicarbonate	11	22–26 mmol/L
Base excess	−18	0 ± 2 mmol/L
Anion gap	[Na$^+$] − [Cl$^-$] − [HCO$_3^-$]	8–16 mmol/L (mEq/L)
Urine analysis		
Urine pH	6	5–7
Urine protein	Negative	Negative
Urine blood	Trace	Negative
Urine nitrites	Negative	Negative
Urine leucocytes	Negative	Negative
Urine glucose	Negative	Negative
Urine ketones	Negative	Negative
Urine chemistry		
Spot urine sodium	31	2–250 mmol/L
Spot urine potassium	7.1	25–125 mmol/L
Spot urine chloride	22	115–240 mmol/L
Urine anion gap	[Na$^+$] + [K$^+$] − [Cl$^-$]	

Conversion factors: For blood gases see Table 15.1.
Urea mmol/L × 2.80 = blood urea nitrogen mg/dL
Creatinine μmol/L × 0.011 = mg/dL

Questions:

1. Why is the patient weak?
2. Why is she breathless?
3. What type of acidosis is present? Is the anion gap high or normal?
4. What is odd about the urine pH?
5. What is the urine anion gap?
6. What is wrong with Mrs Distaff?

Answers:

1. She is weak because of severe hypokalaemia (K^+ = 1.0 mmol/L).
2. She is breathless because of the acidosis (pH = 7.06). The rapid breathing blows off CO_2 (pCO_2 = 4.0 kPa).
3. The base excess of −18 mmol/L indicates a severe metabolic acidosis.
   The anion gap is $[Na^+] - ([Cl^-] + [HCO_3^-]) = 143 - (119 + 11)$ = 13 mmol/L.
   This is a normal anion gap metabolic acidosis.
4. If the kidneys were compensating for the acidosis, the urine pH would be low (acidic). In this patient, the urine pH is inappropriately high (alkaline).
5. The urine anion gap (UAG) = $([Na^+] + [K^+]) - [Cl^-] = (31 + 7) - 22$ = +16 mmol/L. The UAG is positive due to the low urine chloride concentration relative to the two anions. Chloride is accompanied in the urine by ammonium (NH_4^+) so the positive urine anion gap suggests a low urinary NH_4^+. In acidosis, healthy tubules excrete the excess H^+ ions as NH_4^+. Here, ammonium production in the distal tubule is reduced, leading to impaired excretion of H^+ ions in the urine and acidosis.
6. She has acute kidney injury and distal renal tubular acidosis caused by ibuprofen. The acute kidney injury is caused by tubular damage, so there is no proteinuria.

Renal Tubular Acidosis

Abnormalities of the reabsorption of bicarbonate (HCO_3^-) and/or the excretion of hydrogen ions (H^+) by the kidney tubules lead to different types of renal tubular acidosis (RTA) (Table 15.4) [7]. The RTA syndromes are characterized by a relatively normal GFR and a metabolic acidosis with a high serum chloride concentration and normal plasma anion gap (Fig. 15.5) [8]. This contrasts with the acidosis of kidney failure in which the GFR is low, serum chloride concentration is normal or low and there is a high plasma anion gap.

Table 15.4 A summary of the three major types of renal tubular acidosis [7]

Type	Type 1 Distal RTA	Type 2 Proximal RTA	Type 4 Hyperkalaemic RTA
Mechanism	Impaired distal tubule acidification: – Impaired H^+ secretion – Collecting duct permeable to H^+ (back leak) – Impaired distal sodium reabsorption with loss of lumen negative charge (voltage defect) – Impaired basolateral HCO_3^- exit	Impaired proximal tubule bicarbonate reabsorption—often with generalised tubular dysfunction (Fanconi syndrome)	Impaired distal tubule H^+ and K^+ secretion, due to hypoaldosteronism: – Low renin production – Low aldosterone production – Collecting duct resistance to aldosterone action
Features	Often adult with Sjogren's syndrome Preserved GFR Nephrolithiasis and nephrocalcinosis	Typically seen in children with Fanconi syndrome Rickets, osteomalacia	Hyperkalaemia CKD stage 3 or 4 50% diabetic
Serum bicarbonate	10 mmol/L or less	12–20 mmol/L	18–22 mmol/L
Serum potassium	Moderate to severe hypokalaemia	Mild hypokalaemia	High normal to hyperkalaemia
Urine pH in acidosis	>5.5 (e.g. 6.0–6.5)	<5.5	Variable
Therapy	Moderate amounts of alkali (1 mmol/kg/day) as a mix of potassium and sodium alkali	Large amounts of alkali (10 mmol/kg/day) as a potassium salt: potassium citrate	Stop offending agent if possible Diuretic therapy Alkali therapy

There are three main types of RTA—1, 2 and 4. Type 3 is a combination of types 1 and 2, and is now very rare.

Type 1: Distal Renal Tubular Acidosis

In distal RTA (dRTA), a genetic or acquired condition impairs the distal tubule's ability to acidify the urine to a pH <5.5 despite the presence of acidosis. Mechanisms include: a failure of H^+ secretion (classic inherited dRTA); leakage of secreted H^+ back down the concentration gradient into the interstitium (amphotericin); and impaired reabsorption of sodium causing loss of the negative charge in the distal tubular lumen (urinary obstruction).

The more common causes of type 1 distal renal tubular acidosis are listed in Table 15.5.

Table 15.5 Causes of type 1 distal renal tubular acidosis

Genetic
AE1 and H⁺ ATPase defects, with or without nerve deafness (typically presenting in childhood)
Disorders with nephrocalcinosis
Hyperparathyroidism, idiopathic hypercalciuria
Autoimmune diseases
Sjogren's syndrome, systemic lupus erythematosus, primary biliary cirrhosis
Drugs
Non-steroidal anti-inflammatories, amphotericin, toluene (glue sniffing), lithium, amiloride, trimethoprim
Renal diseases affecting the distal tubule
Urinary tract obstruction, medullary sponge kidney, sickle cell disease, kidney transplant rejection

For examples, see patients 15.1 and 15.2

Type 2: Proximal Renal Tubular Acidosis

This is due to impaired reabsorption of bicarbonate by the proximal tubule. It typically occurs in a child with generalised dysfunction of the proximal tubules—the Fanconi syndrome—causing glycosuria, phosphaturia and other defects of reabsorption [9].

Reduced reabsorption of bicarbonate and sodium in the proximal tubule increases the load of bicarbonate on the loop of Henle and distal tubule to above their resorptive capacity. Bicarbonate and sodium are lost into the urine leading to a reduced serum bicarbonate concentration (metabolic acidosis) and volume depletion. The filtered bicarbonate load then falls until a new equilibrium with the resorptive capacity is reached. The increased load of sodium on the distal tubule is reabsorbed in exchange for potassium, leading to a fall in the serum potassium concentration.

The more common causes of type 2 proximal renal tubular acidosis are listed in Table 15.6.

Type 4: Hyperkalaemic Renal Tubular Acidosis

This is the most common type of renal tubular acidosis in adults, distinguished from types 1 and 2 by a raised serum potassium concentration [10]. It occurs in adults with underlying CKD Stages 3 and 4, often with diabetes, and affected patients have low plasma and urinary aldosterone levels, and reduced urinary excretion of ammonium. Serum chloride concentration is raised (Fig. 15.4), making this a normal anion gap metabolic acidosis. The urine pH can fall below 5.5.

In the collecting duct, aldosterone stimulates the insertion of sodium channels (ENaC) into the luminal cell membrane (Fig. 15.2). Positively charged sodium ions

Table 15.6 Causes of type 2 proximal renal tubular acidosis

Isolated (without Fanconi syndrome)
• Genetic—mutations of Sodium-Bicarbonate Co-transporter-1 (NBC1)
• Carbonic anhydrase inhibitors—acetazolamide and others
Renal tubular acidosis with Fanconi syndrome
• Genetic disorders
• Cystinosis, Wilson's disease and other rarer systemic causes
• Multiple myeloma
• Heavy metal poisoning
• Drugs—ifosfamide, antiretrovirals
• Post kidney transplantation

Table 15.7 Causes of type 4 renal tubular acidosis

Mineralocorticoid deficiency
Low renin production
• Hyporeninaemic hypoaldosteronism
• Renal disease damaging juxta-glomerular apparatus
• Non-steroidal anti-inflammatory drugs
• Calcineurin inhibitor drugs: ciclosporin, tacrolimus
Low aldosterone production
• ACE inhibitors
• Angiotensin receptor blockers
• Adrenal insufficiency
• Congenital adrenal hyperplasia
Impaired collecting duct response to aldosterone
• Potassium sparing diuretics—spironolactone, eplerenone, amiloride, triamterene
• Trimethoprim
• Tubulointerstitial disease

(Na^+) diffuse down the concentration gradient into the cell, creating a negative electrical charge in the lumen. This promotes the secretion of cations into the lumen: K^+ via potassium channels (ROMK) and H^+ via the H^+ ATPase. If this process is impaired by a deficiency of aldosterone (hyporeninaemic hypoaldosteronism) or the effect of aldosterone being blocked by drugs, excretion of K^+ and H^+ is reduced, leading to a hyperkalaemic metabolic acidosis.

Reduced glomerular filtration rate is an important factor in this condition; deficiency of aldosterone alone causes only a small drop in the serum bicarbonate concentration. However, the acidosis in type 4 RTA is greater than would be expected from the reduced GFR alone.

The more common causes of type 4 renal tubular acidosis are listed in Table 15.7.

Table 15.8   Causes of a High Anion Gap Metabolic Acidosis (HAGMA)

	Unmeasured anions
Excess acid produced within the body	
Lactic acidosis	L-lactate
Ketoacidosis	β-hydroxybutyrate
Renal failure	Lactate, ketoanions, proteins,
D-lactic acidosis (short bowel syndrome)	D-lactate
Pyroglutamic acidosis (paracetamol—acetaminophen)	Pyroglutamic acid (5-Oxoproline)
Massive rhabdomyolysis	
Excess acid taken into the body	
Aspirin	Ketones, lactate, salicylate
Methanol (ethanol, toluene, paraldehyde)	Formate (other toxins)
Ethylene and propylene Glycols (anti-freeze)	Glycolate, oxalate
Paraldehyde	Organic anion

Pyroglutamic acid, also known as 5-oxoproline, is a metabolite of glutamine (see Patient 15.2). Massive rhabdomyolysis cause acidosis through the release of endogenous acids into the circulation as well through lactic acidosis and kidney failure

High Anion Gap Metabolic Acidosis (HAGMA)

In high anion gap metabolic acidosis, unmeasured anions cause the acidosis (Table 15.8). The mnemonic GOLDMARK is helpful for remembering the various causes [11] - see the bold letters in the table.

The excess acid in lactic acidosis, ketoacidosis and kidney failure is produced within the body, i.e. it is endogenous. Lactic acid accumulates when there is increased production and/or reduced metabolism, most commonly due to circulatory collapse and hypoxia (Table 15.9) (Patient 4.1). A serum lactate concentration of 5 mmol/L or more indicates lactic acidosis—the higher the lactate level, the higher the mortality [12].

Ketoacidosis is a common complication of both type 1 and type 2 diabetes [13]. Excess alcohol, fasting and rare congenital conditions can cause non-diabetic ketoacidosis. Acidosis due to kidney failure is discussed below. High anion gap metabolic acidosis caused by pyroglutamic acid (5-oxoproline) is illustrated by Patient 15.2.

Patient 15.2 Acidosis Linked to Regular Paracetamol (Acetaminophen)
Mrs Goldman, aged 79 years, was in hospital because of cellulitis and a collection of pus in her left calf, being treated with high doses of flucloxacillin. Pain relief was achieved with oral paracetamol (acetaminophen), up to 1 g four times daily. She had a poor appetite and was frail.

After 1 week, the serum potassium dropped to 2.4 mmol/L and remained low despite oral and intravenous potassium supplements.

After 2 weeks of flucloxacillin, Mrs Goldman became breathless at rest. An arterial blood gas analysis indicated a severe metabolic acidosis: pCO_2 = 1.72 kPa; pH = 7.16; $[HCO_3^-]$ = 7.4 mmol/L; Base Excess = −22.4 mmol/L.

The anion gap was high, especially after correcting for the low serum albumin concentration of 20 g/L. Anion gap = $[Na^+] - ([Cl^-] + [HCO_3^-])$ = 146 − (114 + 7) = +25. Corrected anion gap = 25 + (0.25 × (40 − [20]) = +30.

The serum [Mg] was 0.6 mmol/L (1.4 mg/dL), normal range = 0.65–1.05 mmol/L. Metabolic acidosis reduces the active reabsorption of magnesium in the distal tubule, leading to hypomagnesaemia [14].

The urine pH was 5.5–6.0 and the urine anion gap was positive (+30), suggesting inadequate urinary acidification—a type 1 distal renal tubular acidosis (compare with Patient 15.1).

The urine potassium concentration was high (66 mmol/L, compared with the urine sodium concentration of 65 mmol/L), suggesting that excessive potassium losses were contributing to the hypokalaemia.

The cause of the high anion gap was unclear. The serum creatinine and lactate concentrations were normal. The blood ketone concentration was 2 mmol/L, below the threshold of 3.0 mmol/L set for a diagnosis of ketoacidosis.

Initially, she was given small volumes of intravenous 8.4% sodium bicarbonate. This raised the pH but worsened the hypokalaemia, so was stopped. Intravenous fluids containing potassium and magnesium were given.

Her condition progressively weakened, she developed acute kidney injury, bronchopneumonia and, sadly, died. The results of a urine organic acid profile then became available, including a 'grossly increased' level of pyroglutamic acid (5-oxoproline).

Mrs Goldman had many of the common features of pyroglutamic acidosis [15]. Patients typically are malnourished older females receiving prolonged courses of paracetamol and antibiotics, often flucloxacillin, sometimes with kidney failure, who develop the condition many days into a hospital admission. It can also occur with chronic liver disease due to alcohol excess and in pregnancy.

It is a high anion gap metabolic acidosis, often mixed with other acid-base disturbances, in this case distal renal tubular acidosis. Pyroglutamate and flucloxacillin are non-absorbable anions that stimulate secretion of K^+ cations in the distal tubule, leading to hypokalaemia [16].

Chronic paracetamol ingestion is associated with reduced plasma glutathione levels and raised pyroglutamic acid (5-oxoproline) levels in serum and urine. The metabolic acidosis differs from the lactic acidosis seen with liver necrosis following overdosage of paracetamol. When pyroglutamic acidosis is suspected, paracetamol should be stopped and N-acetylcysteine given to replenish glutathione stores while waiting for the results of confirmatory tests.

Table 15.9 The commoner causes of lactic acidosis

Impaired oxygen delivery or utilisation
• Shock
• Sepsis
• Cardiac arrest
• Severe heart failure
• Severe hypoxia
• Severe anaemia
• Carbon monoxide or cyanide poisoning
Increased metabolic rate
• Generalised seizures
• Severe exercise
• Shivering in hypothermia
Impaired metabolism of lactate
• Severe liver failure
Multiple and/or unknown mechanisms
• Diabetes
• Metformin
• Cancer

Aspirin (salicylate) poisoning causes a complex acid-base disturbance. Initially there is a respiratory alkalosis caused by direct stimulation of the respiratory centre in the brainstem by the drug, more noticable in adults. Metabolic acidosis develops later, 24 h or more after ingestion in adolescents or adults and 4–6 h in infants. It is worse in infants than adults and is caused more by accumulation of ketones and lactic acid than by the salicylic acid itself.

Ethylene glycol and methanol are metabolised by alcohol dehydrogenase into glycolic acid and formic acid respectively. This process can be slow, for example the half-life of the conversion of methanol to formic acid is 6–18 h. Therefore, the high anion gap metabolic acidosis can develop as late as 15–20 h after ingestion, when the alcohols themselves can no longer be detected.

Acidosis in Chronic Kidney Disease

As kidney disease progresses, the number of working nephrons declines. To maintain acid-base balance, ammonium excretion per remaining nephron increases, stimulated by increased angiotensin production in the kidney. When the GFR falls below about 45 mL/min/1.73 m^2, total ammonium excretion starts to fall (Fig. 15.6).

Initially, excess H$^+$ ions are buffered by bicarbonate in the extracellular fluid and by tissue buffers and bone. But as GFR falls further, these buffers become saturated, metabolic acidosis develops, and serum bicarbonate falls [17]. The plasma anion gap increases due to unmeasured anions, mainly lactate and ketoanions [18].

30–50% of patients develop metabolic acidosis as eGFR falls to 30–40 mL/min/1.73 m^2. Metabolic acidosis develops at higher levels of eGFR in younger

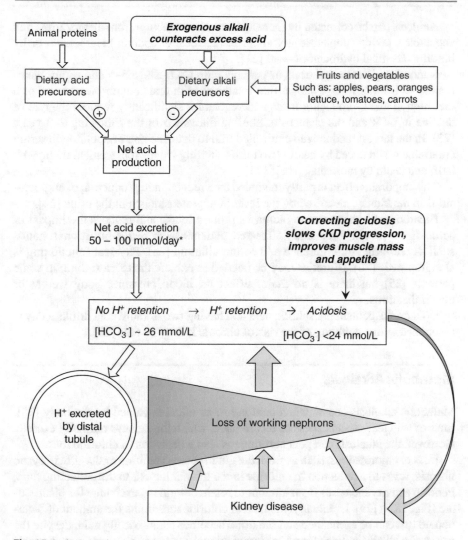

Fig. 15.6 An overview of acid excretion by the kidney, the effects of chronic kidney disease, and the role of treatment to correct acidosis. ∗ Net acid excretion is about 0.8 mmol/kg/day (mEq/kg/day)

patients, and with diabetes mellitus and diseases affecting the tubules, such as obstructive uropathy and interstitial nephritis [19].

The acidosis leads to hyperkalaemia, loss of muscle mass, release of calcium from bone, progression of kidney disease, and an increased risk of mortality [20]. The risk of GFR declining is associated with the level of serum bicarbonate, the lower the level the greater the risk. This association is found over a range of serum bicarbonate that includes normal values above 22 mmol/L (mEq/L).

Acidosis can be corrected by increasing alkali production from dietary fruits and vegetables, taking supplementary alkali in the form of sodium bicarbonate, or by binding intestinal hydrochloric acid [21].

Randomised controlled trials of patients with CKD Stage 3–5 and serum bicarbonate <24 mmol/L have shown that treatment with oral sodium bicarbonate or a diet high in alkali-producing fruits and vegetables significantly reduces the rate of decline in GFR and the chances of starting dialysis over the following 2–3 years [22]. In the largest randomized controlled trial to date, the risk of doubling in serum creatinine was reduced by nearly two thirds, starting kidney replacement therapy by half, and death by more than a half [23].

This important effect is partly mediated by a reduction in production of angiotensin II in the kidney, measured by the level of angiotensinogen in the urine [24].

Bicarbonate treatment also increases protein intake and reduces the impact of acidosis on protein breakdown. Treated patients have better nutritional status, such as mid-arm circumference and serum albumin [25]. Physical functioning is also improves [26]. Diuretics may be needed to excrete the extra sodium in some patients [25] but there is no major effect on blood pressure, body weight or hospitalizations.

Cola drinks contain phosphoric acid and having two or more cola drinks a day is associated with a doubling of the risk of chronic kidney disease [27].

Metabolic Alkalosis

Metabolic alkalosis occurs when acid is lost or alkali is gained by the body [28]. Loss of acid leads to an excess of bicarbonate, which the kidneys normally excrete. However, the alkalosis can persist if there is also a depletion of chloride ions.

Loss of chloride ions, such as from the gut in severe vomiting or the skin in cystic fibrosis, leads to a reduction in chloride in the tubular lumen. In the collecting duct, Pendrin activity increases in an attempt to retain chloride in exchange for bicarbonate (Fig. 15.3) [29]. Eventually, the lack of chloride ions limits the amount of bicarbonate that can be exchanged and the urine becomes paradoxically acid, despite the metabolic alkalosis. Because of sodium depletion, the activity of sodium channels (ENaC) in the collecting duct may increase (Fig. 15.2), leading to an increase in urinary potassium and hypokalaemia.

Patients with mild-to-moderate alkalosis (serum $[HCO_3^-]$ = 30–39 mmol/L) are usually asymptomatic. Patients with more severe alkalosis (serum $[HCO_3^-]$ ≥40 mmol/L) have symptoms related to volume depletion or hypokalaemia [30].

The cause can usually be diagnosed from the history, unless the patient does not admit to persistent vomiting or diuretic use. Hyperaldosteronism may not be symptomatic and, if the patient is not volume depleted, spot urine chloride and potassium measurements can be useful in making the diagnosis.

Treatment depends upon the underlying cause and the severity of the deficits of chloride, sodium, water and potassium. Saline, such as 0.9% sodium chloride which

Table 15.10 Causes of metabolic alkalosis

Chloride depletion
Gastrointestinal loss
• Vomiting or nasogastric suction
• Diarrhoea—villous adenoma
Kidney loss
• Diuretic use—"chloriuretic" diuretics
• Bartter or Gitelman syndromes
Skin loss
• Cystic fibrosis
Potassium depletion
Mineralocorticoid excess
• Primary hyperaldosteronism
• Secondary hyperaldosteronism
• Apparent mineralocorticoid excess
– Liquorice overuse
– Congenital adrenal hyperplasia
– Liddle syndrome
Gain of alkali
Prescribed or over-the-counter alkali— especially with chronic kidney disease
Massive transfusion

has a high chloride concentration, with added potassium may be need. Rarely, intravenous hydrochloric acid (HCl) may be needed.

The more common causes of metabolic alkalosis are listed in Table 15.10.

References

1. Kelly AM. Review article: can venous blood gas analysis replace arterial in emergency medical care. Emerg Med Australas. 2010;22:493–8. https://doi.org/10.1111/j.1742-6723.2010.01344.x.
2. Hamm LL, Nakhoul N, Hering-Smith KS. Acid-base homeostasis. Clin J Am Soc Nephrol. 2015;10:2232–42. https://cjasn.asnjournals.org/content/10/12/2232.long.
3. Berend K. Diagnostic use of base excess in acid-base disorders. N Engl J Med. 2018;378:1419–28. https://doi.org/10.1056/NEJMra1711860.
4. Kraut JA, Madias NE. Serum anion gap: its uses and limitations in clinical medicine. Clin J Am Soc Nephrol. 2007;2(1):162–74. https://doi.org/10.2215/CJN.03020906. https://cjasn.asnjournals.org/content/2/1/162.
5. Batlle D, Ba Aqeel SH, Marquez A. The urine anion gap in context. Clin J Am Soc Nephrol. 2018;13:195–7. https://doi.org/10.2215/CJN.13791217. https://cjasn.asnjournals.org/content/clinjasn/13/2/195.full.pdf.
6. Rastegar M, Nagami GT. Non-anion gap metabolic acidosis: a clinical approach to evaluation. Am J Kidney Dis. 2017;69:296–301. https://www.ajkd.org/article/S0272-6386(16)30515-7/fulltext.
7. Rodriguez SJ. Renal tubular acidosis: the clinical entity. J Am Soc Nephrol. 2002;13:2160–70. https://jasn.asnjournals.org/content/13/8/2160.
8. Soleimani M, Rastegar A. Pathophysiology of renal tubular acidosis: core curriculum 2016. Am J Kidney Dis. 2016;68:488–98. https://www.ajkd.org/article/S0272-6386(16)30039-7/fulltext.

9. Kashoor I, Batlle D. Proximal renal tubular acidosis with and without Fanconi syndrome. Kidney Res Clin Pract. 2019;38:267–81. http://www.krcp-ksn.org/journal/view.html?doi=10.23876/j.krcp.19.056.

10. Batlle D, Arruda J. Hyperkalemic forms of renal tubular acidosis: clinical and pathophysiological aspects. Adv Chronic Kidney Dis. 2018;25:321–33. https://www.ackdjournal.org/article/S1548-5595(18)30100-9/fulltext.

11. Mehta AN, Emmett JB, Emmett M. GOLD MARK: An anion gap mnemonic for the 21st century. Lancet. 2008;372(9642):892. https://doi.org/10.1016/S0140-6736(08)61398-7. https://www.thelancet.com/journals/lancet/article/PIIS0140-6736(08)61398-7/fulltext.

12. Kraut JA, Madias NE. Lactic acidosis. N Engl J Med. 2014;371:2309–19. https://doi.org/10.1056/NEJMra1309483. https://www.nejm.org/doi/full/10.1056/NEJMra1309483.

13. Misra S, Oliver NS. Diabetic ketoacidosis in adults. BMJ. 2015;351:h5660. https://www.bmj.com/content/351/bmj.h5660.long.

14. Nijenhuis T, Renkema KY, Hoenderop JG, Bindels RJ. Acid-base status determines the renal expression of Ca2+ and Mg2+ transport proteins. J Am Soc Nephrol. 2006;17(3):617–26. https://doi.org/10.1681/ASN.2005070732. https://jasn.asnjournals.org/content/17/3/617.long.

15. Hunter RW, Lawson C, Galitsiou E, Gifford F, Neary JJ. Pyroglutamic acidosis in association with therapeutic paracetamol (acetaminophen) use. Clin Med (Lond). 2016;16(6):524–9. https://doi.org/10.7861/clinmedicine.16-6-524. https://www.ncbi.nlm.nih.gov/pmc/articles/PMC6297337/.

16. Amorim JBO, Bailey MA, Musa-Aziz R, Giebisch G, Malnic G. Role of luminal anion and pH in distal tubule potassium secretion. Am J Physiol Renal Physiol. 2003;284:F381–8. https://doi.org/10.1152/ajprenal.00236.2002.

17. Goraya N, Simoni J, Sager LN, Pruszynski J, Wesson DE. Acid retention in chronic kidney disease is inversely related to GFR. Am J Physiol Renal Physiol. 2018;314:F985–91. https://doi.org/10.1152/ajprenal.00463.2017.

18. Abramowitz MK, Hostetter TH, Melamed ML. The plasma anion gap is altered in early kidney disease and associates with mortality. Kidney Int. 2012;82(6):701–9. https://doi.org/10.1038/ki.2012.196. https://www.ncbi.nlm.nih.gov/pmc/articles/PMC3434284/.

19. Moranne O, Froissart M, Rossert J, et al. Timing of onset of CKD-related metabolic complications. J Am Soc Nephrol. 2009;20:164–71. https://jasn.asnjournals.org/content/20/1/164.long.

20. Dobre M, Rahman M, Hostetter TH. Current status of bicarbonate in CKD. J Am Soc Nephrol. 2015;26:515–23. https://doi.org/10.1681/ASN.2014020205. http://jasn.asnjournals.org/content/26/3/515.abstract.

21. Wesson DE, Mathur V, Tangri N, Stasiv Y, Parsell D, Li E, et al. Veverimer versus placebo in patients with metabolic acidosis associated with chronic kidney disease: a multicentre, randomised, double-blind, controlled, phase 3 trial. Lancet. 2019;393(10179):P1417–27. https://www.thelancet.com/journals/lancet/article/PIIS0140-6736(18)32562-5/fulltext?dgcid=raven_jbs_etoc_email.

22. Navaneethan SD, Shao J, Buysse J, Bushinsky DA. Effects of treatment of metabolic acidosis in CKD: a systematic review and meta-analysis. Clin J Am Soc Nephrol. 2019;14(7):1011–20. https://cjasn.asnjournals.org/content/early/2019/06/12/CJN.13091118.abstract.

23. Di Iorio BR, Bellasi A, Raphael KL, Santoro D, Aucella F, Garofano L, Ceccarelli M, Di Lullo L, Capolongo G, Di Iorio M, Guastaferro P, Capasso G, The UBI Study Group. Treatment of metabolic acidosis with sodium bicarbonate delays progression of chronic kidney disease: the UBI Study. J Nephrol. 2019;32(6):989–1001. https://doi.org/10.1007/s40620-019-00656-5. https://link.springer.com/article/10.1007/s40620-019-00656-5.

24. Goraya N, Simoni J, Jo C-H, Wesson DE. Treatment of metabolic acidosis in patients with stage 3 chronic kidney disease with fruits and vegetables or oral bicarbonate reduces urine angiotensinogen and preserves glomerular filtration rate. Kidney Int. 2014;86:1031–8. https://doi.org/10.1038/ki.2014.83. http://www.nature.com/ki/journal/v86/n5/full/ki201483a.html.

25. Dubey AK, Sahoo J, Vairappan B, Haridasan S, Parameswaran S, Priyamvada PS. Correction of metabolic acidosis improves muscle mass and renal function in chronic kidney disease

stages 3 and 4: a randomized controlled trial. Nephrol Dial Transplant. 2020;35(1):121–9. https://doi.org/10.1093/ndt/gfy214.

26. Wesson DE, Mathur V, Tangri N, Stasiv Y, Parsell D, Li E, Klaerner G, Bushinsky DA. Long-term safety and efficacy of veverimer in patients with metabolic acidosis in chronic kidney disease: a multicentre, randomised, blinded, placebo-controlled, 40-week extension. Lancet. 2019;394(10196):P396–406. https://doi.org/10.1016/S0140-6736(19)31388-1. https://www.thelancet.com/journals/lancet/article/PIIS0140-6736(19)31388-1/fulltext.

27. Saldana TM, Basso O, Darden R, Sandler DP. Carbonated beverages and chronic kidney disease. Epidemiology. 2007;18(4):501–6. http://www.ncbi.nlm.nih.gov/pmc/articles/PMC3433753/.

28. Galla JH. Metabolic alkalosis. J Am Soc Nephrol. 2000;11:369–75. https://jasn.asnjournals.org/content/11/2/369.long.

29. Luke RG, Galla JH. It is chloride depletion alkalosis, not contraction alkalosis. J Am Soc Nephrol. 2012;23:204–7. https://jasn.asnjournals.org/content/23/2/204.long.

30. Soifer JT, Kim HT. Approach to metabolic alkalosis. Emerg Med Clin North Am. 2014;32:453–63. https://www.sciencedirect.com/science/article/abs/pii/S0733862714000066?via%3Dihub.

Calcium, Phosphate and Bones: How Bone and Mineral Metabolism is Altered in Kidney Disease

16

As kidney function declines, number of changes occur in the metabolism of bones, minerals and the hormones that affect them [1] (Fig. 16.1).

Minerals and Bones: Interactions Between Magnesium, Phosphate, Calcium, PTH, Vitamin D and FGF-23

Magnesium

Magnesium is predominantly an intracellular cation. Its serum concentration [Mg^{++}] is regulated by changes in excretion by the kidney tubules [2]. It can rise when eGFR falls below 10 mL/min/1.73 m^2 and the remaining tubules are unable to excrete enough magnesium to match dietary intake. This is more likely if the patient is taking laxatives, antacids or phosphate-binding agents that contain magnesium [3].

It can fall with long-term diuretic use. Thiazide diuretics increase magnesium excretion by decreasing its reabsorption in the distal tubule and loop diuretics have a similar effect in the loop of Henle. Magnesium losses from the gut are increased in patients with chronic diarrhoea and malabsorption.

Magnesium normally inhibits the excretion of potassium in the renal tubule. When serum [Mg^{++}] is low, potassium excretion is increased leading to hypokalaemia. Low intracellular magnesium inhibits the release of parathyroid hormone, which in turn causes hypocalcaemia. To correct these abnormalities, sufficient magnesium needs to be given to restore intracellular and serum magnesium, as well as giving potassium and calcium (Patient 16.1).

© Springer Nature Switzerland AG 2020
H. C. Rayner et al., *Understanding Kidney Diseases*,
https://doi.org/10.1007/978-3-030-43027-6_16

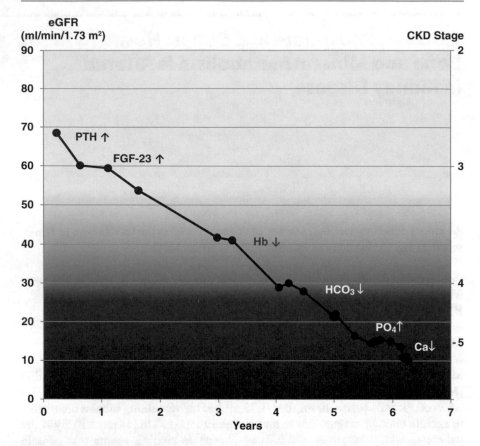

Fig. 16.1 Metabolic abnormalities that occur at different stages of chronic kidney disease. Arrows indicate whether the abnormality is an increase or decrease in the level in blood. Arrows are placed at the typical eGFR below which the level starts to change

Patient 16.1 Replace Magnesium to Correct Calcium

Mr. Jones, aged 79 years, had had lengths of bowel removed 50 and 20 years previously because of Crohn's disease. He also suffered from congestive cardiac failure. He presented to hospital on 18th April with low blood pressure and acute kidney injury (Fig. 16.2).

Serum [Ca++] was 1.36 mmol/L (5.4 mg/dL). Despite giving intravenous calcium gluconate, 4 days later the serum [Ca++] had fallen to 1.33 mmol/L (5.3 g/dL). The serum [Mg++] had also fallen from 0.6 to 0.4 mmol/L (1.4 to 0.96 mg/dL).

Intravenous magnesium sulfate was added to the calcium gluconate replacement; the blood pressure rose and serum [Ca++] steadily increased. His eGFR improved and he was discharged from hospital on 6th May taking oral calcium and magnesium supplements.

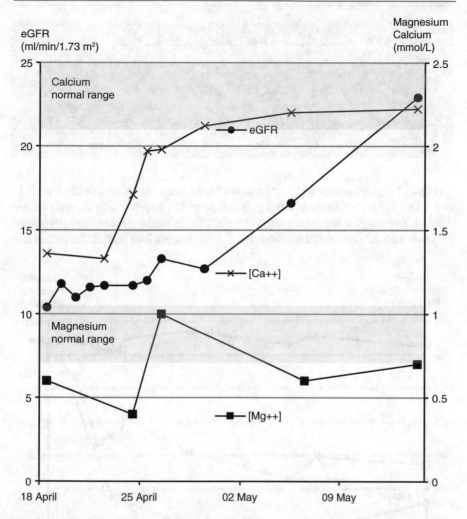

Fig. 16.2 Trends in eGFR and serum calcium and magnesium concentrations. Calcium is corrected for serum albumin. To convert units: [Ca++] 2.5 mmol/L = 10.0 mg/dL; [Mg++] 1 mmol/L = 2.4 mg/dL. [Mg++] normal range = 0.65–1.05 mmol/L

Phosphate

Serum phosphate is derived mainly from the breakdown of phosphorylated proteins. As GFR declines, the ability to excrete phosphate decreases. Excretion eventually fails to balance production and serum phosphate concentration $[(PO_4)^{3-}]$ increases. 30% of patients with a GFR less than 20 mL/min/1.73 m² have a raised serum phosphate (Patient 16.2).

Patient 16.2 Progressive Abnormalities of Mineral Metabolism in Kidney Disease

Mr. Jordan, a fit 65-year-old white man, had IgA nephropathy. His eGFR declined by more than 15 mL/min/1.73 m² per year. Initially the serum parathyroid hormone (PTH) increased, followed by a rise in serum phosphate and fall in serum calcium (Fig. 16.3). He did not take any calcium or vitamin D supplements during this time.

High phosphate levels are associated with cardiovascular adverse events and all-cause mortality, both in the general population and in patients with chronic kidney disease. Even higher levels that are still within the laboratory reference range show these associations. Potential mechanisms for the associations include abnormalities

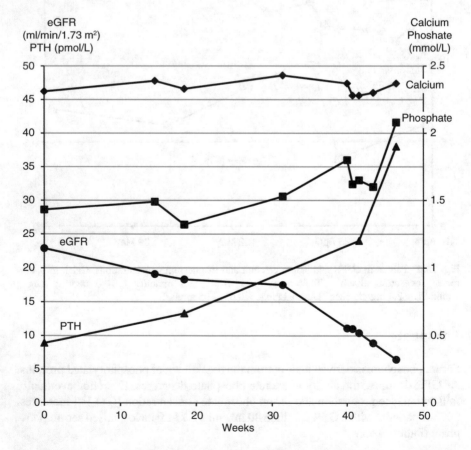

Fig. 16.3 Trends in serum parathyroid hormone (PTH), phosphate and calcium concentrations as GFR declines. To convert units: PTH 50 pmol/L = 470 pg/mL; phosphate 2 mmol/L = phosphorus 6.2 mg/dL; calcium 2.5 mmol/L = 10.0 mg/dL

of the function of arteries, such as calcification and stiffness, and of small blood vessels, such as capillary dilatation measured in the skin and retina [4].

Calcium, Parathyroid Hormone, Vitamin D and FGF-23

Figure 16.3 shows how parathyroid hormone (PTH) increases as GFR decreases. The main function of PTH is to regulate the serum calcium concentration. A fall in serum calcium is detected by the calcium-sensing receptors on the chief cells of the parathyroid glands, triggering an increase in PTH production and secretion. PTH stimulates calcium absorption from the gut and release from bone. The basic elements of the feedback control of serum calcium and phosphate are shown in Fig. 16.4.

PTH concentration increases in response to a fall in serum calcium. But Mr Jordan's calcium did not decrease, so why was the PTH high? PTH production by the parathyroid glands is suppressed by calcium and activated vitamin D (Fig. 16.4); the main cause of the increase in PTH is a decrease in vitamin D activity.

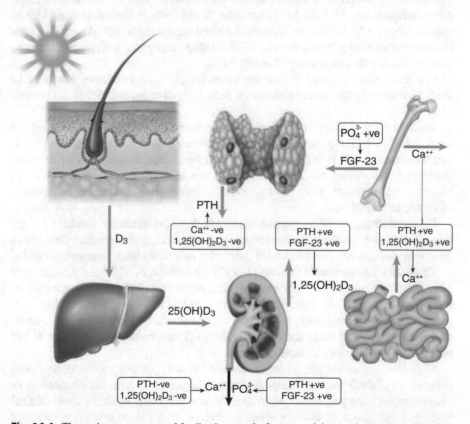

Fig. 16.4 The main components of feedback control of serum calcium and phosphate. The grey arrows indicate release of substances into the circulation. The wide black arrow indicates excretion into the urine. Feedback is shown in boxes, either negative (suppression) or positive (stimulation). D_3 = vitamin D_3. $1,25(OH)_2D_3$ = calcitriol

Vitamin D

Vitamin D_3 (cholecalciferol) is synthesized in the deeper layers of the skin and absorbed from the gut. In the liver it is converted to the storage form of vitamin D_3, 25(OH)-vitamin D_3. This is activated by 1-hydroxylation to $1,25(OH)_2$-vitamin D_3 (calcitriol) in many tissues, but mainly in the kidneys.

Chronic kidney disease leads to reduced calcitriol production through a number of mechanisms [5]. Firstly, patients often lack sufficient 25(OH)-vitamin D_3 from diet and sun exposure, especially in dark skinned races. Secondly, reduced GFR and damage to tubular cells limits the capacity for 25(OH)-vitamin D_3 to be hydroxylated in the kidney cortex.

Thirdly, high serum phosphate levels stimulate the release of factors that increase urinary phosphate excretion, called phosphatonins. These include fibroblast growth factor-23 (FGF-23), which is produced by bone osteoblasts. FGF-23 is filtered by glomeruli and bound to α-Klotho in proximal tubules, where it suppresses phosphate reabsorption. FGF-23 levels increase in the early stages of chronic kidney disease (Fig. 16.1), leading to increased phosphate excretion so that serum phosphate concentration remains normal. FGF-23 also suppresses 1-alpha-hydroxylase activity, leading to a deficiency of calcitriol.

Children with X-linked hypophosphataemia produce excessive amounts of FGF-23 leading to low serum phosphate, deficiency of calcitriol, rickets and osteomalacia [6].

Because PTH production is normally suppressed by vitamin D_3, low levels of calcitriol allow PTH production to increase, so called secondary hyperparathyroidism. The increased PTH in turn stimulates 1-alpha-hydroxylase activity in the proximal tubules, boosting calcitriol production and increasing osteoclast activity in bone to release calcium. Both these actions mitigate against a fall in serum calcium, as shown in Patient 16.2.

Calcitriol increases the absorption of calcium from the intestines and from kidney tubules. It is also required for the coupling of osteoblast and osteoclast function in bone remodelling. Persistent calcitriol deficiency eventually leads to hypocalcaemia.

The interactions between vitamin D_3, PTH, phosphate, FGF-23 and other factors are complicated, and the major changes that occur in kidney disease are incompletely understood [7, 8]. Interventions to manipulate individual parts of this complex system do not have easily predictable effects. Studies often use the blood levels of different factors to study the effects of drugs. These surrogate outcomes do not necessarily translate into clinical outcomes.

High levels of serum phosphate are associated with adverse outcomes and most patients on dialysis take a phosphate-binding agent to reduce the absorption of phosphate from the gut. However, to date there is no strong evidence from clinical trials that this treatment is more effective than placebo [9], or that using different types of phosphate-binders leads to different outcomes [10].

Drugs that mimic the effect of calcium by binding to the calcium-sensing receptor can be used to suppress PTH levels. PTH concentration is used as a surrogate outcome to measure the effectiveness of treatment. However, the benefits in terms of clinical outcomes relating to cardiovascular and bone disease, which is what matters to patients, are not clear [11].

Observational studies in the general population show associations between low serum levels of vitamin D and adverse outcomes. To date, trials in patients without clinical features of vitamin D deficiency have not shown any benefit from vitamin D supplementation [12].

Why Is Vitamin D Activated in the Kidneys?

It may seem odd that the kidneys are the main site of activation of vitamin D in the body. The reason for this is explained by the selective pressure of evolution.

Free vitamin D is a steroid molecule and so can diffuse freely across cell membranes. To avoid it being lost from the circulation and to control its uptake into cells, it is almost all bound to a plasma protein called Vitamin D-Binding Protein (DBP). DBP is small (58 kDa, compared to albumin 66.5 kDa) and is filtered by the glomerulus in significant amounts.

If filtered vitamins were lost into the urine, severe vitamin D deficiency, hypocalcaemia and bone disease would develop. This can be produced experimentally in genetically modified mice and occurs naturally in some types of Fanconi syndrome [13].

To avoid this loss, filtered 25(OH)-vitamin D_3 bound to DBP is taken up by proximal tubular cells. Once inside the mitochondria of these cells, the 25(OH)-vitamin D_3 is hydroxylated to the active form, calcitriol, which is then bound to DBP and released into the circulation. By combining the conservation and activation of vitamin D into one uptake process in the kidneys, survival is ensured using the minimum amount of metabolic energy.

Hyperparathyroidism

Progressive enlargement of the parathyroid glands tends to occur in patients with long-standing chronic kidney disease. Vitamin D supplements and dietary phosphate binders are used to suppress PTH and slow the enlargement. Persistently high PTH levels increase bone turnover; the volume of unmineralised bone is increased and osteoclasts and osteoblasts multiply—so called renal osteodystrophy. Features of renal osteodystrophy can be seen on X-rays of the hands (Fig. 16.5).

The bone structure is weakened and fractures easily (Patient 16.3).

Patient 16.3 Severe Hyperparathyroidism
Mrs Bibi had advanced chronic kidney disease due to kidney stones for over 25 years. For the last 10 years she had been treated with haemodialysis. The serum alkaline phosphatase had progressively risen to over 1000 IU/L

(normal range 30–130) and parathyroid hormone to 452 pmol/L (normal range 1.6–6.9) (= 4262 pg/mL). She had declined parathyroid surgery.

She was admitted with severe pain in the legs. A plain X-ray was taken (Fig. 16.6). Soon afterwards, she suffered a pathological fracture of the femur.

A year later, she was admitted with difficulty speaking and swallowing. A CT scan of the skull showed thickening and abnormal texture of the bones, particularly affecting the jaw and facial bones. At the base of the skull, at the right antero-lateral aspect of the foreman magnum, there was a 2.1 × 3.7 cm brown tumour. This is composed of fibrous tissue and unmineralised woven bone, and is coloured brown by haemosiderin deposition. It had caused pressure on the spinal cord and lower cranial nerves (Fig. 16.7).

High PTH levels combined with persistent hyperphosphataemia in CKD stages 4 and 5 leads to the deposition of calcium and phosphate in blood vessels and other tissues. This contributes to the increased risk of cardiovascular disease.

Parathyroidectomy

Prolonged stimulation of the parathyroid glands can lead to one or more parathyroid hormone-producing cells becoming unresponsive to the suppressive effect of serum calcium. One cell in each gland may multiply to form an adenoma made up of

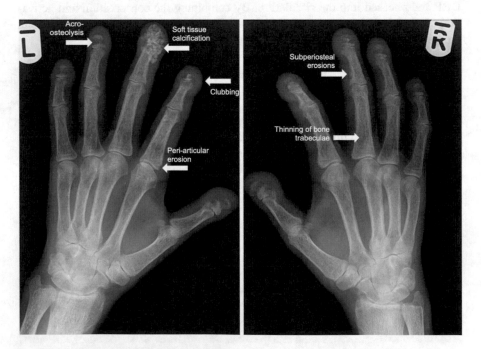

Fig. 16.5 Changes in the hands caused by tertiary hyperparathyroidism

Fig. 16.6 Plain X-ray showing severe renal osteodystrophy affecting the femur, tibia and fibula. The bone texture is very abnormal with loss of mineral density, destruction of the normal trabeculae and subperiosteal erosions. There is calcification in the femoral artery (*arrow*)

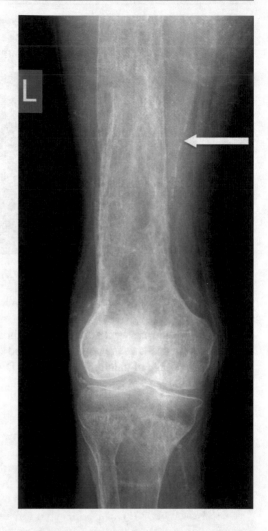

clones of cells. These adenomata are autonomous, i.e. they secrete large amounts of PTH despite the serum calcium being normal. Eventually the very high PTH levels cause the serum calcium to increase—so called tertiary hyperparathyroidism (Patients 16.3 and 16.4).

Whereas drugs that lower PTH do not provide clear clinical benefits in patients on dialysis [10], parathyroidectomy—the surgical removal of all the enlarged glands—is associated with a 20–43% reduction in mortality in patients with severe hyperparathyroidism [14–16].

After parathyroidectomy, there is a sudden drop in PTH and osteoclast activity. Bone mineral resorption and release of calcium stops but bone formation continues. Large quantities of calcium re-enter the skeleton from the blood—the 'hungry bone' syndrome. Rapid and severe hypocalcaemia can occur, the severity being proportional to the pre-operative alkaline phosphatase, which reflects the 'appetite' of the bones.

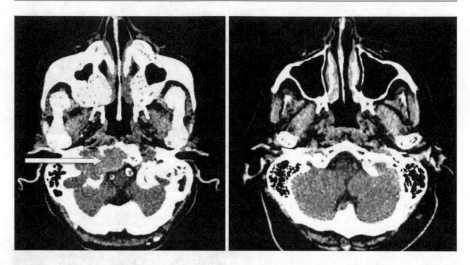

Fig. 16.7 CT scan of the base of the skull showing (*left*) massive hypertrophy of the facial bones and a tumour at the foramen magnum compressing the brain stem (*arrow*). There is also calcification in the vertebral and scalp arteries. A normal scan is shown for comparison (*right*)

Over the following weeks the alkaline phosphatase rises as osteoblast activity increases; it then falls as the bones are satiated with calcium. This trend can be used to guide the dosage of calcium and vitamin D supplements to keep the serum calcium within the normal range (Patient 16.4).

Patient 16.4 The Effects of Parathyroidectomy on Calcium Metabolism

Sally had been on dialysis for 10 years. Despite treatment with the calcimimetic drug cinacalcet, her hyperparathyroidism had progressed to a tertiary stage, i.e. hypercalcaemia with a high PTH. She had aching pains in her hips, knees and feet.

In November 2011, what appeared to be four enlarged parathyroid glands were surgically removed. However, histological examination showed one to be lymphoid tissue. Her serum calcium and PTH remained elevated.

A nuclear medicine parathyroid subtraction scan was performed. In this procedure, a radioisotope, technetium 99m pertechnetate, is injected and taken up by the thyroid gland. This is followed by an injection of technetium 99m sestamibi that is taken up by both thyroid and parathyroid glands (Fig. 16.8).

Subtracting one scan from the other reveals the parathyroid gland (Fig. 16.9).

In August 2012, a further operation was performed to remove the fourth gland. The effect on her blood results is shown in Fig. 16.10.

Removal of the remaining overactive gland led to an abrupt drop in serum PTH, calcium and phosphate. The alkaline phosphatase initially rose and then exponentially declined as bone turnover returned to a normal rate.

In September, 6 weeks after the operation, when alkaline phosphatase approached the normal range (30–130 IU/L), the dose of elemental calcium and then of 1α(OH)-vitamin D$_3$ (alfacalcidol) was reduced to avoid hypercalcaemia. Subsequent adjustments in the dose of alfacalcidol were too large, causing swings in serum calcium outside the normal range.

A stable equilibrium was reached 6 months after the operation. Sally's bone pains resolved and she felt generally much better.

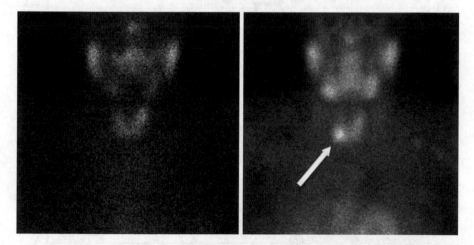

Fig. 16.8 Technetium 99m (99mTc) pertechnetate scan (left) showing the thyroid gland and laryngeal bones. Technetium 99m sestamibi (MIBI) scan (right) shows a hot spot at the lower pole of the right lobe of thyroid (arrow)

Fig. 16.9 99mTc + MIBI subtraction scan showing a hot spot (arrow) consistent with a right lower pole parathyroid adenoma

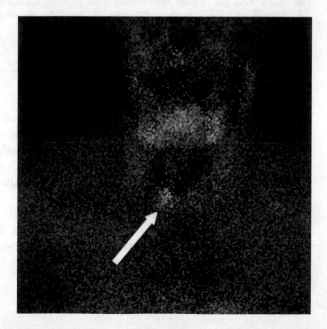

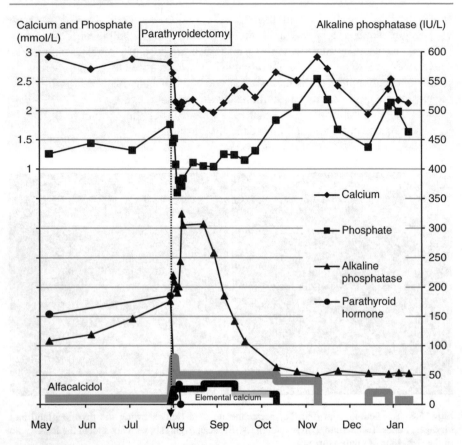

Fig. 16.10 Changes in bone biochemistry after parathyroidectomy. To convert units: calcium 2.5 mmol/L = 10.0 mg/dL; phosphate 2 mmol/L = phosphorus 6.2 mg/dL; PTH 300 pmol/L = 2800 pg/mL

Hypercalcaemia

It takes years for hypercalcaemia to develop as a result of kidney failure, as in Sally's case (Patient 16.4). If serum calcium is raised when kidney disease is first discovered, the hypercalcaemia is likely to be due to another disease.

High serum calcium, particularly over 3 mmol/L (12 mg/dL), reduces GFR by causing vasoconstriction within the kidney [17]. It can also reduce the ability of the tubules to concentrate urine and so cause dehydration.

The first thing to check is the medication list. Hypercalcaemia may be caused by excessive calcium and vitamin D treatment. Thiazide diuretics reduce calcium excretion by the distal tubule and can cause mild hypercalaemia.

Diseases which cause hypercalcaemia can also reduce GFR in other ways. These are listed in Table 16.1.

Table 16.1 Causes of hypercalcaemia that also affect kidney function

	Cause of hypercalcaemia	Cause of reduced GFR other than hypercalcaemia
Malignancy (Patient 16.5)	Calcium released from bone by osteolytic deposits and/or PTH-related peptide	Urinary tract obstruction
Primary hyperparathyroidism	PTH-producing adenoma not suppressed by serum calcium	Kidney stones Nephrocalcinosis
Multiple myeloma	Calcium released from bone by osteolytic deposits	Casts of paraprotein blocking tubules
Sarcoidosis (Patient 16.6)	1,25(OH)$_2$-vitamin D$_3$ produced by granulomas	Granulomas infiltrating the kidney interstitium

Patient 16.5 Hypercalcaemia Due to Malignancy Causing Acute Kidney Injury

Mrs Reynolds, aged 60 years, was admitted to hospital with pain in the left hip. She had had a squamous cell carcinoma of the mouth treated with chemo-radiotherapy a year previously. Three months before admission, serum urea and electrolytes were normal.

Laboratory results on admission showed acute kidney injury and severe hypercalcaemia (Table 16.2)

A urinary tract ultrasound scan was normal.

Plain X-ray of the left femur and pelvis showed a lytic lesion in the inferior pubic ramus (Fig. 16.11), confirmed by CT scan (Fig. 16.12). Biopsy showed it to be a secondary deposit.

Patient 16.6 Hypercalcaemia Due to Sarcoidosis Causing Acute Kidney Injury

Ian, a 38-year-old businessman, first presented to his GP having felt generally tried and unwell for a few weeks. He was noted to have red eyes and swollen lymph nodes. It was thought he most likely had a viral infection but his kidney function was reduced, eGFR = 30 mL/min/1.73 m². This improved to 60 mL/min/1.73 m² over the subsequent 10 weeks and he felt much better. He was referred to the haematology clinic for assessment of the lymphadenopathy.

The serum calcium level was elevated, 2.71 mmol/L (10.8 mg/dL). An ultrasound scan showed normal-sized kidneys but very prominent pyramids (Fig. 16.13).

A CT scan of the thorax and abdomen revealed widespread bulky lymph-adenopathy in the neck, chest and upper abdomen, particularly the anterior mediastinum (Fig. 16.14).

Sarcoidosis was considered likely but lymphoma needed to be excluded, so a lymph node biopsy was performed. Histology showed tightly packed small granulomas composed of epithelioid histiocytes with no necrosis. The residual lymphoid tissue consisted of lymphocytes and mature plasma cells with no atypical cells. These features are consistent with sarcoidosis (Fig. 16.15).

The serum angiotensin-converting enzyme (ACE) was markedly raised at 226 IU/L (normal range 20–70). ACE is produced by granulomas and a raised level combined with other clinical features supports a diagnosis of sarcoidosis.

Ian was feeling completely well. However, serial eGFR measurements showed that his kidney function was worsening again. He was therefore started on 10 mg of prednisolone per day. Over the subsequent months, his serum ACE steadily declined to normal, the size of the lymph nodes in his chest reduced slightly on a repeat CT scan, and serum calcium and kidney function returned to normal (Fig. 16.16).

Table 16.2 Results of blood tests taken on admission to hospital

		Normal range	Non-SI units
Sodium	139 mmol/L	133–146	139 mEq/L
Potassium	3.5 mmol/L	3.5–5.3	3.5 mEq/L
Urea	31.2 mmol/L	2.5–7.8	BUN 87 mg/dL
Creatinine	475 µmol/L	64–111	5.4 mg/dL
eGFR	8 mL/min/1.73 m^2		
Albumin	29 g/L	35–50	2.9 g/dL
Calcium (corrected for serum albumin)	4.12 mmol/L	2.20–2.60	16.5 mg/dL
Phosphate	2.00 mmol/L	0.80–1.50	Phosphorus 6.2 mg/dL
Alkaline phosphatase	71 IU/L	30–130	

Fig. 16.11 Plain X-ray of the left femur and pelvis showing a lytic lesion in the inferior pubic ramus

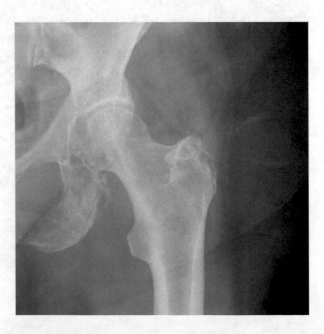

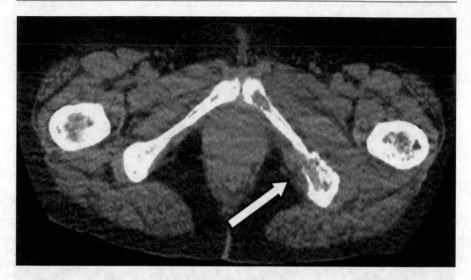

Fig. 16.12 CT scan showing a soft-tissue swelling beside the lesion, consistent with a metastatic deposit (arrow)

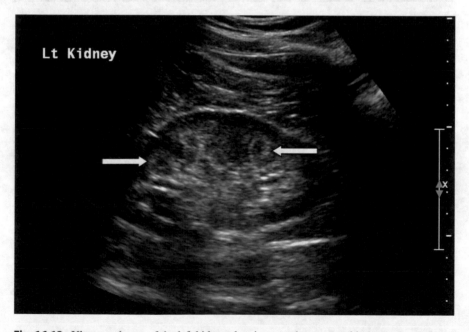

Fig. 16.13 Ultrasound scan of the left kidney showing prominent pyramids (arrows), consistent with infiltration or possible papillary necrosis

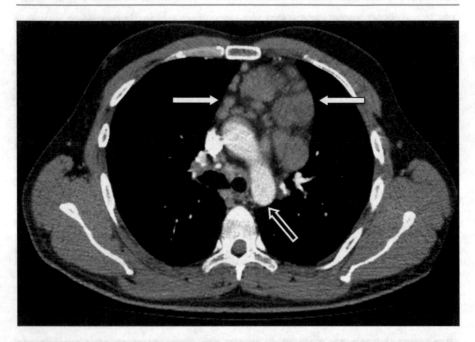

Fig. 16.14 Contrast CT scan section at the level of the aortic arch (enhanced with contrast, black arrow) showing massively enlarged lymph nodes in the anterior mediastinum (white arrows)

Fig. 16.15 Light micrograph of the excised lymph node showing compact coalescing granulomas with intervening lymphoid tissue. Haematoxylin and eosin ×200

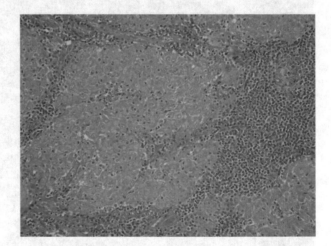

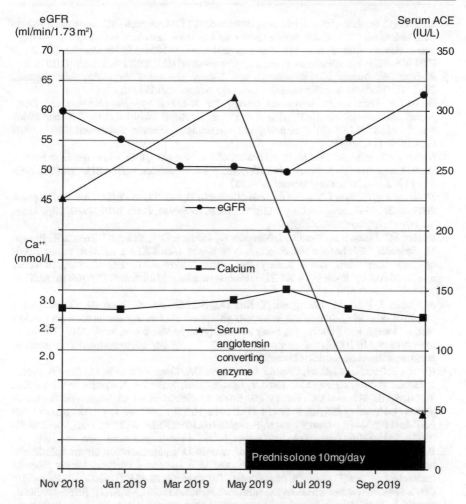

Fig. 16.16 Changes in eGFR, serum calcium and serum ACE with steroid therapy in sarcoidosis. To convert units: calcium 2.5 mmol/L = 10.0 mg/dL

References

1. Moranne O, Froissart M, Rossert J, et al. Timing of onset of CKD-related metabolic complications. J Am Soc Nephrol. 2009;20:164–71. https://jasn.asnjournals.org/content/20/1/164.long.
2. Swaminathan R. Magnesium metabolism and its disorders. Clin Biochem Rev. 2003;24(2):47–66. https://www.ncbi.nlm.nih.gov/pmc/articles/PMC1855626/.
3. Cunningham J, Rodríguez M, Messa P. Magnesium in chronic kidney disease stages 3 and 4 and in dialysis patients. Clin Kidney J. 2012;5(Suppl 1):i39–51. https://doi.org/10.1093/ndtplus/sfr166.2. https://www.ncbi.nlm.nih.gov/pmc/articles/PMC4455820.

4. Ginsberg C, Houben AJHM, Malhotra R, Berendschot TTJM, Dagnelie PC, Kooman JP, Webers CA, Stehouwer CDA, Ix JH. Serum phosphate and microvascular function in a population-based cohort. Clin J Am Soc Nephrol. 2019;14(11):1626–33. https://doi.org/10.2215/CJN.02610319. https://cjasn.asnjournals.org/content/early/2019/09/19/CJN.02610319.full.

5. Al-Badr W, Martin KJ. Vitamin D and kidney disease. Clin J Am Soc Nephrol. 2008;3(5):1555–60. http://cjasn.asnjournals.org/content/3/5/1555.full.

6. Perwad F, Portale AA. Burosumab therapy for X-linked hypophosphatemia and therapeutic implications for CKD. Clin J Am Soc Nephrol. 2019;14(7):1097–9. https://doi.org/10.2215/CJN.15201218. https://cjasn.asnjournals.org/content/clinjasn/early/2019/06/05/CJN.15201218.full.pdf.

7. Blaine J, Chonchol M, Levi M. Renal control of calcium, phosphate, and magnesium homeostasis. Clin J Am Soc Nephrol. 2015;10(7):1257–72. https://doi.org/10.2215/CJN.09750913. http://cjasn.asnjournals.org/content/10/7/1257.full.

8. Naveh-Many T, Silver J. The Pas de Trois of vitamin D, FGF23, and PTH. J Am Soc Nephrol. 2017;28(2):393–5. https://doi.org/10.1681/ASN.2016090944. Epub 2016 Nov 2. https://jasn.asnjournals.org/content/28/2/393.long.

9. Palmer SC, Gardner S, Tonelli M, Mavridis D, Johnson DW, Craig JC, French R, Ruospo M, Strippoli GF. Phosphate-binding agents in adults with CKD: a network meta-analysis of randomized trials. Am J Kidney Dis. 2016;68(5):691–702. https://doi.org/10.1053/j.ajkd.2016.05.015. Epub 2016 Jul 22. https://www.ajkd.org/article/S0272-6386(16)30253-0/fulltext.

10. Spoendlin J, Paik JM, Tsacogianis T, Kim SC, Schneeweiss S, Desai RJ. Cardiovascular outcomes of calcium-free vs calcium-based phosphate binders in patients 65 years or older with end-stage renal disease requiring hemodialysis. JAMA Intern Med. 2019;179:741–9. https://doi.org/10.1001/jamainternmed.2019.0045. https://jamanetwork.com/journals/jamainternalmedicine/article-abstract/2732117.

11. EVOLVE Trial Investigators, Chertow GM, Block GA, Correa-Rotter R, Drüeke TB, Floege J, Goodman WG, Herzog CA, Kubo Y, London GM, Mahaffey KW, Mix TC, Moe SM, Trotman ML, Wheeler DC, Parfrey PS. Effect of cinacalcet on cardiovascular disease in patients undergoing dialysis. N Engl J Med. 2012;367(26):2482–94. https://doi.org/10.1056/NEJMoa1205624. https://www.nejm.org/doi/10.1056/NEJMoa1205624?url_ver=Z39.88-2003&rfr_id=ori:rid:crossref.org&rfr_dat=cr_pub%3dwww.ncbi.nlm.nih.gov.

12. Bolland MJ, Grey A, Avenell A. Effects of vitamin D supplementation on musculoskeletal health: a systematic review, meta-analysis, and trial sequential analysis. Lancet Diabetes Endocrinol. 2018;6(11):847–58. https://doi.org/10.1016/S2213-8587(18)30265-1. Epub 2018 Oct 4. https://www.thelancet.com/journals/landia/article/PIIS2213-8587(18)30265-1/fulltext.

13. Negri AL. Proximal tubule endocytic apparatus as the specific renal uptake mechanism for vitamin D-binding protein/25-(OH)D3 complex. Nephrology. 2006;11:510–5. http://onlinelibrary.wiley.com/enhanced/doi/10.1111/j.1440-1797.2006.00704.x/.

14. Goldenstein PT, Elias RM, do Carmo LPDF, Coelho FO, Magalhaes LP, et al. Parathyroidectomy improves survival in patients with severe hyperparathyroidism: a comparative study. PLoS One. 2013;8(8):e68870. https://doi.org/10.1371/journal.pone.0068870. http://journals.plos.org/plosone/article?id=10.1371/journal.pone.0068870.

15. Komaba H, Taniguchi M, Wada A, Iseki K, Tsubakihara Y, Fukagawa M. Parathyroidectomy and survival among Japanese hemodialysis patients with secondary hyperparathyroidism. Kidney Int. 2015;88(2):350–9. https://doi.org/10.1038/ki.2015.72. Epub 2015 Mar 18. http://www.nature.com/ki/journal/v88/n2/full/ki201572a.html.

16. Ivarsson KM, Akaberi S, Isaksson E, Reihnér E, Rylance R, Prütz KG, Clyne N, Almquist M. The effect of parathyroidectomy on patient survival in secondary hyperparathyroidism. Nephrol Dial Transplant. 2015;30(12):2027–33. https://doi.org/10.1093/ndt/gfv334. Epub 2015 Sep 15. https://www.ncbi.nlm.nih.gov/pmc/articles/PMC4832998/.

17. Levi M, Ellis MA, Berl T. Control of renal hemodynamics and glomerular filtration rate in chronic hypercalcemia. Role of prostaglandins, renin-angiotensin system, and calcium. J Clin Invest. 1983;71(6):1624. http://dm5migu4zj3pb.cloudfront.net/manuscripts/110000/110918/JCI83110918.pdf.

Immunology: Serological Tests That Help Diagnose Kidney Diseases

Do the Right Test on the Right Patient

The kidney is vulnerable to damage by the immune system [1]. The high blood flow rate through glomeruli exposes them to immunologically active cells. Antibodies and lymphocytes can attack vascular endothelial cells. Antigen-antibody complexes and complement molecules are trapped within the filtration barrier, and taken into mesangial cells and podocytes by endocytosis. Antibodies can be generated against antigens expressed in the glomerular basement membrane or on podocytes. Cell injury, inflammation and repair responses cause a wide range of kidney diseases [2] and many glomerular diseases are treated with immunosuppressive drugs [3].

Immunological tests on serum can help distinguish between different conditions with similar clinical presentations. It is tempting to tick a number of boxes on the blood test request form to check for immune-mediated disease—a kidney disease 'immunology screen'. However, this may not be a wise move.

There is a danger of a false positive result with any screening test. The likelihood that a positive result will be 'false' is dependent upon the pre-test probability—the prior odds that the patient actually has the disease in question.

For example, the chances of an anti-nuclear antibody (ANA) test being positive in a healthy older person can be as high as one in five. The chance that an older person with slowly progressive chronic kidney disease with minimal proteinuria has systemic lupus erythematosus (SLE) is perhaps one in a thousand. So, if 1000 such patients with chronic kidney disease are screened, for every one true positive there will be 200 false positives. In other words, the test has a 0.5% chance of being correct.

Serum IgA levels are elevated in a high proportion of patients with IgA nephropathy. A raised level can be useful supportive evidence in a patient with other typical features of IgA nephropathy. However, serum IgA is elevated in many other conditions including chronic infection and so is not useful for making a diagnosis on its own [4].

© Springer Nature Switzerland AG 2020
H. C. Rayner et al., *Understanding Kidney Diseases*,
https://doi.org/10.1007/978-3-030-43027-6_17

The risk of ignoring these laws of probability is that you will be led along a path of ever-more invasive tests to exclude a serious cause for the abnormal result. For example, immunoglobulins and a protein electrophoresis are often assayed in patients with chronic kidney disease to 'exclude' multiple myeloma. In older people it is not uncommon to find a small amount of monoclonal paraprotein. This raises the possibilities that the paraprotein is the cause of the kidney disease, a monoclonal gammopathy of renal significance (MGRS), and that the patient would benefit from chemotherapy [5]. More commonly, the paraprotein is unrelated to the kidney disease and is a monoclonal gammopathy of uncertain significance (MGUS). You may be left with the dilemma of whether to exclude monoclonal protein-related kidney disease by performing a kidney biopsy.

The following sections describe the most commonly used immunological tests along with the clinical features that indicate when they are likely to be useful for making a diagnosis.

Immunoglobulins, Protein Electrophoresis, Free Light Chains in Serum and Urine

Clinical features:
1. Multiple myeloma with myeloma kidney
   - Anaemia
   - Declining GFR
   - Minimal proteinuria on dipstick testing but raised urine protein:creatinine ratio
   - Bone pain with normal alkaline phosphatase
   - Hypercalcaemia
2. Amyloidosis
   - Nephrotic-range proteinuria or nephrotic syndrome
   - Hypotension
   - Heart failure
   - Bruising

Paraproteins are immunoglobulins produced by a proliferating clone of B lymphocytes or plasma cells. They can be deposited within glomeruli and cause a range of diseases, such as monoclonal Ig deposition disease (MIDD), proliferative glomerulonephritis with monoclonal Ig deposits (PGNMID), and C3 glomerulopathy. The deposits are organised in characteristic structures in amyloidosis, immunotactoid glomerulopathy, fibrillary glomerulonephritis, and cryoglobulinaemic glomerulonephritis [6]. Treatment of these conditions involves using drugs that act on the clone producing the monoclonal protein, such as the proteasome inhibitor bortezomib [7].

Free light chains are smaller than albumin and freely filtered by glomeruli. Their serum concentration is therefore dependent upon GFR and patients with reduced GFR have increased serum levels of polyclonal free light chains. The levels are further increased by inflammation and are associated with an increased risk of progression of chronic kidney disease and of mortality [8].

The ratio of kappa to lambda light chain concentrations is used to identify a monoclonal excess of one type of chain. An abnormal ratio is not proof of clonality; further tests are needed to prove a monoclonal plasma cell disorder.

Monoclonal free light chains in the urine (Bence Jones protein) are not detected by dipstick testing but the laboratory urine protein assay does detect them. A specific assay for free light chains is the most sensitive test to use [9].

Multiple Myeloma

The kidneys can be damaged in patients with myeloma through a range of mechanisms. Hypercalcaemia has a direct effect on GFR through vasoconstriction. Filtered free light chains are reabsorbed by proximal tubular cells and can cause cell injury. If light chains are in large amounts, they may combine with uromodulin to form casts that obstruct the tubules (Fig. 17.1).

With treatment to reduce the amount of monoclonal protein in the serum, the casts can clear and kidney function can improve (Patient 17.1).

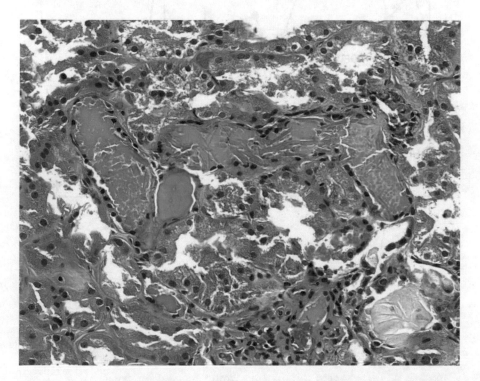

Fig. 17.1 Light micrograph of a section of a kidney biopsy from a patient with multiple myeloma showing occlusion of distal tubules by casts formed of uromodulin and monoclonal light chains. The casts are fractured and surrounded by epithelial cells. Haematoxylin and eosin ×200

Patient 17.1 Myeloma Kidney

Mrs Drake suffered repeated relapses of her myeloma over the course of 4 years, shown by rises in the concentration of monoclonal protein (Fig. 17.2).

During the first relapse in 2008 her kidney function was not affected.

During the second and third relapses in 2009 and 2010 her eGFR declined as the paraprotein level rose. Both times, further treatment led to a decline in paraprotein and recovery in eGFR.

Sadly her disease continued to progress and became unresponsive to treatment after 2010. She died in 2011.

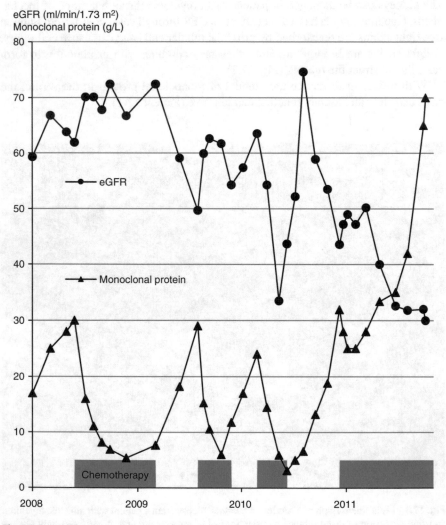

Fig. 17.2 eGFR mirrors the rises and falls in the concentration of monoclonal protein in a patient with multiple myeloma

Amyloidosis

Systemic amyloidosis refers to a group of conditions in which a small subunit of a plasma protein undergoes polymerisation and is deposited in the tissues as a fibril with a beta-pleated sheet configuration.

Examples of the proteins that can form amyloid deposits are:

- Immunoglobulin light chain (25 kDa)—AL amyloidosis in plasma cell dyscrasia
- Serum amyloid A (12 kDa)—AA amyloidosis in chronic inflammation
- Beta-2 microglobulin (12 kDa)—Dialysis amyloidosis

The kidneys can be affected by deposition of amyloid protein in vessel walls and glomerular membranes (Figs. 17.3 and 17.4). This disrupts the filtration barrier, allowing proteinuria that is often heavy enough to cause the nephrotic syndrome.

Amyloid protein may also affect systemic arteriolar walls and the autonomic nerve fibres that mediate vasoconstriction. This causes postural hypotension and can reduce kidney blood flow.

Treatment of immunoglobulin light chain AL amyloidosis uses chemotherapy to suppress the production of the light chains. The quicker and more completely they are suppressed, the better the prognosis [10].

Anti-nuclear Antibody, Anti-dsDNA Antibody

Clinical features:
Systemic lupus erythematosus (SLE) nephritis

Nephritic syndrome:
- Proteinuria ++ or greater
- Microscopic ++ or greater
- Macroscopic haematuria with turbid urine due to casts
- Worsening GFR over weeks or months

About half of people with SLE have kidney involvement, this proportion being higher in men and in black races. The pattern of kidney disease is very variable, ranging from asymptomatic urine abnormalities to acute nephritis and nephrotic syndrome. A biopsy is required to characterise the type of kidney disease. Histological appearances are grouped into six classes, each associated with different clinical features and requiring different treatment [12].

Class 1
- Histology: Normal light microscopy; mesangial immune complexes by immuno-fluorescence microscopy.
- Clinical features: None related to the kidney.

Fig. 17.3 Light micrographs of a section of a kidney biopsy from a patient with amyloidosis stained with Congo red. (**a**) amyloid, coloured red, is deposited throughout the glomerulus and in the wall of an arteriole (*top left*). (**b**) anomalous colours are displayed when the specimen is examined between a crossed polarizer and analyser [11]. ×200

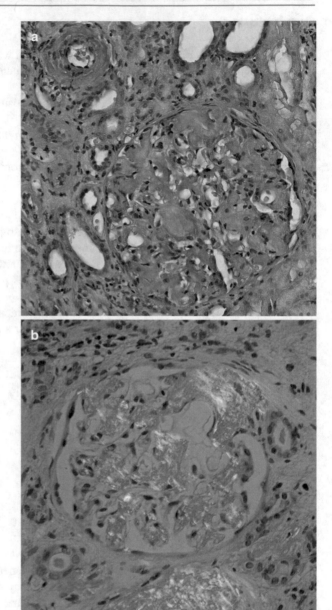

Fig. 17.4 Electron micrograph showing amyloid fibrils (*star*) deposited in the glomerular basement membrane

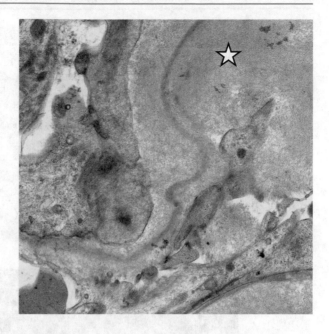

Class 2
- Histology: Mesangial immune complexes/ mesangial cell proliferation.
- Clinical features: Haematuria; low-grade proteinuria; reduced GFR.

Class 3
- Histology: Mesangial and subendothelial immune complexes/segmental endo-capillary proliferation in <50% of glomeruli.
- Clinical features: Haematuria; proteinuria seen in most patients; nephrotic syndrome not unusual; reduced GFR.

Class 4
- Histology: Mesangial and subendothelial immune complexes/segmental or global endocapillary proliferation in ≥50% of glomeruli.
- Clinical features: Haematuria; proteinuria seen in most patients; nephrotic syndrome not unusual; reduced GFR.

Class 5
- Histology: Numerous subepithelial immune complexes in >50% of glomerular capillaries.
- Clinical features: Proteinuria, often nephrotic range; haematuria possible; usually normal GFR.

Class 6
- Histology: Glomerulosclerosis in >90% of glomeruli.
- Clinical features: Advanced chronic kidney disease; proteinuria and hematuria often present.

Patient 17.2 Lupus Nephritis Causing Nephrotic Syndrome
A 23-year-old woman who was known to have systemic lupus erythematosus presented with a 4-week history of swelling of the face and abdomen. Investigations revealed: eGFR = 70 mL/min/1.73 m². Urine protein:creatinine ratio = 811 mg/mmol (8000 mg/g). Serum albumin = 16 g/L (1.6 g/dL).

Complement C3 = 0.36 g/L (Normal Range 0.75–1.65); Complement C4 = 0.06 g/L (NR 0.14–0.54). ANA titre = 1600. DNA abs (Crithidia) Positive. dsDNA abs = 282 IU/mL (NR 0.5–9.9).

A kidney biopsy was performed (Fig. 17.5).

Immunofluorescence studies of the biopsy showed membranous and mesangial deposits of C1q, C3, and IgA, M and G. These appearances are a mixture of lupus nephritis Classes 4 and 5.

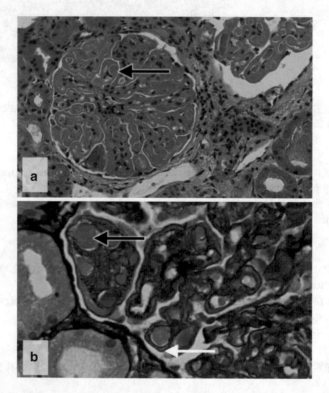

Fig. 17.5 Light micrographs of a section of a kidney biopsy from a woman with systemic lupus erythematosus. (**a**) The glomerulus shows global endocapillary hypercellularity due to a proliferation of mesangial, inflammatory and endothelial cells. There is marked thickening of the glomerular basement membrane, which has a 'wire-loop' appearance due to subendothelial immune deposits. Hyaline thrombi composed of immune deposits are present in the capillary lumina (black arrow). Haematoxylin and eosin, ×200. (**b**) Silver stain showing intraluminal hyaline thrombi (black arrow) and reduplication of the glomerular basement membrane (white arrow). Methenamine silver ×400

Complement C3 and C4

Clinical features:
 Glomerulonephritis

Nephritic syndrome:
- Proteinuria ++ or greater
- Microscopic ++ or greater
- Macroscopic haematuria with turbid urine due to casts
- Worsening GFR over days, weeks or months

Components of the complement cascade (Fig. 17.6) are consumed in a range of auto-immune disorders. The glomerulus is particularly susceptible to complement-mediated damage [13].

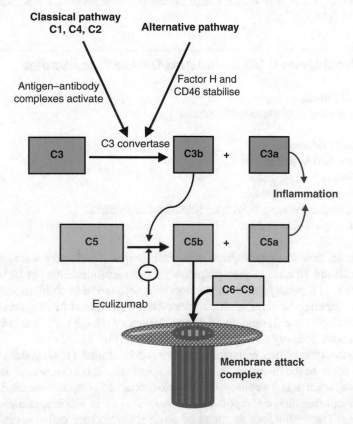

Fig. 17.6 The main elements of the complement cascade. Immune complexes activate the classical pathway, lowering levels of both C3 and C4. When the alternative pathway is activated, typically C3 is low but C4 is normal. Factor H and CD46 inhibit the alternative pathway C3 convertase. If they are defective, the alternative pathway is overactive and leads to cell damage by the generation of membrane attack complexes (C5b-9). Eculizumab blocks C5 cleavage and is used to control overactivity of the alternative pathway in atypical haemolytic uraemic syndrome (aHUS)

Immune complexes of antibody and antigen are deposited in the glomeruli where they can fix complement and cause glomerulonephritis. Deposits of the C3 component of complement are the common feature of a category of glomerulonephritis called C3 glomerulopathy [14].

Serum C3 and C4 levels are reduced in patients with nephritis associated with SLE and cryoglobulinaemia. This suggests activation of the classical and alternative pathways. C4 levels may be unreliable for monitoring SLE nephritis because genetic deficiencies of C4 are relatively common and cause a low C4 without disease.

C3 is usually decreased more than C4 in patients with C3 glomerulopathy, dense deposit disease (DDD), post-streptococcal glomerulonephritis, bacterial endocarditis glomerulonephritis and cholesterol crystal embolism. This suggests activation of the alternative pathway.

The drop in C3 found in children with post-streptococcal glomerulonephritis is usually short lasting. If the level of C3 remains low for longer than 8 weeks, the autoantibody 'C3 nephritic factor' that blocks the regulation of C3 activation may be present [15].

Anti-streptolysin O (ASO) and Anti-DNAse B Antibodies

Clinical features:
  Post-streptococcal glomerulonephritis

Nephritic syndrome:
• Oedema and hypertension
• Proteinuria ++ or greater
• Microscopic ++ or greater
• Macroscopic haematuria with turbid urine due to casts
• Worsening GFR over days

Although rare in industrialized countries, in the developing world there are between 10 and 30 cases of post-streptococcal glomerulonephritis per 100,000 people per year. It typically follows a streptococcal sore throat in children and the skin infection impetigo in older adults. Antibodies are generated in response to infections with Group A and sometimes Group C Streptococci. C3 levels are low because the alternative pathway of complement is activated (Fig. 17.6).

The onset of nephritis with smoky brown-red haematuria is classically 2 weeks after the onset of the infection, in contrast to the haematuria that occurs at the time of the sore throat in IgA nephropathy. Streptococcal antigens are deposited between the basement membrane and podocytes, where they form immune complexes with antibodies. These stimulate an influx of acute inflammatory cells—a proliferative glomerulonephritis (Fig. 17.7).

As well as anti-streptolysin O (ASO) antibodies, anti-hyaluronidase (AHase), anti-streptokinase (ASKase), anti-nicotinamide-adenine dinucleotidase (anti-NAD) and anti-DNAse B antibodies may be detected. ASO, anti-DNAse B, anti-NAD, and

Fig. 17.7 Section of a kidney biopsy from a patient with nephritis following a streptococcal sore throat. There is global endocapillary hypercellularity with infiltration of neutrophils and mononuclear cells and obliteration of the peripheral glomerular capillary loops. This glomerulus is representative of all in the specimen, i.e. the glomerulonephritis is diffuse and proliferative

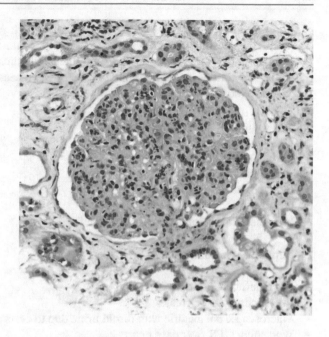

AHase titers are commonly elevated after a pharyngeal infection. Only the anti-DNAse B and AHase titers are typically increased after a skin infection. The rise in ASO titre may be blunted by antibiotic therapy.

The prognosis varies with age; in children kidney function usually returns to normal whereas the elderly may have persistent chronic kidney disease and a mortality rate of up to 25% [16].

Anti-neutrophil Cytoplasmic Antibody (ANCA)

Immunofluorescence
- Cytoplasmic or C-ANCA
- Perinuclear or P-ANCA, either typical or atypical

Enzyme-linked immunosorbent assay (ELISA)
- Anti-myeloperoxidase (MPO)
- Anti-proteinase 3 (PR3)

   Clinical features:
   Systemic vasculitis with glomerulonephritis

- PR3-ANCA (usually C-ANCA) is associated with Granulomatosis with Polyangiitis (GPA, formerly Wegener's granulomatosis)

- MPO-ANCA (usually P-ANCA) is associated with Microscopic Polyangiitis (MPA) and Eosinophilic GPA (EGPA, formerly Churg-Strauss syndrome)
- Atypical-ANCA (negative for MPO and PR3 antibodies) occurs in many inflammatory conditions including inflammatory bowel disease and rheumatoid arthritis, and in some infections.

Vasculitic illness lasting a few weeks:

- Fevers, malaise, weight loss
- Arthralgia, purpuric rash
- ENT symptoms, haemoptysis,
- Uveitis
- Mononeuritis multiplex

Nephritic syndrome:

- Proteinuria ++ or greater
- Microscopic ++ or greater
- Macroscopic haematuria with turbid urine due to casts
- Worsening GFR over days or weeks

Patients with ANCA-associated vasculitis may have one or more features of a vasculitic illness in different combinations, giving rise to different disease subtypes [17]. The diseases also tend to relapse and remit over time. Some patients have both ANCA and anti-GBM antibodies and show features of both diseases [18].

Serum is tested for ANCA by immunofluorescence, and for anti-PR3 and anti-MPO by enzyme-linked immunosorbent assay (ELISA). The results of the ELISA test are quantitative and more specific for different disease subtypes.

ANCA antibodies bind to antigens in neutrophils and monocytes [19]. The cells are activated and cluster at sites of inflammation where they release webs of fibres called Neutrophil Extracellular Traps (NETs), which normally capture and kill micro-organisms. The cells damage the endothelium of blood vessels and cause fibrinoid necrosis (Fig. 17.8) [20].

Patient 17.3 ANCA Positive, Anti-PR3 Positive Vasculitis

Mr Grantham, a 70-year-old retired businessman, became increasingly unwell over a few months with lethargy, fever, joint pains, weight loss and painful numbness in his feet. There was blood +++ and protein +++ on the urine dipstick test. His eGFR fell from 70 mL/min/1.73 m^2 to 30 over 1 week.

His C-reactive protein (CRP) was high (99 mg/L). The ANCA test was positive with a cytoplasmic pattern (c-ANCA). Proteinase 3 (PR3) antibodies were present at 91 IU/mL (Normal Range 0.2–1.9). Myeloperoxidase (MPO) antibodies were not increased (0.2 IU/mL, NR 0.2–3.4).

A kidney biopsy showed a focal segmental glomerulonephritis with necrosis and crescents (Fig. 17.9). There was no significant deposition of immunoglobulins or complement, consistent with a pauci-immune glomerulonephritis.

He was treated with intravenous methylprednisolone followed by daily oral prednisolone and intravenous cyclophosphamide every 3 weeks. His symptoms settled and the PR3 antibody titre and CRP fell quickly. His eGFR rose over the following months (Fig. 17.10). Cyclophosphamide was changed to azathioprine as maintenance immunosuppression. Apart from some painful neuropathy in his feet he felt well.

In March 2016 Mr Grantham had a superficial spreading melanoma completely removed from his back. The risk of malignancy prompted azathioprine to be stopped in November 2016. In January 2017 he became unwell with fever, tiredness and loss of appetite. He suspected the vasculitis was returning. PR3 titre rose to 63 and azathioprine was restarted. In April 2017 he became more short of breath. CRP rose to 177 and a diagnosis of lung vasculitis was made. The disease was brought back under control with increased doses of prednisolone and azathioprine.

Not all ANCA antibodies are pathogenic. Some are non-specific markers of inflammatory disease and their presence does not necessarily mean that the patient has vasculitis. c-ANCA with PR3 on ELISA testing can rarely be found in

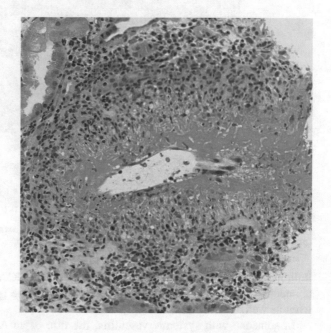

Fig. 17.8 Vasculitis with fibrinoid necrosis of a renal artery. There is destruction of the vessel wall which is replaced by pink fibrin. Mixed inflammatory cells surround and focally infiltrate the vessel wall. Haematoxylin and eosin ×200

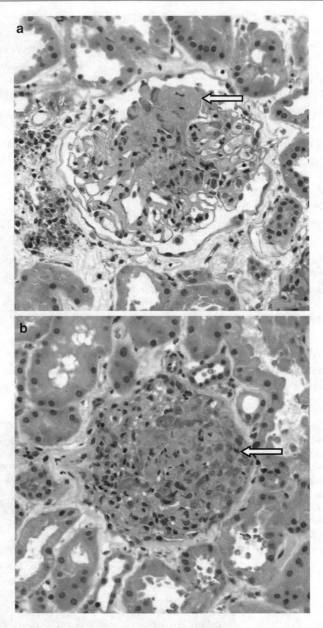

Fig. 17.9 Glomeruli showing (**a**) segmental necrotising lesion (*arrow*) and (**b**) cellular crescent (*arrow*). Haematoxylin and eosin ×200

inflammatory conditions without vasculitis [21]. p-ANCA with MPO is found in connective tissue diseases, autoimmune diseases of the gastrointestinal tract and liver, as well as with infections [22].

In someone with systemic vasculitis, the titre of an ANCA antibody is not a direct measure of disease activity. A rising titre indicates an increased risk of relapse

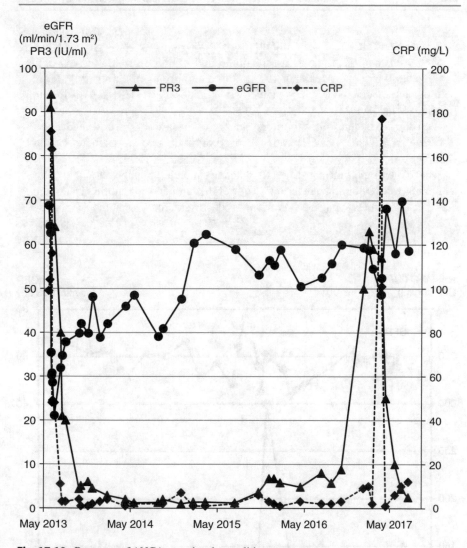

Fig. 17.10 Response of ANCA-associated vasculitis to treatment

of the kidney disease but should not be used alone to guide immunosuppressive treatment. Less than half of patients with a rising titre suffer a clinical relapse within the next year. On the other hand, a negative ANCA is reassuring as the risk of relapse is very low [23].

If someone has a past history of vasculitis and the immunosuppression has been reduced or stopped, it is helpful to compare any new symptoms with the original vasculitic illness to decide if the disease has come back (compare Patients 17.3 and 17.4).

Patient 17.4 ANCA Positive, Anti-MPO Positive Vasculitis

Mr Austin had been taking prednisolone and azathioprine for microscopic polyangiitis for many years. In 2012, routine monitoring of the anti-MPO titre showed a sudden increase associated with a modest rise in CRP but no drop in eGFR (Fig. 17.11).

Although he felt well, a thorough search for disease activity revealed a new nodule in the lung on a CT scan. The dose of prednisolone was increased for 3 months.

Two years later the anti-MPO titre steadily increased but he remained completely well, with no change in CRP or eGFR and no proteinuria. Treatment was not increased but he was monitored closely for symptoms of disease activity.

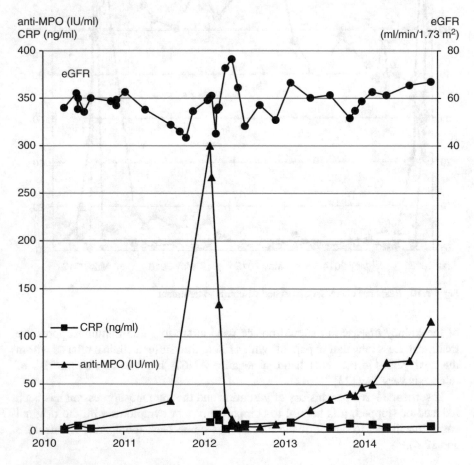

Fig. 17.11 Periods of acute and progressive increase in the titre of anti-MPO antibody that were not associated with a decline in eGFR

Anti-glomerular Basement Membrane Antibody (Anti-GBM ab)

Clinical features:
    Anti-GBM disease (Goodpasture's syndrome)

Acute nephritic syndrome:
- Proteinuria ++ or greater
- Microscopic ++ or greater
- Macroscopic haematuria with turbid urine due to casts
- Worsening GFR over days

Alveolar haemorrhage with haemoptysis

Anti–glomerular basement membrane (anti-GBM) disease is a rare small vessel vasculitis. Autoantibodies bind to an autoantigen in the basement membranes of capillaries in the kidneys and lungs. Environmental factors such as infection may trigger the disease in genetically susceptible individuals [24].

Patients with anti-GBM disease are usually very ill. The diagnosis should be confirmed urgently by testing serum for anti-GBM antibodies and, if there is doubt about the diagnosis, by kidney biopsy (Figs. 17.12 and 17.13). Intensive immuno-suppressive therapy including plasma exchange is indicated for kidney disease and lung haemorrhage.

Fig. 17.12 Kidney biopsy from a patient with anti-GBM disease showing two glomeruli, each with a large crescent filling Bowman's space around the collapsed glomerular tuft. Upper panel—haematoxylin and eosin; lower panel—silver ×130

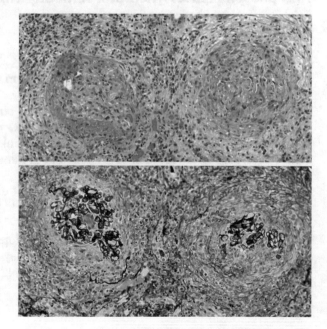

Fig. 17.13 Glomerulus stained with fluorescent-labelled anti-IgG from a patient with anti-GBM disease. The continuous linear staining indicates that IgG antibody has bound all along the glomerular basement membrane. Bowman's space around the glomerular tuft is filled with a crescent. (Image provided by Professor Agnes Fogo)

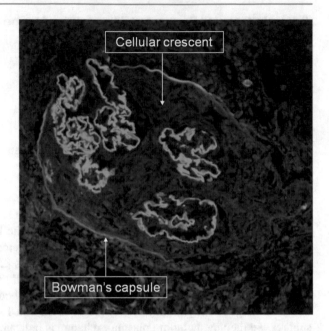

Anti-phospholipase A$_2$ Receptor Antibody (Anti-PLA$_2$R ab)

Clinical features:
   Membranous nephropathy (MN)

• Nephrotic-range proteinuria or nephrotic syndrome, in adults

The majority of patients with primary MN have circulating autoantibodies against the M-type phospholipase A$_2$ receptor (PLA$_2$R) which is located on normal podoctyes [25]. The function of the PLA$_2$R is unknown. The protein was named according to the location of its gene but in humans it does not actually bind PLA$_2$.

Some patients with idiopathic MN without PLA$_2$R antibodies have circulating autoantibodies against thrombospondin type-1 domain-containing 7A (THSD7A) [26].

A positive PLA$_2$R antibody test is diagnostic of idiopathic MN in adults with nephrotic syndrome. It may avoid the need for a kidney biopsy in such patients, especially if the eGFR is normal (>60 mL/min/1.73 m^2) [27].

About 20% of patients with MN on kidney biopsy have secondary MN, caused by infections (hepatitis B and C, HIV, parasites, leprosy, syphilis, hydatid disease, sarcoid), malignancy (the commonest being lung cancer), autoimmune diseases (the commonest being SLE), alloimmune diseases (in a kidney transplant, graft versus host disease), or drugs and toxins (such as NSAIDs, COX2 inhibitors, gold, d-penicillamine, mercury). Patients with secondary MN are negative for anti-PLA$_2$R antibody.

PLA$_2$R antibody titres are very helpful for monitoring the disease and planning treatment. If the antibody is absent there is a good chance the disease will go into remission spontaneously [28]. If the titre goes negative with treatment there is a good chance that proteinuria will decline over the following months. Conversely, if the titre rises after treatment is stopped there is a high chance the disease will relapse [29].

Immune complexes of PLA$_2$R antigen and IgG$_4$ are formed in the space between the glomerular basement membrane and the podocytes. Their presence stimulates the membrane to thicken around them (Fig. 17.14) forming 'spikes' seen by light microscopy with a silver stain (Fig. 17.15) and electron microscopy (Fig. 17.16).

Fig. 17.14 Glomerulus affected by membranous nephropathy. Glomerular capillary membranes are thickened. The inset shows the thickness of normal membranes for comparison. Haematoxylin and eosin ×400

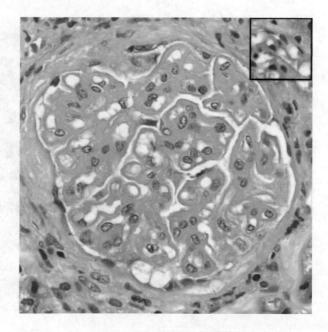

Fig. 17.15 External surfaces of the capillary loops have spikes protruding from them. The spikes are separated by spaces containing immune deposits that do not take up the silver stain. Some sections of the glomerular basement membrane are thickened and contain holes where deposits have been enclosed within the membrane (*inset*). Silver ×400

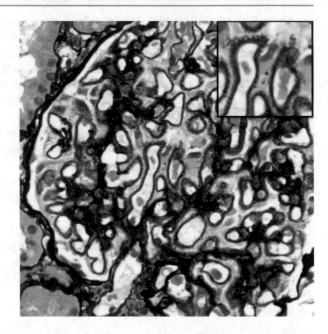

Fig. 17.16 Subepithelial immune deposits between the glomerular basement membrane and a podocyte with spikes of membrane between adjacent deposits. Electron micrograph ×13,000

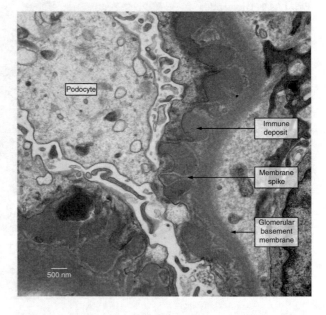

References

1. Yatim KM, Lakkis FG. A Brief Journey through the immune system. CJASN CJN.10031014. https://doi.org/10.2215/CJN.10031014. http://cjasn.asnjournals.org/content/early/2015/04/06/CJN.10031014.full.
2. Kitching AR, Hutton HL. The players: cells involved in glomerular disease. Clin J Am Soc Nephrol. 2016;11(9):1664–74. https://doi.org/10.2215/CJN.13791215. Epub 2016 Apr 12. http://cjasn.asnjournals.org/cgi/pmidlookup?view=long&pmid=27073196.
3. Jefferson JA. Complications of immunosuppression in glomerular disease. Clin J Am Soc Nephrol. 2018;13(8):1264–75. https://doi.org/10.2215/CJN.01920218. Epub 2018 Jul 24. https://cjasn.asnjournals.org/content/13/8/1264.long.
4. Maeda A, Gohda T, Funabiki K, Horikoshi S, Shirato I, Tomino Y. Significance of serum IgA levels and serum IgA/C3 ratio in diagnostic analysis of patients with IgA nephropathy. Clin Lab Anal. 2003;17(3):73–6. http://onlinelibrary.wiley.com/doi/10.1002/jcla.10071/abstract;jsessionid=A271E49EC0DF8F1FF6196265F755FA83.f02t02.
5. Rosner MH, Edeani A, Yanagita M, Glezerman IG, Leung N, American Society of Nephrology Onco-Nephrology Forum. Paraprotein-related kidney disease: diagnosing and treating monoclonal gammopathy of renal significance. Clin J Am Soc Nephrol. 2016;11(12):2280–7. Epub 2016 Aug 15. https://cjasn.asnjournals.org/content/11/12/2280.long.
6. Motwani SS, Herlitz L, Monga D, Jhaveri KD, Lam AQ, American Society of Nephrology Onco-Nephrology Forum. Paraprotein-related kidney disease: glomerular diseases associated with paraproteinemias. Clin J Am Soc Nephrol. 2016;11(12):2260–72. Epub 2016 Aug 15. https://cjasn.asnjournals.org/content/11/12/2260.long.
7. Leung N, Drosou ME, Nasr SH. Dysproteinemias and Glomerular Disease. Clin J Am Soc Nephrol. 2018;13(1):128–39. https://doi.org/10.2215/CJN.00560117. Epub 2017 Nov 7. https://cjasn.asnjournals.org/content/13/1/128.long.
8. Ritchie J, Assi LK, Burmeister A, Hoefield R, Cockwell P, Kalra PA. Association of serum Ig free light chains with mortality and ESRD among patients with nondialysis-dependent CKD. CJASN CJN.09660914; published ahead of print March 30, 2015. https://doi.org/10.2215/CJN.09660914. http://cjasn.asnjournals.org/content/early/2015/03/30/CJN.09660914.
9. McTaggart MP, Lindsay J, Kearney EM. Replacing urine protein electrophoresis with serum free light chain analysis as a first-line test for detecting plasma cell disorders offers increased diagnostic accuracy and potential health benefit to patients. Am J Clin Pathol. 2013;140(6):890–7. https://doi.org/10.1309/AJCP25IHYLEWCAHJ. https://academic.oup.com/ajcp/article/140/6/890/1761562.
10. Rezk T, Lachmann HJ, Fontana M, Sachchithanantham S, Mahmood S, Petrie A, Whelan CJ, Pinney JH, Foard D, Lane T, Youngstein T, Wechalekar AD, Bass P, Hawkins PN, Gillmore JD. Prolonged renal survival in light chain amyloidosis: speed and magnitude of light chain reduction is the crucial factor. Kidney Int. 2017;92(6):1476–83. https://doi.org/10.1016/j.kint.2017.05.004. Epub 2017 Jul 18. https://www.kidney-international.org/article/S0085-2538(17)30328-9/fulltext.
11. Howie AJ, Brewer DB, Howell D, Jones AP. Physical basis of colors seen in Congo red-stained amyloid in polarized light. Lab Invest. 2008;88(3):232–42. https://doi.org/10.1038/labinvest.3700714. Epub 2007 Dec 31. http://www.nature.com/labinvest/journal/v88/n3/full/3700714a.html.
12. Almaani S, Meara A, Rovin BH. Update on lupus nephritis. Clin J Am Soc Nephrol. 2017;12(5):825–35. https://doi.org/10.2215/CJN.05780616. Epub 2016 Nov 7. https://cjasn.asnjournals.org/content/12/5/825.long.
13. Thurman JM, Nester CM. All things complement. Clin J Am Soc Nephrol. 2016;11(10):1856–66. https://doi.org/10.2215/CJN.01710216. Epub 2016 Jun 23. https://cjasn.asnjournals.org/content/11/10/1856.long.

14. Fakhouri F, Frémeaux-Bacchi V, Noël LH, Cook HT, Pickering MC. C3 glomerulopathy: a new classification. Nat Rev Nephrol. 2010;6(8):494–9. https://doi.org/10.1038/nrneph.2010.85. Epub 2010 Jul 6. http://www.nature.com/nrneph/journal/v6/n8/full/nrneph.2010.85.html.
15. Paixão-Cavalcante D, López-Trascasa M, Skattum L, Giclas PC, Goodship TH, Rodríguez de Córdoba S, Truedsson L, Morgan BP, Harris CL. Sensitive and specific assays for C3 nephritic factors clarify mechanisms underlying complement dysregulation. Kidney Int. 2012;82:1084–92. https://doi.org/10.1038/ki.2012.250. http://www.nature.com/ki/journal/v82/n10/full/ki2012250a.html.
16. Rodriguez-Iturbe B, Musser JM. The current state of poststreptococcal glomerulonephritis. JASN. 2008;19:1855–64. https://doi.org/10.1681/ASN.2008010092. http://jasn.asnjournals.org/content/19/10/1855.full
17. Jennette JC, Nachman PH. ANCA glomerulonephritis and vasculitis. Clin J Am Soc Nephrol. 2017;12(10):1680–91. https://doi.org/10.2215/CJN.02500317. https://cjasn.asnjournals.org/content/12/10/1680.long.
18. McAdoo SP, Tanna A, Hrušková Z, Holm L, Weiner M, Arulkumaran N, Kang A, Satrapová V, Levy J, Ohlsson S, Tesar V, Segelmark M, Pusey CD. Patients double-seropositive for ANCA and anti-GBM antibodies have varied renal survival, frequency of relapse, and outcomes compared to single-seropositive patients. Kidney Int. 2017;92(3):693–702. https://doi.org/10.1016/j.kint.2017.03.014. PubMed PMID: 28506760; PubMed Central PMCID: PMC5567410. https://www.ncbi.nlm.nih.gov/pmc/articles/PMC5567410/#__ffn_sectitle.
19. Jennette JC, Falk RJ. ANCAs are also antimonocyte cytoplasmic autoantibodies. Clin J Am Soc Nephrol. 2014;10:4–6. https://doi.org/10.2215/CJN.11501114. http://cjasn.asnjournals.org/content/10/1/4.short.
20. Schoenermarck U, Csernok E, Gross WL. Pathogenesis of anti-neutrophil cytoplasmic antibody-associated vasculitis: challenges and solutions. Nephrol Dial Transplant. 2014;30:i46–52. https://doi.org/10.1093/ndt/gfu398. http://ndt.oxfordjournals.org/content/30/suppl_1/i46.abstract.
21. Knight A, Ekbom A, Brandt L, Askling J. What is the significance in routine care of c-ANCA/PR3-ANCA in the absence of systemic vasculitis? A case series. Clin Exp Rheumatol. 2008;26(3 Suppl 49):S53–6. https://www.clinexprheumatol.org/article.asp?a=3375.
22. Antonelou M, Perea Ortega L, Harvey J, Salama A. Anti-myeloperoxidase antibody positivity in patients without primary systemic vasculitis. Clin Exp Rheumatol. 2019;37 Suppl 117(2):86–9. https://www.clinexprheumatol.org/abstract.asp?a=12869.
23. Kemna MJ, Damoiseaux J, Austen J, Winkens B, Peters J, van Paassen P, Tervaert JWC. ANCA as a predictor of relapse: useful in patients with renal involvement but not in patients with non-renal disease. JASN. 2015;26:537–42. https://doi.org/10.1681/ASN.2013111233. http://jasn.asnjournals.org/content/26/3/537.abstract.
24. McAdoo SP, Pusey CD. Anti-glomerular basement membrane disease. Clin J Am Soc Nephrol. 2017;12(7):1162–72. https://doi.org/10.2215/CJN.01380217. https://cjasn.asnjournals.org/content/12/7/1162.long.
25. McQuarrie EP. Anti-phospholipase A2 receptor antibodies in primary membranous nephropathy-10 key points. Nephrol Dial Transplant. 2018;33(2):212–3. https://doi.org/10.1093/ndt/gfx366. https://academic.oup.com/ndt/article/33/2/212/4834145.
26. Tomas NM, Beck LH, Meyer-Schwesinger C, Seitz-Polski B, Ma H, Zahner G, Dolla G, Hoxha E, Helmchen U, Dabert-Gay A-S, Debayle D, Merchant M, Klein J, Salant DJ, Stahl RAK, Lambeau G. Thrombospondin type-1 domain-containing 7A in idiopathic membranous nephropathy. N Engl J Med. 2014;371:2277–87. https://doi.org/10.1056/NEJMoa1409354.
27. Bobart SA, De Vriese AS, Pawar AS, Zand L, Sethi S, Giesen C, Lieske JC, Fervenza FC. Noninvasive diagnosis of primary membranous nephropathy using phospholipase A2 receptor antibodies. Kidney Int. 2019;95(2):429–38. https://doi.org/10.1016/j.kint.2018.10.021. https://www.kidney-international.org/article/S0085-2538(18)30822-6/fulltext.
28. Hoxha E, Harendza S, Pinnschmidt HO, Tomas NM, Helmchen U, Panzer U, Stahl RA. Spontaneous remission of proteinuria is a frequent event in phospholipase A2 receptor antibody-negative patients with membranous nephropathy. Nephrol Dial Transplant.

2015;30(11):1862–9.   https://doi.org/10.1093/ndt/gfv228.   https://academic.oup.com/ndt/article/30/11/1862/2459994.

29. De Vriese AS, Glassock RJ, Nath KA, Sethi S, Fervenza FCA. Proposal for a serology-based approach to membranous nephropathy. J Am Soc Nephrol. 2017;28(2):421–30. https://doi.org/10.1681/ASN.2016070776. Epub 2016 Oct 24. https://jasn.asnjournals.org/content/28/2/421.long.

Image the Urinary Tract: Strengths and Weaknesses of Different Radiology Modalities

18

Ultrasound

The most common modality for imaging the urinary tract is plain ultrasound (Figs. 18.1 and 18.2).

Abnormal Appearances on Kidney Ultrasound Scans

Changes to the ultrasound appearance are seen in both acute and chronic kidney disease. Cellular infiltration, interstitial oedema, sclerosis of glomeruli and fibrosis all non-specifically increase the reflectivity to ultrasound and the 'brightness' of the image. This is most easily judged by comparing the reflectivity of the cortex with the adjacent liver. The scan report may describe 'increased cortical echogenicity' or 'loss of cortico-medullary differentiation'.

The kidney may shrink in volume as chronic damage progresses and ultimately it can be hard to distinguish the kidney from the surrounding tissues (Fig. 18.3). Localised damage and scarring may make the outline of the kidney irregular (Fig. 18.4).

A common incidental finding that may cause unnecessary concern is an angiomyolipoma (Fig. 18.5). These benign tumours are only clinically relevant when they are unusually large. Multiple angiomyolipomas are found in tuberous sclerosis, usually in both kidneys. They can become very large and when >4 cm in diameter there is a risk of major bleeding from minor trauma.

Cysts are a frequent incidental finding and may cause concern to the patient and doctor (Fig. 18.6). They may be multiple, large and in both kidneys. Patients with end-stage kidney disease often develop cysts in their small kidneys—acquired cystic disease—which uncommonly can progress to carcinoma. Centrally located, parapelvic cysts are found in Fabry disease.

Cysts are classified according to the presence of internal membranes (septa), calcification and solid structures within them—the Bosniak classification [1]. If the

© Springer Nature Switzerland AG 2020
H. C. Rayner et al., *Understanding Kidney Diseases*,
https://doi.org/10.1007/978-3-030-43027-6_18

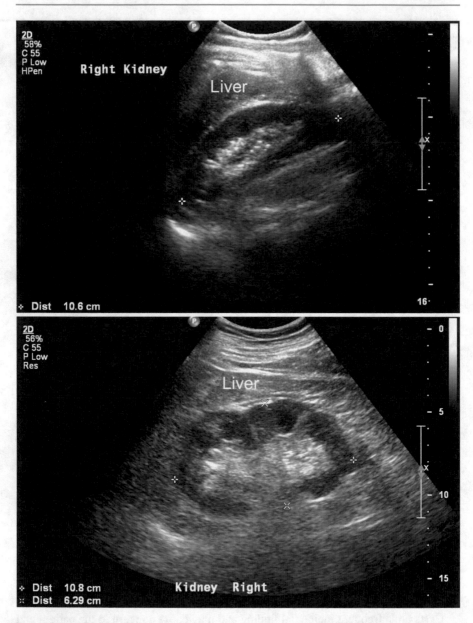

Figs. 18.1 and 18.2 Ultrasound scans of normal kidneys. The cortex is of the same or lower echogenicity (reflectivity) than the liver or spleen. The liver lies immediately superior to the right kidney. The centrally placed sinus fat is of greater echogenicity than both the cortex and the liver and spleen

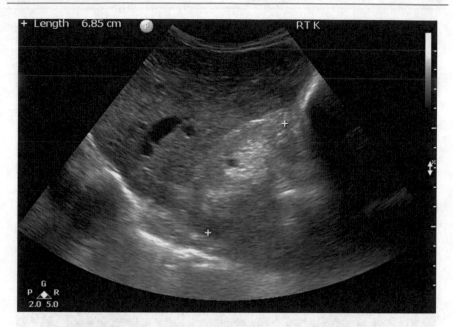

Fig. 18.3 Ultrasound scan of a small (6.85 cm in length) chronically damaged right kidney. The cortex is thinned and appears brighter than the liver, which lies above it. Both cortex and medulla are hyperechoic, making it hard to distinguish between them

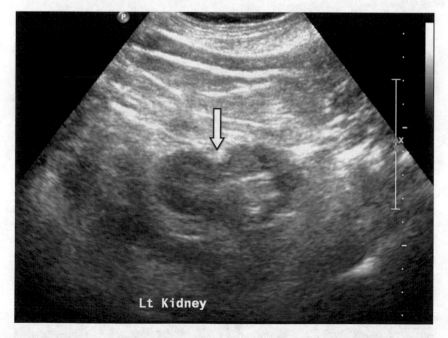

Fig. 18.4 Ultrasound of a shrunken left kidney showing a large cortical scar at the mid-pole *(arrow)*

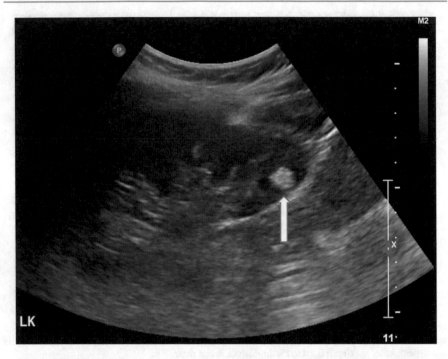

Fig. 18.5 Ultrasound scan of a left kidney showing a single 1 cm diameter angiomyolipoma (arrow)

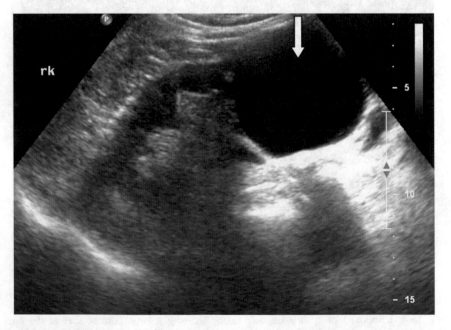

Fig. 18.6 Ultrasound scan of a right kidney containing a simple thin walled cyst on the lower pole, 6.2 cm in diameter (*arrow*). Otherwise the kidney is normal in appearance

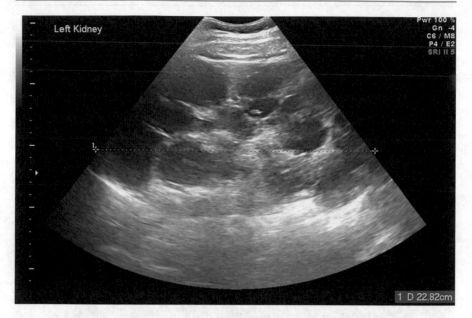

Fig. 18.7 Ultrasound scan of a grossly enlarged autosomal dominant polycystic kidney (22.8 cm in length) that was easily felt on physical examination

cysts have a thin wall and do not contain septa, calcification or solid structures, they are benign and of no clinical significance. In particular, they do not cause pain unless they become infected or there is bleeding into them.

In autosomal dominant polycystic kidney disease the cysts are more numerous, the kidneys become enlarged and the remaining tissues are distorted (Fig. 18.7). Cysts may also be found in the liver and spleen [2].

Urinary Tract Obstruction

Ultrasound is the first modality to use for detecting obstruction to urinary flow at any level of the urinary tract. In a hydronephrotic kidney, dilation of the sinuses and calyces is seen as a branching fluid space within the echogenic central sinus area (Figs. 18.8, 18.9 and 18.10). Centrally located cysts can mimic this appearance.

Patient 18.1 Retroperitoneal Fibrosis
Mr Castle, aged 60, went to donate blood and was found to be anaemic, Hb = 108 g/L (10.8 g/dL). He had been tired over the previous 3 weeks but other than some back pain had no symptoms. His eGFR was found to be 11 mL/min/1.73 m^2 so he was referred to hospital urgently. He had no past or family history of kidney disease. The blood pressure was 196/119 mmHg and

an ECG showed left ventricular hypertrophy. Urine albumin:creatinine ratio was normal, 1.8 mg/mmol (16 mg/g). CRP was raised, 71 mg/L.

The report on an urinary tract ultrasound scan (Figs. 18.11 and 18.12) stated: "minimal fullness of the collecting system is noted bilaterally, otherwise both kidneys appear normal in size and echopattern. Kidney lengths: Right 10.7 cm, Left 10.4 cm. No scarring or obvious calculi seen."

Doppler ultrasound studies showed normal kidney blood flow but there was considerable atheroma lining the anterior wall of the aorta, measuring 1.27 cm in antero-posterior depth (Fig. 18.13).

The medical team interpreted the ultrasound scan report as indicating that there was no obstruction and he was referred to the renal medicine team. They reviewed the images and suspected bilateral hydronephrosis. A repeat scan confirmed hydronephrosis and bilateral nephrostomies were inserted.

Nephrostogram studies showed dilated pelvicalyceal systems in both kidneys with medial deviation and narrowing of both ureters from L4 inferiorly (Fig. 18.14). This suggested bilateral extrinsic compression due to retroperitoneal fibrosis.

Stents were passed down the ureters via the nephrostomies and Mr Castle's kidney function returned to normal over the following 6 weeks.

A CT urogram showed soft tissue around the aorta attached to the ureters, extending down to the common iliac arteries (Fig. 18.15).

These appearances are typical of retroperitoneal fibrosis, which is an inflammatory reaction to atheromatous material that has leaked out from the aorta into the surrounding retroperitoneal space [3].

He was treated with prednisolone and his back pain improved. The CRP returned to normal, 6 mg/L, and his anaemia resolved, Hb 141 g/L (14.1 g/dL). A subsequent CT scan confirmed that the tissue had reduced in volume.

Retroperitoneal fibrosis is a relapsing condition; up to half of patients have a disease recurrence over 15 years. This is more likely if antinuclear antibodies are present at diagnosis and less likely if they are treated with prednisolone and/or tamoxifen [4].

Dilatation of the collecting system in a kidney does not necessarily mean that it is obstructed. In the last trimester of pregnancy, normal kidneys can appear moderately hydronephrotic due to the pressure of the uterus and the effects of progesterone. A transplanted kidney usually has a dilated intrarenal collecting system. If there is doubt, an isotope renogram is required that shows the flow of urine.

Figs. 18.8–18.10 Ultrasound scans of the right and left kidneys and bladder in a patient with chronic bladder outlet obstruction. Both kidneys show gross hydronephrosis. The bladder is distended and the wall is thickened (1.84 cm) with an irregular trabeculated surface. In a man, these appearances are usually caused by prostatic enlargement. These images are from a woman with a urethral stricture. If the obstruction occurred very recently, the kidneys may appear normal on ultrasound with no visible hydronephrosis. If a patient has clinical features that suggest obstruction, even a suggestion of dilatation of the collecting system should prompt further studies (Patient 18.1)

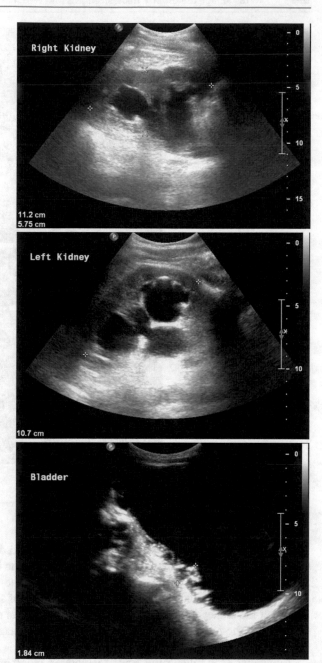

Figs. 18.11 and 18.12 Ultrasound scans of Mr Castle's kidneys

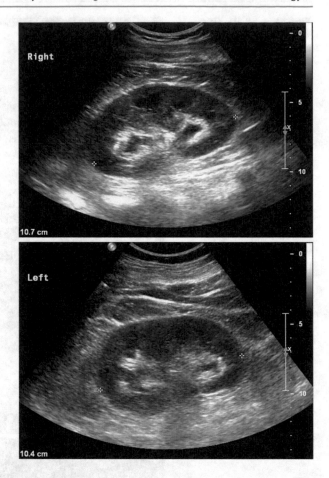

Isotope Renography

There are two types of isotope kidney scan—static and dynamic. Static scans are taken to show the size of the kidneys and how evenly the isotope is distributed. An isotope is used that is concentrated and retained in the kidney, technetium 99m dimercaptosuccinic acid (DMSA). If there is an area of scarring in one kidney or failure of the kidney to develop (agenesis), the isotope is not taken up. The DMSA scan is also the reference technique for showing the relative function between the two kidneys.

A dynamic scan follows the flow of isotope in blood into the kidneys and out of them in the urine. The patient receives an intravenous dose of the radioisotope technetium-99m mercaptoacetyltriglycine (MAG3) that is concentrated in the kidneys and excreted in the urine. The trace of radioactivity is called a MAG3 renogram. The MAG3 can be used like DMSA to produce a static scan (Figs. 18.16 and 18.17).

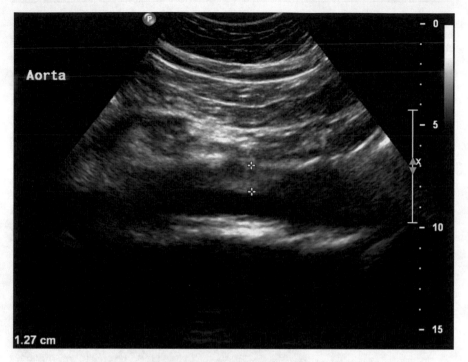

Fig. 18.13 Ultrasound scan of Mr Castle's aorta. Markers indicate atheroma in front of the anterior wall of the aorta, measuring 1.27 cm in antero-posterior depth

Radioactivity is counted to track the flow of isotope in urine out of the kidney (Fig. 18.18). Intravenous diuretic, furosemide, is given to maximise the flow of urine and accentuate any obstruction (Fig. 18.19).

The anatomical site of the obstruction is identified using an X-ray contrast study (Fig. 18.20).

Computed Tomography

When imaging a patient who presents with suspected renal colic, it is common practice to perform a non-contrast CT urogram rather than an ultrasound scan (Figs. 18.21 and 18.22).

CT is more sensitive than ultrasound for calculi and allows other organs and blood vessels to be assessed on the same scan, theoretically increasing the diagnostic yield. However, skilled ultrasound scanning can be of additional value, such as to locate a stone at the distal end of the ureter [5] (Fig. 18.23).

On a plain X-ray, stones vary in their opacity to the X-rays. Stones containing calcium (calcium oxalate, calcium phosphate) or struvite (magnesium ammonium phosphate) are opaque. Stones containing sulphur (cystine) are semi-opaque. Stones composed of uric acid, xanthine or pure matrix (coagulated mucoid material) are radiolucent [6].

Fig. 18.14 Antegrade nephrostogram study showing dilated pelvicalyceal systems in both kidneys. The lower ureters are deviated medially and compressed by retroperitoneal fibrotic tissue

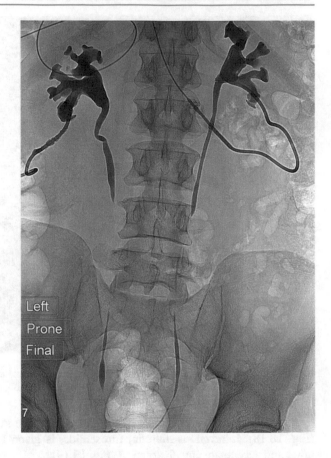

No contrast is required with a CT scan because even radiolucent stones are visible, apart from the very rare pure matrix stones. This avoids any risk of contrast-induced nephropathy.

In patients with macroscopic haematuria but no colic, a soft tissue lesion is much more likely than a stone and so contrast is required.

CT is also good for visualising gas within and around the urinary tract. Gas can be produced in the urine of patients with diabetes from the fermentation of glucose by bacteria, usually *Eschericia coli* or *Klebsiella pneumoniae.* This causes a severe form of kidney infection - emphysematous pyelonephritis (Fig. 18.24) [7].

The Risks and Benefits of Using Contrast Media

To increase the differentiation between structures on an X-ray, radio-contrast medium is injected intravenously. The iodine in the medium attenuates the X-rays and creates a contrast in density between blood vessels and tissues, and areas with high and low blood flows (Figs. 18.25 and 18.26).

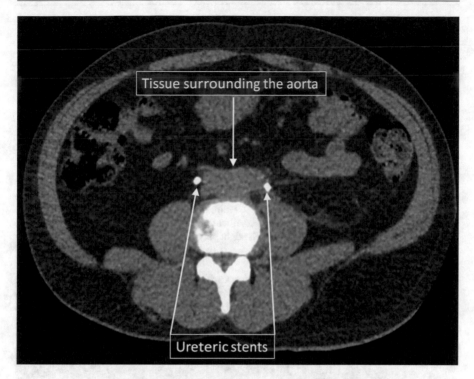

Fig. 18.15 CT urogram showing soft tissue around the aorta attached to the ureters that are identified by the radio-opaque stents within them

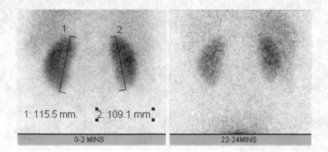

Fig. 18.16 Static scans from a normal 99m Tc MAG3 renogram. The kidneys are of normal size and shape: left (1) = 115.5 mm, right (2) 109.1 mm. The isotope is homogeneously distributed on the scan taken during the first 2 min. The level of radioactivity has declined symmetrically on the scan taken between 22 and 24 min

Media vary in their iodine content and this affects their osmolality; high-osmolar media have a higher ratio of iodine atoms to dissolved particles.

Patients with risk factors for acute kidney injury such as chronic kidney disease, diabetes mellitus, congestive heart failure, and older age are at risk of contrast-induced nephropathy (CIN, or CI-AKI) (Fig. 18.27) [8]. The injury is caused by

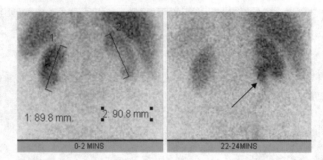

Fig. 18.17 A 99m Tc MAG3 renogram with intravenous furosemide in a patient with a right hydronephrosis and hydroureter on an ultrasound scan. Both kidneys have a normal shape but thin cortex and are smaller than normal: left (1) = 89.8 mm, right (2) = 90.8 mm; c.f. Fig. 18.16. On the scan taken in the first 2 min there is less uptake of isotope on the right (2) than the left (1). On the 22–24 min scan there is increased activity in the right pelvicalyceal system in keeping with ureteric obstruction (arrow)

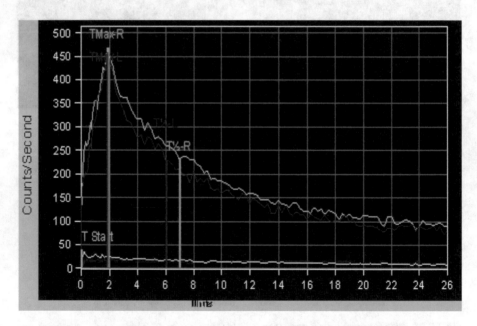

Fig. 18.18 A normal MAG3 renogram. There is rapid symmetrical uptake (TMax = 2 min, normal <6 min) and excretion of the isotope (T½ left = 6 min, T½ right = 7 min, normal <15 min)

vasoconstriction in the outer medulla of the kidney. This region normally has a limited blood supply so as not to wash away the urea concentration gradient. It is therefore vulnerable to ischaemic damage. Contrast agents may also have direct toxic effects on tubular cells.

The risk of CIN is greater with increasing volumes of contrast medium and with high- rather than low-osmolar contrast medium. Intravenous isotonic (0.9%) saline given before and after the radio-contrast study reduces the risk of CIN [9].

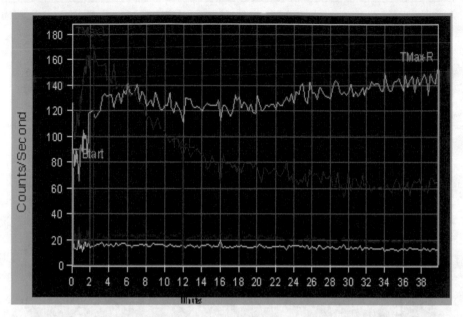

Fig. 18.19 MAG3 renogram in a patient with right hydroureter. Maximum uptake of the isotope is reduced in both kidneys compared to the normal scan (see Fig. 18.18) due to reduced GFR (TMax left = 170 counts/second, right = 150, normal = 450). The left kidney excretion curve (*TMaxL and T½L in red*) is within normal limits (T½ = 12 min, normal <15 min). The right kidney curve (*TMax-R in yellow*) shows slower uptake and no decline, indicating obstruction to urinary flow

Fig. 18.20 Retrograde urogram shows a filling defect in the right ureter due to a ureteric tumour that is causing hydroureter, i.e. dilatation of the ureter above it

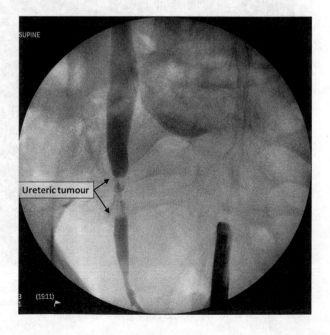

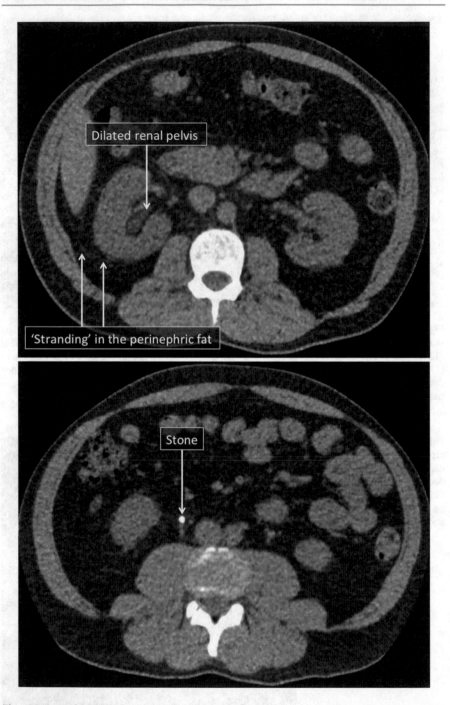

Figs. 18.21 and 18.22 Non-contrast CT scan showing hydronephrosis of the right kidney caused by a stone impacted in the ureter. There is 'stranding' in the fat around the kidney due to increased pressure in the collecting system causing leakage of fluid

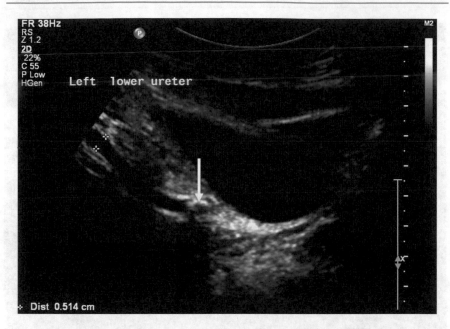

Fig. 18.23 Ultrasound scan showing echogenic stone (arrow) at the distal end of the ureter next to the bladder

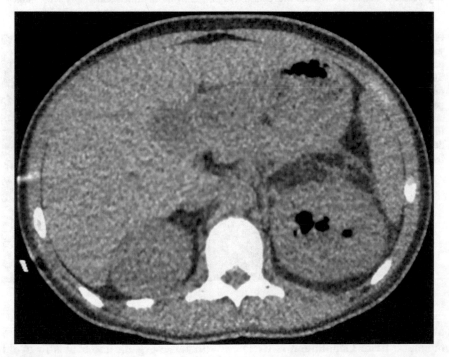

Fig. 18.24 CT scan showing gas within the collecting system of an enlarged left kidney in a patient with emphysematous pyelonephritis

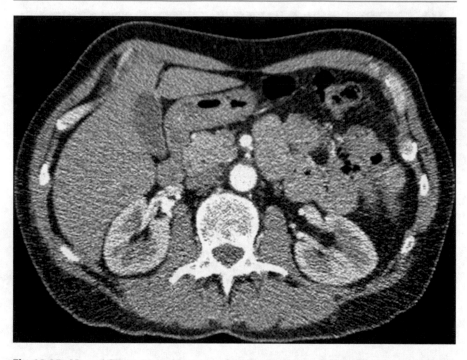

Fig. 18.25 Normal CT urogram with contrast, highlighting the arterial blood supply to the kidneys

Fig. 18.26 CT urogram with contrast from a patient with chronic atrial fibrillation who suddenly developed severe left loin pain. There are segmental areas of low attenuation throughout the left kidney due to infarcts caused by emboli

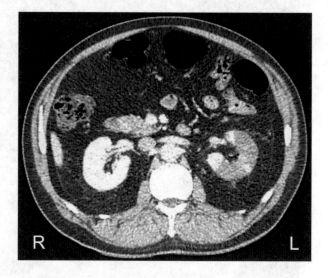

In magnetic resonance imaging, contrast medium containing the element gadolinium is used. It is para-magnetic and so affects the behaviour of tissue in the magnetic field. Gadolinium is chelated with large organic molecules to avoid toxicity from the gadolinium ions. The complexes are hyperosmolar and excreted

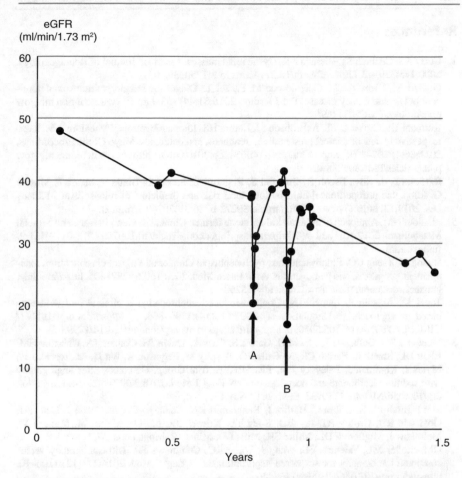

Fig. 18.27 Progressive decline in eGFR in a 60-year-old man with diabetes. At the time labeled A he underwent an abdominal CT scan with contrast. An acute drop in eGFR followed. At the time labeled B he underwent a coronary angiogram. An identical drop in eGFR occurred. Both episodes of contrast-induced nephropathy had the same severity of injury and time course for recovery. The underlying chronic decline in GFR was not affected in this patient

by glomerular filtration. If gadolinium-contrast is used in patients with low GFR, the persistently high levels of contrast can stimulate a fibrosing reaction in the tissues under the skin and in other organs - nephrogenic systemic fibrosis (NSF). This debilitating and potentially fatal condition is untreatable. Hence a strict GFR limit of >30 mL/min/1.73 m^2 is applied to the use of contrast containing gadolinium [8].

References

1. Curry NS, Cochran ST, Bissada NK. Cystic renal masses. American Journal of Roentgenology. 2000;175:339–42. https://doi.org/10.2214/ajr.175.2.1750339.
2. Gradzik M, Niemczyk M, Gołębiowski M, Pączek L. Diagnostic imaging of autosomal dominant polycystic kidney disease. Pol J Radiol. 2016;81:441–53. https://www.ncbi.nlm.nih.gov/pmc/articles/PMC5031169/.
3. Kermani TA, Crowson CS, Achenbach SJ, Luthra HS. Idiopathic retroperitoneal fibrosis: a retrospective review of clinical presentation, treatment, and outcomes. Mayo Clinic Proceedings. 2011;86(4):297–303. https://doi.org/10.4065/mcp.2010.0663. http://www.ncbi.nlm.nih.gov/pmc/articles/PMC3068889/.
4. Raffiotta F, da Silva Escoli R, Quaglini S, Rognoni C, Sacchi L, Binda V, Messa P, Moroni G. Idiopathic retroperitoneal fibrosis: long-term risk and predictors of relapse. Am J Kidney Dis. 2019;13. https://www.ajkd.org/article/S0272-6386(19)30740-1/fulltext.
5. Maalouf NM. Approach to the adult kidney stone former. Clinical Reviews in Bone and Mineral Metabolism. 2012;10(1):38–49. http://link.springer.com/article/10.1007/s12018-011-9111-9/fulltext.html.
6. Huang JJ, Tseng CC. Emphysematous pyelonephritis: clinicoradiological classification, management, prognosis, and pathogenesis. Arch Intern Med. 2000;160(6):797–805. http://archinte.jamanetwork.com/article.aspx?articleid=485260.
7. Tepel M, Aspelin P, Lameire N. Contrast-induced nephropathy: a clinical and evidence-based   approach.   Circulation.   2006;113(14):1799–806.   https://doi.org/10.1161/CIRCULATIONAHA.105.595090. http://circ.ahajournals.org/content/113/14/1799.full.
8. Weisbord SD, Gallagher M, Jneid H, Garcia S, Cass A, Thwin SS, Conner TA, Chertow GM, Bhatt DL, Shunk K, Parikh CR, McFalls EO, Brophy M, Ferguson R, Wu H, Androsenko M, Myles J, Kaufman J, Palevsky PM, PRESERVE Trial Group. Outcomes after angiography with sodium bicarbonate and acetylcysteine. N Engl J Med. 2018;378(7):603–14. https://doi.org/10.1056/NEJMoa1710933. Epub 2017 Nov 12.
9. Smith-Bindman R, Aubin C, Bailitz J, Bengiamin RN, Camargo CA Jr, Corbo J, Dean AJ, Goldstein RB, Griffey RT, Jay GD, Kang TL, Kriesel DR, Ma OJ, Mallin M, Manson W, Melnikow J, Miglioretti DL, Miller SK, Mills LD, Miner JR, Moghadassi M, Noble VE, Press GM, Stoller ML, Valencia VE, Wang J, Wang RC, Cummings SR. Ultrasonography versus computed tomography for suspected nephrolithiasis. N Engl J Med. 2014;371(12):1100–10. https://doi.org/10.1056/NEJMoa1404446.

Should We Do a Kidney Biopsy? Balancing the Diagnostic Benefits Against the Clinical Risks

19

No guidelines or consensus statements have been issued by specialist organisations to help clinicians decide when to perform a kidney biopsy. Therefore, the following comments are our personal views, inevitably coloured by our clinical experiences.

'Primum Non Nocere': First, Do No Harm

Most nephrologists know of patients who have come to serious harm as a result of a kidney biopsy. Even with ultrasound guidance, it is not possible to guide the needle to avoid blood vessels (Figs. 19.1 and 19.2). Hence, every kidney biopsy causes bleeding; the question is how much. Published reports of adults [1] and children [2] report a rate of blood transfusion of 1 in every 100 biopsies. Fatality is rarer, 1 in 2500 biopsies [1], but must be considered in the decision whether to perform a biopsy and when obtaining the patient's consent.

Kidney histology is fascinating and beautiful. However, curiosity about what will be found is, on its own, insufficient justification to perform a kidney biopsy. Remember the old saying: 'Curiosity killed the cat'. If you cannot answer positively the question: "How will the result of this biopsy affect the treatment plan *and* the likely outcome for the patient?" you should reconsider whether to seek the patient's consent.

There are three main reasons to perform a biopsy: diagnosis; prognosis and research. A kidney biopsy on its own does not make a diagnosis. Although its status is often elevated to a higher level, it is just one more test that contributes to the clinical and laboratory information used to make a diagnosis. The interpreting the histological appearances is subjective and is done in the context of the clinical information.

Fig. 19.1 Think twice
before you do a
kidney biopsy

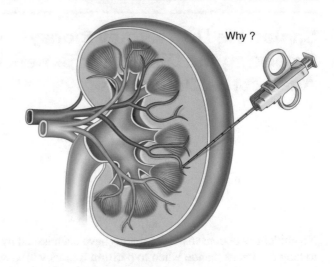

Fig. 19.2 Light
micrograph of a section
through a kidney biopsy
specimen showing the wall
of a muscular artery.
Haematoxylin and eosin ×4

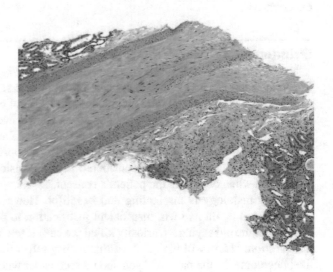

A diagnosis can often be made with sufficient confidence to begin treatment based upon clinical features and the results of other tests. The biopsy can then be deferred until the response to that treatment has been assessed.

Histology may sometimes provide a more precise prognosis, but the amount of proteinuria and the trend in eGFR are often sufficient. The histological appearances are often an unreliable guide to prognosis.

Performing a biopsy for academic purposes beyond the individual patient's needs requires explicit consent, as for a fully-fledged research study.

Conventional criteria for performing a biopsy are based upon the likelihood of finding a treatable disease [3]. They include:

- Proteinuria more than 1 g per day (PCR >100 mg/mmol, >1000 mg/g)
- eGFR declining over weeks or months, with or without haematuria and proteinuria
- Systemic illness with evidence of kidney involvement where a tissue diagnosis is needed

Exclusion criteria are based upon the likelihood of finding irreversible damage. They include:

- Reduced kidney size with thin cortical width on ultrasound scan
- eGFR declining over years

The risk of bleeding is greater in patients who have:

- uncontrolled high blood pressure
- high serum urea
- anaemia
- low platelets or abnormal clotting
- anticoagulant or antiplatelet therapy

The final decision whether to perform a biopsy rests with the patient. They may feel strongly that they want a definitive diagnosis of their condition, even if there is no treatment. Uncertainty about the diagnosis may affect their ability to get insurance or a job, such as joining the armed forces. Proof that there is no glomerular disease may be as helpful for a patient as finding a histological abnormality.

Is It Diabetic Nephropathy?

The 'to biopsy or not to biopsy' dilemma often arises in people with diabetes. As diabetes is so common, it is possible that the patient also has an unrelated kidney disease.

The first step is to image the kidneys with an ultrasound scan. Diabetic nephropathy does not affect the ultrasound appearances, other than sometimes increasing the echogenicity of the cortex so that the differentiation between the cortex and medulla is reduced.

If the ultrasound scan is normal, the following questions are helpful:

1. How long has the patient been diabetic?

   Nephropathy usually only develops once the patient has been diabetic for over 10 years. However, it can be difficult to estimate how long diabetes has been present as type 2 diabetes can remain asymptomatic for many years. The likelihood of finding diabetic nephropathy in the biopsy specimen is greater if there has been a long period of poor glucose control [4].

2. Does the patient have type 1 or type 2 diabetes?

   A kidney biopsy is much less likely to reveal pathology other than diabetic nephropathy in someone with type 1 rather than type 2 diabetes [5].

3. Has there been a change in the rate of decline in GFR?

   A typical rate of decline in GFR in someone with diabetic nephropathy is 3 mL/min/1.73 m^2 per year [6]. However, in patients with poorly controlled blood pressure or a long history of poor glucose control the decline can be faster than 10 mL/min/1.73 m^2 per year.

   As a rule of thumb, the slower the rate of decline, the less likely the loss will be reversible. A sudden change in the rate of decline is a sign that there may be a new and possibly treatable pathology (Patients 19.1 and 19.2).

4. Is there proteinuria or haematuria?

   A patient with reduced GFR due to diabetic nephropathy will usually (but not invariably [7]) have proteinuria with an albumin:creatinine ratio greater than 30 mg/mmol (300 mg/g). Conversely, there is usually no microscopic haematuria, or at most a trace. If there is no protein or both blood and protein on a urine dipstick test, there may be pathology other than diabetic nephropathy.

5. Is the patient hypertensive?

   Diabetic nephropathy with proteinuria leads to sodium and water retention and high blood pressure. If the patient has normal blood pressure on no antihypertensive treatment, it may not be diabetic nephropathy.

6. Are there other complications of diabetes?

   The microvascular and macrovascular effects of diabetes are usually not confined to the kidneys [8]. Patients with diabetic nephropathy usually have retinopathy [3] and often cardiovascular or peripheral vascular disease as well.

7. Are there blood tests indicating inflammation?

   Diabetic nephropathy is not an inflammatory disease. If the level of C-reactive protein (CRP) is increased and there is no obvious infection or other cause, the inflammation may be related to a kidney disease. Other immunological tests such as serum immunoglobulins and auto-antibodies can provide further information, although low titres of anti-nuclear and anti-cytoplasmic antibodies may be unrelated to kidney disease.

Patient 19.1 Crescentic Glomerulonephritis

Mr. Reynolds had had insulin-treated type 2 diabetes for 20 years. Despite good glucose and blood pressure control, his eGFR was progressively declining. He was otherwise well with only background diabetic retinopathy and no cardiovascular disease.

At a routine check-up, his eGFR was found to have dropped much further than expected from the previous trend (Fig. 19.2). The urine dipstick test showed blood and protein. CRP was 1 mg/L; anti-myeloperoxidase and proteinase 3 ANCA antibodies were not detected.

Stopping the ACE inhibitor treatment did not lead to any improvement. A kidney biopsy was performed. The specimen showed a crescentic glomerulonephritis.

He responded well to treatment with cyclophosphamide and prednisolone and his eGFR increased to near its previous level (Fig. 19.3).

Patient 19.2 Interstitial Nephritis

Mrs. Clarkson had type 2 diabetes, well controlled with metformin. She was troubled by gastro-oesophageal reflux and started taking a proton-pump inhibitor (PPI), omeprazole, for her symptoms. Six months later, her eGFR started to decline rapidly. Her urine contained no blood or protein. Her kidneys looked normal on an ultrasound scan. Full blood count (including eosinophils), CRP and immunological tests were normal.

A kidney biopsy showed acute interstitial nephritis, most likely caused by the PPI (Fig. 19.4).

The PPI was replaced by an H2-receptor antagonist (ranitidine) and she was treated with 30 mg prednisolone per day.

Her GFR steadily improved, although her glucose control became so erratic on the corticosteroids that she temporarily required insulin. She was left with some residual loss of kidney function (Fig. 19.5).

Kidney Biopsy in Nephrotic Syndrome and Vasculitis

The role of kidney biopsy in the diagnosis and assessment of some kidney diseases has changed as specific serological tests have become available.

Patients with the nephrotic syndrome and normal kidney function who are positive for anti-phospholipase A_2 receptor antibody (PLA_2R Ab) and have no evidence of an underlying cause can be assumed to have idiopathic membranous nephropathy without a biopsy [9].

Fig. 19.3 Fall in eGFR
due to crescentic
glomerulonephritis and rise
following treatment

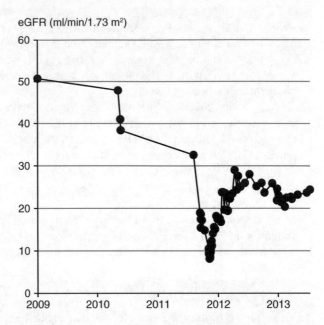

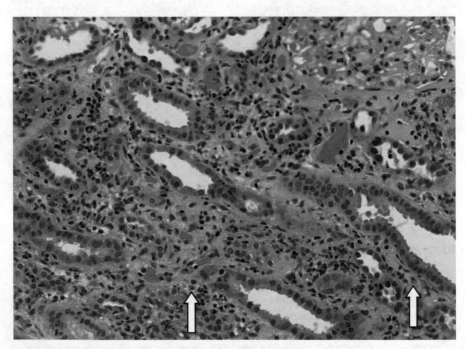

Fig. 19.4 Kidney biopsy section showing typical appearances of interstitial nephritis. There is an infiltration of inflammatory cells between the tubules, mainly lymphocytes with some eosinophils (*arrows*). The glomerulus (*top right*) is normal. Haematoxylin and eosin ×200

Fig. 19.5 Fall in eGFR due to interstitial nephritis and rise following treatment

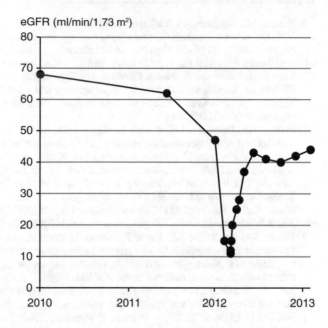

If a patient has typical clinical features of kidney vasculitis with a positive anti-PR3 or MPO ANCA and no evidence of a secondary vasculitis or false-positive ANCA, a biopsy may be delayed [10]. There are no biopsy features that guide the choice or duration of therapy.

Similarly, if the anti-GBM antibody titre is high and there are typical features of Goodpasture's syndrome, the biopsy may be deferred. It can be done later to investigate progressive disease or an atypical response to treatment. The practice of delaying the biopsy until after induction treatment is used in the management of lupus nephritis [11].

References

1. Hogan JJ, Mocanu M, Berns JS. The native kidney biopsy: update and evidence for best practice. Clin J Am Soc Nephrol. 2016;11(2):354–62. https://doi.org/10.2215/CJN.05750515. Epub 2015 Sep 2. https://cjasn.asnjournals.org/content/clinjasn/11/2/354.full.pdf.
2. Varnell CD Jr, Stone HK, Welge JA. Bleeding complications after pediatric kidney biopsy: a systematic review and meta-analysis. Clin J Am Soc Nephrol. 2019;14(1):57–65. https://doi.org/10.2215/CJN.05890518. Epub 2018 Dec 6. https://cjasn.asnjournals.org/content/clinjasn/14/1/57.full.pdf.
3. Dhaun N, Bellamy CO, Cattran DC, Kluth DC. Utility of renal biopsy in the clinical management of renal disease. Kidney Int. 2014;85(5):1039–48. https://doi.org/10.1038/ki.2013.512. Epub 2014 Jan 8. http://www.nature.com/ki/journal/v85/n5/full/ki2013512a.html.
4. Pallayova M, Mohammed A, Langman G, Taheri S, Dasgupta I. Predicting non-diabetic renal disease in type 2 diabetic adults: the value of glycated hemoglobin. J Diabetes Complications. 2015;29(5):718–23. https://doi.org/10.1016/j.jdiacomp.2014.12.005. pii: S1056-8727(14)00401-2. http://www.ncbi.nlm.nih.gov/pubmed/25633572.

5. Sharma SG, Bomback AS, Radhakrishnan J, Herlitz LC, Stokes MB, Markowitz GS, D'Agati VD. The modern spectrum of renal biopsy findings in patients with diabetes. Clin J Am Soc Nephrol. 2013;8:1718–24. https://www.ncbi.nlm.nih.gov/pmc/articles/PMC3789339/.
6. Ruggenenti P, Porrini EL, Gaspari F, Motterlini N, Cannata A, Carrara F, Cella C, Ferrari S, Stucchi N, Parvanova A, Iliev I, Dodesini AR, Trevisan R, Bossi A, Zaletel J, Remuzzi G, GFR Study Investigators. Glomerular hyperfiltration and renal disease progression in type 2 diabetes. Diabetes Care. 2012;35(10):2061–8. Epub 2012 Jul 6. http://care.diabetesjournals.org/content/35/10/2061.long.
7. Perkins BA, Ficociello LH, Roshan B, Warram JH, Krolewski AS. In patients with type 1 diabetes and new-onset microalbuminuria the development of advanced chronic kidney disease may not require progression to proteinuria. Kidney Int. 2010;77(1):57–64. https://doi.org/10.1038/ki.2009.399. http://www.nature.com/ki/journal/v77/n1/full/ki2009399a.html.
8. Klessens CQ, Woutman TD, Veraar KA, Zandbergen M, Valk EJ, Rotmans JI, Wolterbeek R, Bruijn JA, Bajema IM. An autopsy study suggests that diabetic nephropathy is underdiagnosed. Kidney Int. 2016;90(1):149–56. https://doi.org/10.1016/j.kint.2016.01.023. Epub 2016 Apr 9. https://www.kidney-international.org/article/S0085-2538%2816%2900313-6/fulltext.
9. Bobart SA, De Vriese AS, Pawar AS, Zand L, Sethi S, Giesen C, Lieske JC, Fervenza FC. Noninvasive diagnosis of primary membranous nephropathy using phospholipase A2 receptor antibodies. Kidney Int. 2019;95(2):429–38. https://doi.org/10.1016/j.kint.2018.10.021. https://www.kidney-international.org/article/S0085-2538(18)30822-6/fulltext.
10. Jayne D. Vasculitis-when can biopsy be avoided? Nephrol Dial Transplant. 2017;32(9):1454–6. https://doi.org/10.1093/ndt/gfx248. https://academic.oup.com/ndt/article/32/9/1454/4110253.
11. Hill GS, Delahousse M, Nochy D, Rémy P, Mignon F, Méry J-P, Bariéty J. Predictive power of the second renal biopsy in lupus nephritis: significance of macrophages. Kidney Int. 2001;59:304–16. https://www.sciencedirect.com/science/article/pii/S0085253815474666.

Kidney Stone Disease: A Link Between Nephrology and Urology

Kidney stones are common; about 9% of the United States population will develop kidney stones at some time. They are more common in men than women, although the incidence in women is rising faster than in men. Between countries, their prevalence varies from 2 to 20%, the highest being in men in the United Arab Emirates and Saudi Arabia [1].

The prevalence of stones has increased by 70% in the last 30 years, especially in children and young adults. Antibiotics may be one reason for this [2]. The type and relative number of bacteria in the gut are different in patients with and without kidney stones. Antibiotics alter the gut's bacterial balance and reduce oxalate breakdown by organisms such as *Oxalobacter formigenes*. The risk of stones is nearly doubled in the year following the use of common oral antibiotics [3].

Fifty-nine percent of stones are made of calcium oxalate, with or without small amounts of calcium phosphate. A further 10% are made predominantly of calcium phosphate. Seventeen percent are uric acid stones, 12% struvite or infection stones, and the remaining 2% are cystine (caused by cystin*uria*, not cystin*osis*) and other stones.

Most kidney stones are the result of a genetic predisposition compounded by environmental and lifestyle factors, such as a low fluid intake, a diet high in protein, salt, refined sugar and oxalate, and cola drinks. Stones are associated with type 2 diabetes, obesity, dyslipidaemia, and hypertension. Without a change in these factors, up to 40% of patients will form a second stone within 3 years of the first [1].

Other predisposing conditions include primary hyperparathyroidism, hypercalciuria and hypercalcaemia, and urinary tract infection. Inflammatory bowel disease (Fig. 20.1) and gastric bypass surgery used to treat morbid obesity lead to increased oxalate absorption in the gut.

Loss of fluid and alkali from an ileostomy leads to low volumes of acidic urine in which crystals are more likely to precipitate. Prolonged immobilization leads to loss of calcium from bones into the urine.

© Springer Nature Switzerland AG 2020
H. C. Rayner et al., *Understanding Kidney Diseases*,
https://doi.org/10.1007/978-3-030-43027-6_20

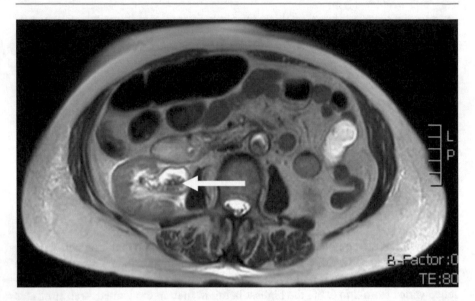

Fig. 20.1 MRI scan performed to investigate inflammatory bowel disease showing an incidental finding of a stone in the right kidney. T2 weighted image in which fluid appears white (note CSF in spinal canal). Stone (white arrow) appears black surrounded by white urine in the right renal pelvis

How Stones Form

The standard theory of stone formation is that, first, crystals precipitate in supersaturated urine. How these crystals stick to the urothelium to allow stones to form is not clear.

One theory is that deposits of apatite (calcium phosphate), known as Randall's plaques, form under the epithelium in areas where the ionic concentration is very high. A more recent theory is that molecules on the luminal surface of collecting duct epithelial cells cause crystals to stick and be taken up by endocytosis, where they are degraded or transported into the interstitium, perhaps to form Randall's plaques. As the plaques grow, they erode through the epithelium into the lumen, where calcium oxalate crystals stick to them and form stones.

Investigating Someone with a Kidney Stone

Patients with kidney stones typically present with renal colic—waves of severe pain radiating from the loin to the groin. Less common is pain restricted to the loin. There may also be visible haematuria, vomiting and sometimes fever. Stones can sometimes be discovered as an incidental finding in someone without symptoms.

The first step in the investigation [4] is to use imaging to look for any structural abnormality that is causing stasis of urine, such as pelvi-ureteric junction

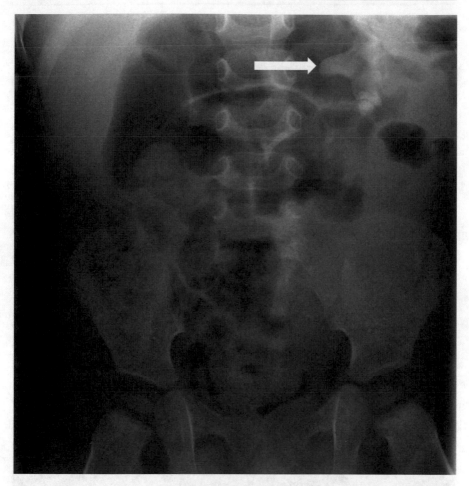

Fig. 20.2 Staghorn calculus (arrow) in the left kidney of a 3-month-old infant with congenital pelvi-ureteric junction obstruction. Note the unfused femoral heads

obstruction (Fig. 20.2), medullary sponge kidney (Fig. 20.3), horseshoe kidney (Fig. 20.4), or enterocystoplasty.

Next, the chemical composition of the stone should be identified, ideally by analysis of the stone itself. Ask the patient to try to catch the stone by passing urine through a tea strainer when they have colic.

A basic metabolic screen then includes serum urea and electrolytes, glucose, chloride, bicarbonate, uric acid, calcium, phosphate, magnesium, parathyroid hormone and vitamin D. This is to identify conditions such as diabetes, renal tubular acidosis, primary hyperparathyroidism and vitamin D toxicity. A high uric acid level is more relevant if the eGFR is normal; uric acid is excreted by glomerular filtration and so the level is inevitably high if the GFR is low.

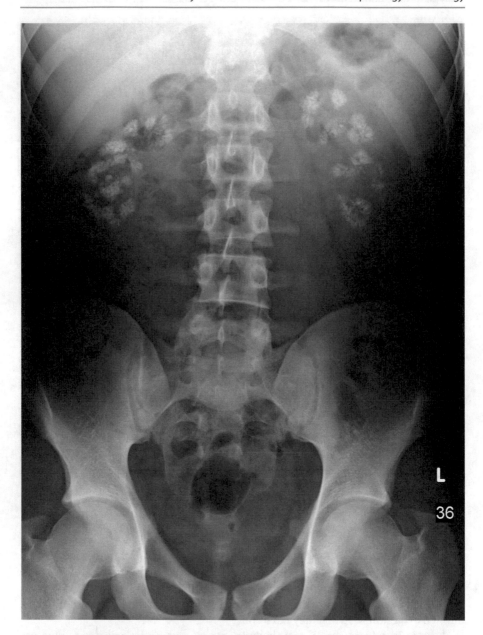

Fig. 20.3 Nephrocalcinosis due to medullary sponge kidney

As discussed in detail in Chap. 12, a negative urine dipstick for leukocytes and nitrites rules out infection, whereas a urine culture is needed to confirm infection. Urea-splitting organisms like *Proteus* sp., *Klebsiella* sp. and *Pseudomonas* sp. generate ammonium and produce struvite stones composed of ammonium-magnesium-phosphate. These stones are also caused by chronic laxative abuse, which stimulates ammonia production.

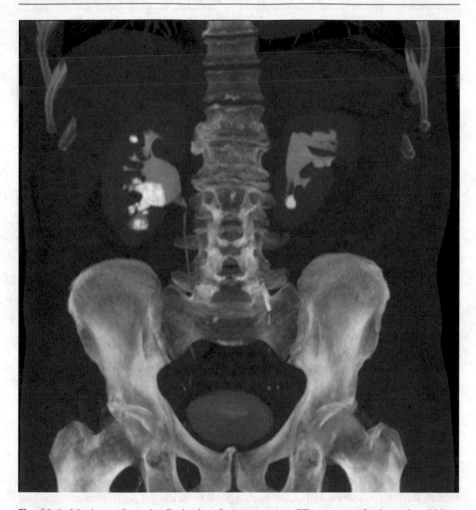

Fig. 20.4 Maximum Intensity Projection from a contrast CT urogram of a horseshoe kidney showing lower pole calculi (white) caused by impaired drainage of the renal pelvices. The ureters pass in front of the bridge of tissue between the two sides of the horseshoe, leading to partial obstruction of both pelvi-ureteric junctions

Patients aged under 25 years or with multiple or bilateral stones, uric acid stones, staghorn calculi (Fig. 20.5), nephrocalcinosis, a single kidney, or a history of recurrent stones should have more detailed metabolic tests, unless there is another obvious cause. A spot fasting sample of urine is tested for pH, electrolytes, protein, and cysteine. Retinol-binding protein and N-acetylglucosamine are measured if a proximal tubulopathy such as Fanconi syndrome or Dent's disease is suspected. 24-h urine collections are analyzed more thoroughly [1].

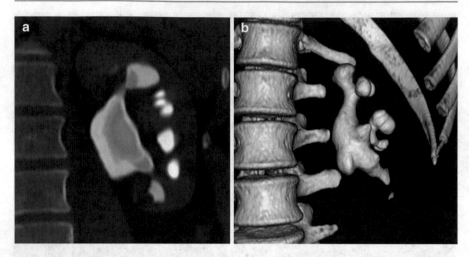

Fig. 20.5 (**a**) Coronal reconstruction from a CT urogram showing a staghorn calculus as a lower density (darker) filling defect within the excreted contrast (lighter). (**b**) 3D reformatted image from a non-contrast CT showing the staghorn calculus alone

Management of Kidney Stone Disease

Fluid and Diet

An increase in fluid intake and modification of the diet underpin the treatment of all types of kidney stones [5]. A urine volume of at least 2 L a day halves the rate of stone recurrence. Fluid intake should mainly be water, and tea or coffee should be taken with some milk to bind free oxalate.

Paradoxically, a low dietary calcium intake increases the risk of calcium oxalate stones, through an increase in oxalate absorption from the gut [6]. Calcium stone risk is reduced by having an adequate dietary calcium intake and avoiding excess sodium, protein, fat and oxalate. Oxalate-rich foods include spinach, rhubarb, beetroot, soya beans and tofu, nuts, peanut butter, okra, yams, sesame seeds, tahini and chocolate.

Replacing animal protein with fresh fruit and vegetables reduces urate excretion, alkalinizes the urine and increase urinary citrate excretion, which is a potent inhibitor of calcium oxalate and calcium phosphate stone formation. Beer increases urate excretion due to it containing the purine guanosine; wine has a much smaller effect.

Medication

Thiazide diuretics can reduce calcium oxalate stone formation by up to 70% in patients with idiopathic hypercalciuria. Allopurinol can be used in those with hyperuricaemia or hyperuricosuria. Citrate supplements can be tried but are often hard to tolerate.

Cystine stones are treated by reducing the concentration of free cystine in the urine and increasing its solubility. 4–5 L of fluid a day are required, including a drink during the night. If the 24-h urine cystine concentration remains <2000 mol/L, chelation therapy with D-penicillamine or tiopronin is used, ideally lowering the concentration to <500 mol/L. D-penicillamine can cause agranulocytosis and proteinuria, and needs careful dose adjustment.

Surgery

Surgical management of kidney stones depends on their size and site, symptoms and signs of obstruction, local expertise, and the patient's preference. About 70% of <5 mm ureteric stones and 50% of >5 and <10 mm stones will pass spontaneously. This is helped by alpha-blocker drugs, which increase stone passage by up to 30%. Ureteric stones larger than 10 mm should be removed endoscopically if pain persists despite intramuscular diclofenac or pethidine, or if there is obstruction (Fig. 20.6).

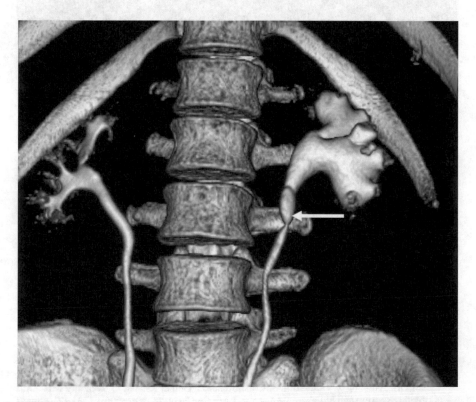

Fig. 20.6 CT urogram 3D reconstruction showing hydronephrosis caused by a stone (arrow) lodged in the left ureter. Iodinated contrast excreted in urine is shown in white. The kidney parenchyma is not visible

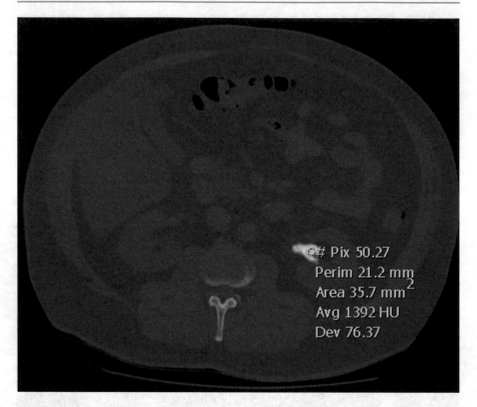

Fig. 20.7 CT scan showing a stone in the left renal pelvis with a radiological density of 1392 Hounsfield units (HU). Stones with a density >1000 HU are less likely to be successfully cleared with lithotripsy

Stones lodged within the kidney can be managed by shock wave lithotripsy, laser removal, or percutaneous nephrolithotomy. The density of the stone on a CT scan can guide the likely success of lithotripsy; denser stones are less likely to be cleared [7] (Fig. 20.7).

References

1. Johri N, Cooper B, Robertson W, Choong S, Rickards D, Unwin R. An update and practical guide to renal stone management. Nephron Clin Pract. 2010;116(3):c159–71. https://doi.org/10.1159/000317196. Epub 2010 Jul 2. https://www.karger.com/Article/Pdf/317196.
2. Nazzal L, Blaser MJ. Does the receipt of antibiotics for common infectious diseases predispose to kidney stones? A cautionary note for all health care practitioners. J Am Soc Nephrol. 2018;29:1590–2. https://doi.org/10.1681/ASN.2018040402.
3. Tasian GE, Jemielita T, Goldfarb DS, Copelovitch L, Gerber JS, Wu Q, Denburg MR. Oral antibiotic exposure and kidney stone disease. J Am Soc Nephrol. 2018;29(6):1731–40. https://doi.org/10.1681/ASN.2017111213. Epub 2018 May 10. https://jasn.asnjournals.org/content/jnephrol/29/6/1731.full.pdf.

4. Mabillard HR, Tomson CRV. Investigation and management of renal stone disease. Nephrol Dial Transplant. 2017;32(12):1984–6. https://doi.org/10.1093/ndt/gfx306. https://academic.oup.com/ndt/article/32/12/1984/4626877.

5. Zisman AL. Effectiveness of treatment modalities on kidney stone recurrence. CJASN. 2017;12(10):1699–708. https://doi.org/10.2215/CJN.11201016. https://cjasn.asnjournals.org/content/clinjasn/12/10/1699.full.pdf.

6. Borghi L, Schianchi T, Meschi T, Guerra A, Allegri F, Maggiore U, Novarini A. Comparison of two diets for the prevention of recurrent stones in idiopathic hypercalciuria. N Engl J Med. 2002;346:77–84. https://www.nejm.org/doi/10.1056/NEJMoa010369?url_ver=Z39.88-2003&rfr_id=ori:rid:crossref.org&rfr_dat=cr_pub%3dwww.ncbi.nlm.nih.gov.

7. Reynolds LF, Kroczak T, Pace KT. Indications and contraindications for shock wave lithotripsy and how to improve outcomes. Asian J Urol. 2018;5(4):256–63. https://doi.org/10.1016/j.ajur.2018.08.006. https://www.ncbi.nlm.nih.gov/pmc/articles/PMC6197584/.

Make a Plan: When and How to Prepare for End-Stage Kidney Disease

21

Once you have made a diagnosis of kidney disease, the next step is to agree a treatment plan with the patient. This chapter explains how to estimate a patient's prognosis and plan their kidney treatment.

Understanding Risk

Patients with a low eGFR and proteinuria have increased risks of both end-stage kidney disease and death, the latter largely due to cardiovascular disease. Damage to the endothelial cells in glomeruli that causes albuminuria reflects damage to the endothelium of blood vessels elsewhere in the body. These include the vasa vasorum that provide the blood supply to the walls of larger arteries. This may explain the link between albuminuria, uraemia and cardiovascular disease [1]. Measuring albuminuria or proteinuria is a useful way of measuring the health of someone's blood vessels and with it their risks of kidney failure and death.

Kidney Failure Risk

The risk of developing kidney failure can be estimated from the patient's age, eGFR and the level of proteinuria. Although the type of disease does play a part, when considering people with the same pathological condition the prognosis is largely determined by these three factors.

Data from a community mass-screening programme in Japan shows how the risk of kidney failure increases with the level of proteinuria [2]. Even small amounts are significant; having + proteinuria on a dipstick test increases the risk of end-stage kidney failure by 1.9 times in men and 2.4 times in women.

© Springer Nature Switzerland AG 2020
H. C. Rayner et al., *Understanding Kidney Diseases*,
https://doi.org/10.1007/978-3-030-43027-6_21

Mortality Risk

Figure 21.1 shows the relative risk of death for people in four age categories according to the level of eGFR and albuminuria.

In each chart, the columns show someone's risk of death compared to someone of the same age with normal kidney function and no albuminuria. One can draw a number of conclusions from these charts. Firstly, the lower the eGFR and the greater the albuminuria, the greater is the risk of death. eGFR and albuminuria each increases the risk in its own right. This applies to all age categories, implying that reduced eGFR and albuminuria are not inevitable features of ageing but represent markers of disease.

Secondly, the increase in relative risk is large, especially in the youngest age category. Someone aged 18–54 years with an eGFR of 15–29 and no albuminuria is 12 times more likely to die over the next 5.8 years than someone with an eGFR 75–89. Similarly, someone with a urine albumin:creatinine ratio > 34 mg/mmol (ACR >300 mg/g, dipstick ++ or more) but normal eGFR is nearly four times more likely to die. Combining the two factors increases the risk nearly 20 times.

Thirdly, the relative risk of death associated with reduced eGFR and albuminuria gets smaller with age. However, as the underlying risk of death in the reference group increases with age, the effect of reduced eGFR and albuminuria on the number of people dying per year is greater in the older age groups.

Association or Causation?

It is important to remember that measurements of the risk of death *associated with* eGFR and albuminuria do not mean that reduced kidney function or albuminuria in some way *cause* the deaths, or that increasing eGFR or reducing albuminuria will necessarily reduce the risk of death. Proving causation requires an interventional study, such as a randomised controlled trial, rather than an observational study.

The effect of reduced eGFR on outcomes has been studied in kidney donors. When one of their kidneys is removed, donors go from normal kidney function to CKD Stage 2 or 3. Does this reduced eGFR increase their risk of future cardiovascular disease? The answer seems to be 'yes, slightly'. Comparing Canadian kidney donors with the healthiest segment of the general population there is no increase in the risk of major cardiovascular events over the next 10 years [4]. However, left ventricular mass does increase during the 12 months after nephrectomy [5] and donors have twice the risk of developing high blood pressure or pre-eclampsia in pregnancy (11% versus 5%) [6]. The risk of developing kidney failure over the 15 years after donation is also increased by between 3.5 and 5.3 times, although the absolute risk remains very low (0.24% among black men, 0.15% among black women, 0.06% among white men, and 0.04% among white women) [7].

Studies in animal models of more advanced kidney disease suggest a causal link between reduced kidney function and heart disease such as left ventricular hypertrophy. The kidney tubular epithelium is the main producer of a protein called Klotho,

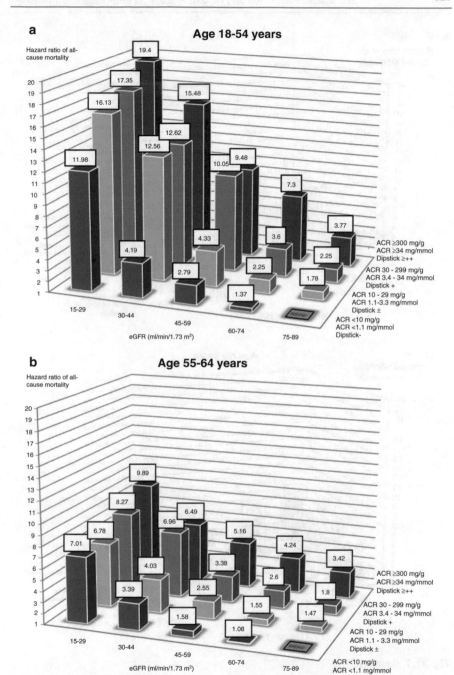

Fig. 21.1 Risk of mortality associated with eGFR and albuminuria by age category (**a**) 18–54 years, (**b**) 55–64 years, (**c**) 65–74 years, (**d**) 75+ years. The reference category is eGFR = 75–89 mL/min/1.73 m² with urine dipstick showing no proteinuria or an albumin:creatinine ratio <1.1 mg/mmol (<10 mg/g). (Drawn using data from [3])

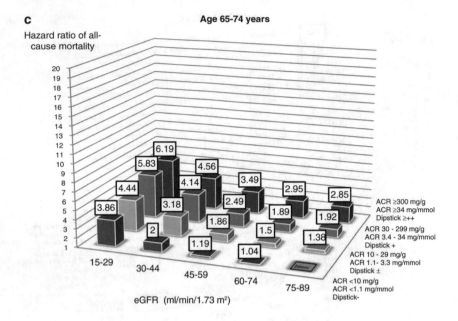

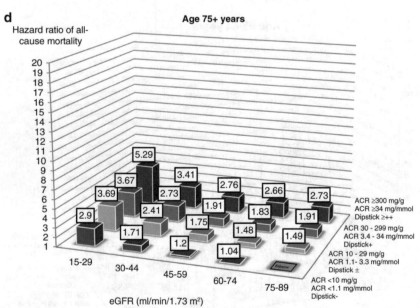

Fig. 21.1 (continued)

named after the Greek mythological figure Clotho who spins the thread of life. It is released into the circulation like a hormone and has anti-aging properties. In chronic kidney disease, levels of Klotho are reduced and so too is its cardioprotective effect [8].

Knowing about your risk of dying is only useful if something can be done about it. The opportunity to alter the natural history of disease is more limited as people get older. Nonetheless, lowering blood pressure to a target of 150/80 mmHg in people aged over 80 years who are otherwise well reduces the rate of death, stroke and heart failure within 1–2 years [9]. On the other hand, over-aggressive treatment of blood pressure in elderly people with other comorbidities increases the risk of falls and harm.

Finally, the wishes of the patient must be taken into account when deciding how much attention to give to these risk factors. An elderly person suffering from a number of long-term conditions may give a much higher priority to improving the quality of their life than its length.

Competing Risks: Dialysis or Death?

Studies of populations of patients with chronic kidney disease show that, for a given level of eGFR, the risk of dying before dialysis is needed increases with age (Fig. 21.2).

When analyzing data on a population of patients to study factors associated with starting dialysis or dying, it is important to use a method that allows for the fact that these two outcomes are not independent. Survival analyses measure the time between a patient entering the study and the event of interest. Patients who die during the follow up period are censored.

Censoring requires two conditions to be met for it to be statistically valid. The first condition is that the event of interest would eventually be observed in all

Fig. 21.2 Competing risks of end-stage kidney disease (ESKD) and death according to age and eGFR for people with chronic kidney disease. (Based upon [10, 11])

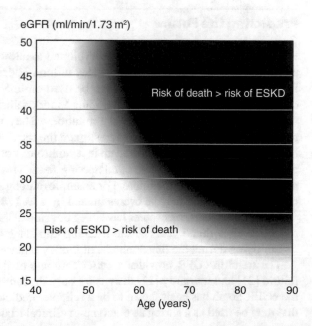

participants if the study lasted long enough. In a study where the event is starting dialysis, this is not the case; kidney failure cannot occur after death, and the opposite outcome 'death without kidney failure' cannot occur after dialysis has been started.

The second condition is that censoring is unrelated to an individual patient's prognosis. Again, this is not the case; a patient who dies is likely to have health issues that would have led to them starting dialysis earlier than someone who does not die. Statistical methods are available that account for these competing risks [12].

The Gender Paradox

The worldwide number of men with reduced kidney function has been estimated to be 336 million, whereas the estimated number of women is 417 million, a ratio of 0.81. Conversely, an estimated 1.7 million men are treated with dialysis and 0.4 million have a functioning kidney transplant, compared with only 1.3 million and 0.3 million women respectively, ratios of 1.3 [13].

The explanation for why a higher prevalence of women have chronic kidney disease but men are more likely to have dialysis or a kidney transplant is elusive. It is a phenomenon replicated in many other aspects of health, which has been summarized in the phrase "women get sick and men die" [14]. It raises concern that women are being discriminated against in the provision of kidney replacement therapy. However, the ratio of men to women receiving kidney replacement therapy has been remarkably stable over long periods of time and across multiple countries, making a biological explanation more likely [15].

Predicting the Future

Risk prediction equations have been developed to allow individual patients to estimate their likelihood of developing kidney failure. The most popular are the Kidney Failure Risk Equations [16] which can be used on-line at kidneyfailurerisk.com to calculate the percentage risk of developing kidney failure over 2 and 5 years.

These equations have important limitations. They were developed from large population databases and may underestimate the risk for the selected population of higher risk patients being followed up in a nephrology clinic [17]. Secondly, they do not fully allow for the problem of competing risks. This is increasingly relevant for predictions further into the future. For example, among men at high-risk, the 5-year risk of kidney failure may be overestimated by 27% (78% versus 51%) [18].

For older patients, risk scores have been developed that give an assessment of the risk of death within 5 years before reaching end-stage kidney disease [19] and the risk of dying during the first 3 months of kidney replacement therapy [20].

The trend in eGFR provides a better estimate of the risk of end-stage kidney failure [21] and mortality [22] than using only the latest eGFR value. The slope of the eGFR graph has been shown to be a reliable predictor of longer-term outcomes that may be used as a surrogate outcome in clinical trials [23].

Changes in albuminuria are also predictive of the risk of kidney failure and death. Compared to patients with a stable urine albumin:creatinine ratio (ACR), a four-fold increase in ACR is associated with three-fold greater risk of kidney failure over 3 years. Conversely, a four-fold decrease in ACR is associated with a one third lower risk [24].

Complex analytical techniques can be applied to serial values to predict risk [25] and the kidney failure risk equations have evolved to incorporate changes in eGFR over time [26].

Predictions of percentage risk are helpful for identifying categories of people who may benefit from more intensive assessment and treatment. However, these risk estimates do not help an individual patient who wants to know if and when a significant event, such as starting dialysis, is likely to happen. In most chronic medical conditions, we can only offer an individual patient a probability of what might happen in the future. With kidney disease, we can often also make a prediction of when.

Prognostication: "Be Prepared"

Many patients who attend the kidney clinic are anxious that they may need to start dialysis soon. A key part of the doctor's role is to provide as good an estimate of the patient's prognosis as possible.

Patients and kidney specialists are generally overly pessimistic about the future [27]. When doctors in an outpatient nephrology clinic were asked the 'surprise' question, "Would you be surprised if this patient died in the next 12 months?" about patients over 60 years of age with CKD Stages 4 and 5 not on dialysis, only 27% of those about whom the doctor answered 'no' actually died during the follow up period [28].

There is a long tradition of using a graph of kidney function to predict when a patient may need to start dialysis. In the past, a plot of the reciprocals of the serum creatinine values was used [29] but the data points did not relate directly to the GFR and so it was hard to identify the time when dialysis would be needed. The eGFR graph overcomes these problems (Patient 21.1).

Patient 21.1 Projection of the eGFR Graph to Predict the Need for Dialysis
Mr. Arnold had been followed regularly in the clinic for his kidney disease. Over a 9-year period, his eGFR had declined by 15 mL/min/1.73 m^2 (Fig. 21.3).

To predict the future, a trendline was projected on the chart (Fig. 21.4).

If Mr. Arnold's loss of kidney function continued at the same rate, he would reach an eGFR of 10 mL/min/1.73 m^2 at the age of 97 years. He was very relieved to know that he did not need to worry about having dialysis for the foreseeable future.

The eGFR graph can be used as a screening tool to identify patients in the community at high risk of progressive kidney disease who would benefit from a

Fig. 21.3 Decline in eGFR by approximately 1.5 mL/min/1.73 m² per year

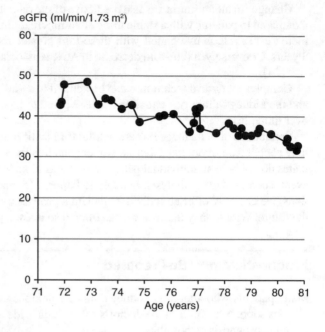

Fig. 21.4 Projection of the trendline to eGFR = 10 mL/min/1.73 m²

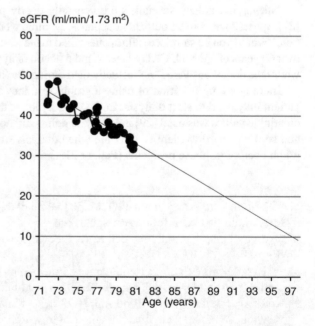

specialist assessment [30]. This system has been implemented in many pathology laboratories through a national project in the United Kingdom [31].

When the trendline on the eGFR graph indicates that someone is likely to need dialysis, care should be planned accordingly. We can learn how to do this from the example of another condition in which health needs are predictable—pregnancy.

Ante-natal classes are provided to help parents prepare for an event that will transform their lives. Like having a baby, kidney failure and dialysis can disrupt your sleep and leave you feeling exhausted. Like bringing up a child, dialysis limits your freedom and continues week-in, week-out for years.

Education and care of patients with advanced kidney failure is provided by a team of professionals, coordinated around the needs of the patient. They address issues that also feature in ante-natal classes, such as:

- Choice of medical treatment
- Symptom control and self-care
- Keeping physically active
- Psychological support
- Involvement of carers and relatives

A comprehensive geriatric assessment [32] should be included in the care plan of older patients with chronic kidney disease [33].

The decision about when to transfer care to the multidisciplinary team is determined by the time needed to prepare for dialysis or a kidney transplant. In pregnancy there are 9 months to prepare; in kidney failure a year is ideal, possibly longer if a transplant is the preferred option. Asking the 'surprise' question is helpful: "Would you be surprised if this patient needed to start dialysis within the next year?"

The eGFR graph helps answer this question. The rate of decline in eGFR varies between patients so there is no single value of eGFR when planning should start. Instead, projecting the eGFR graph forwards to 10 mL/min/1.73 m^2 will give an estimate of the time remaining (Fig. 21.5).

Fig. 21.5 Examples of differences in the rate of decline of eGFR between three patients. Transfer to the multi-professional team occurred at different levels of eGFR to allow at least a year for preparation for transplantation or dialysis

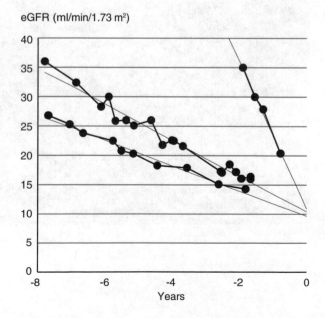

It is wise to have a lower limit of 15 mL/min/1.73 m^2 for referral. When the remaining kidney function is this low, an unpredictable acute illness can bring forward the need for dialysis. When a transplant is planned as the first kidney replacement therapy, it is usually carried out when eGFR falls below 15 mL/min/1.73 m^2 to reduce the risk of unplanned dialysis.

The following story (Patient 21.2) illustrates the kinds of problems that may be addressed during the period of preparation.

Patient 21.2 Planning Dialysis

Mr. Fielding was a 72-year-old retired businessman who divided his time between the family home in Birmingham and a business in Wales. His type 2 diabetes was well treated with insulin but his blood pressure was not well controlled. He reported home systolic blood pressure readings between 165 and 170 mmHg despite taking four antihypertensive drugs.

His kidney function had steadily deteriorated through the late 1990s due to progressive diabetic nephropathy. At a clinic visit in February 2003 his eGFR graph predicted that he would reach end-stage kidney failure in 2005 (Fig. 21.6).

We talked at length about what type of dialysis he would wish to have, a kidney transplant being inappropriate because of angina. In the end he settled on peritoneal dialysis, which would suit his need to return to Wales at regular intervals to manage the business. As he had had no previous abdominal surgery, the peritoneal dialysis catheter could be inserted under a local anaesthetic nearer the time.

A year later, the graph showed that his eGFR had declined as predicted to 15 mL/min/1.73 m^2 (Fig. 21.7).

His care was transferred to the multi-disciplinary predialysis clinic where he could see the specialist nurses, dietitian, anaemia nurse, social worker and consultant at the same visit.

Because of his reduced GFR, his insulin requirements had declined and he was having hypoglycaemia at night. His insulin dose was reduced accordingly. Otherwise, he was asymptomatic and it was agreed not to make further preparations for dialysis for the time being. However, he decided that the time had come for him to sell up the business in Wales.

By 2006, he had become more breathless due to anaemia and was treated with erythropoietin. Then, tragically, his wife became very ill. Having sold the business, Mr. Fielding was able to devote himself to caring for his wife. She sadly died in late 2006.

During this time, his eGFR had been stable, confounding our predictions that he would need dialysis (Fig. 21.8). He was not critical of us; indeed, he was grateful that we had helped him make the decision to sell his business in Wales as this had enabled him to care for his wife throughout her illness.

After the death of his wife, Mr. Fielding's physical and emotional health declined. His eyesight deteriorated and he moved into sheltered accommodation. It became clear that haemodialysis would be more suitable for him than peritoneal dialysis. An arteriovenous fistula was formed in his left forearm in September 2008. An operation in March 2009 improved the blood flow so that the fistula could be cannulated when the time came to start dialysis.

In 2009, 4 years later than predicted, he became more symptomatic of kidney failure. His eGFR reached 7.1 mL/min/1.73 m², urea 44.9 mmol/L (126 mg/dL), calcium 2.17 mmol/L (8.7 mg/dL), phosphate 2.82 mmol/L (8.7 mg/dL), venous bicarbonate 15.1 mmol/L (mEq/L) (Fig. 21.9).

Dialysis was started as a routine outpatient procedure using his arteriovenous fistula.

Fig. 21.6 Projected decline in eGFR using a trendline

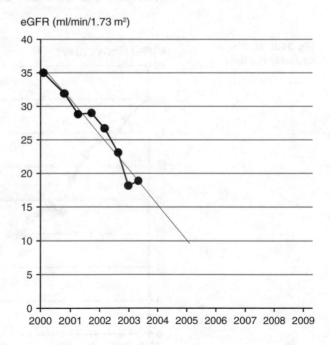

Fig. 21.7 Continued
decline in eGFR along the
projected trendline

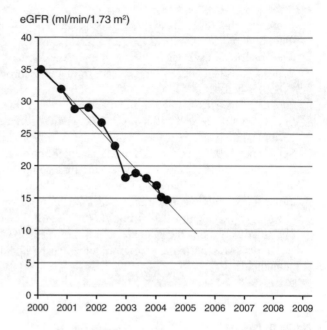

Fig. 21.8 Slowing of
decline in eGFR

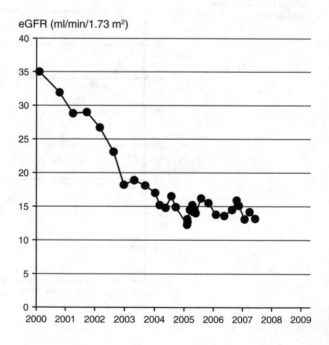

Fig. 21.9 eGFR decline to the start of dialysis

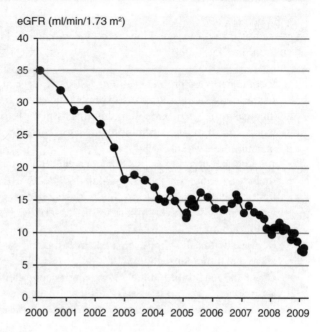

Writing Letters to Patients

Good Medical Practice guidance from the governing body for doctors in the UK, the General Medical Council, states that doctors should:

• Give patients the information they want or need in a way they can understand
• Support patients in caring for themselves to improve and maintain their health

The letter written following an outpatient consultation is a great opportunity to support patients in managing their own health. This is best achieved by writing the letter directly to the patient, a practice recommended by the Academy of Medical Royal Colleges [34]. A copy of this letter is sent to the patient's General Practitioner.

The letter should answer all the questions the patient asks about their condition and its treatment. Your answers should be understandable and accurate. Writing letters that have both of these qualities takes practice. In Chap. 23 we have listed some of the questions more commonly asked by kidney patients. You can use them as exercises for practicing writing letters to patients and compare our suggested answers with your own.

Some tips for writing good letters to kidney patients. For a more detailed discussion see [35]:

- List the patient's problems and diagnoses in a list at the start of the letter
- In the body of the letter, use simpler words with the same meaning as medical terms, e.g. 'kidney' rather than 'renal'. Explain any jargon. Avoid words that may be misinterpreted, e.g. 'chronic' may be interpreted as meaning 'really bad'
- Avoid acronyms such as AKI, CKD and ESKD
- Include a medication list using English rather than Latin (e.g. bd) and highlight any changes, e.g. 'furosemide **increased** to 80 mg twice a day'
- Use graphs wherever you can to describe changes in results, e.g. eGFR, albumin
- Remove words and phrases that add little meaning and keep sentences short
- Have one topic per paragraph
- Check the readability of the letter using a score such as the Flesch Reading Ease Score.

Choosing Treatment: Transplant, Haemodialysis, Peritoneal Dialysis or No Dialysis?

For most patients with end-stage kidney disease it is easy to make the decision to have kidney replacement therapy. For fitter, younger patients, the best outcomes come from having a transplant from a living donor before dialysis is needed—a preemptive transplant. This can be a kidney alone or, for some patients with diabetes, a kidney and a pancreas.

If dialysis is felt to be the right choice, is there any difference between haemodialysis or peritoneal dialysis? Studies have not shown a consistent survival advantage for either type of dialysis. Peritoneal dialysis offers greater independence but imposes a greater responsibility on the patient. Those patients who have dialysis at home, either peritoneal or haemodialysis, have a better quality of life compared to patients having in-centre dialysis.

The eventual decision should be determined mainly by the patient's choice. Some patients find written or web-based information helpful, such as at www.nhs.uk/conditions/Dialysis/Pages/Introduction.aspx.

For some patients the decision whether or not to have dialysis is more difficult. The burden of the treatment may outweigh its benefits. The journey back and forth to the dialysis unit three times every week can be exhausting. Patients may feel unwell during the treatment and tired for hours afterwards [36].

Patients with cognitive impairment may be made more confused by dialysis. Patients who are older, frail or with multiple co-morbidities may consider the quality of their remaining life to be more important than its length and choose to have their symptoms controlled with conservative care rather than start or continue with dialysis [37].

When Should Dialysis Be Started?

Dialysis should be started when the benefits outweigh the harm and inconvenience. The 'Initiating Dialysis Early And Late' (IDEAL) study reassures us that starting dialysis earlier than this is not beneficial in adults [38]. In the trial, the start of dialysis was delayed by an average of 6 months in the later start group, eGFR falling to 7.2 mL/min/1.73 m^2 compared to 9.0 in the early start group. An observational study suggests that an early start is also not beneficial for children [39].

In the UK, the mean eGFR at the start of dialysis in adults is 7.5 mL/min/1.73 m^2. This is much lower than in the US, a difference only partly explained by differences between UK and US patients.

Oedema, both pulmonary and peripheral, which cannot be controlled with high doses or a combination of diuretics, is a common reason to start dialysis. Increasing tiredness, loss of appetite and finally nausea may prompt the start.

A rise in serum phosphate and fall in serum bicarbonate, in addition to a high urea and low eGFR, are useful signs that the true GFR is low enough to warrant dialysis (Patient 21.3).

Patient 21.3 Starting Dialysis by Symptoms Rather Than Numbers

Mr. Shaw was a retired man aged 70 years. He felt well and was able to do all his usual activities. He had a good appetite and ate well. He took regular exercise and had not lost any body weight or muscle bulk.

He was taking sodium bicarbonate 1 g twice daily, alfacalcidol 0.25 μg daily, erythropoietin and no dietary phosphate binders. He had chosen to have haemodialysis and had a functioning arterio-venous fistula in his left forearm.

He was seen monthly in clinic. His eGFR had declined from 7.5 to 5.0 mL/min/1.73 m^2 over last 12 months. Table 21.1 shows his blood results.

Despite the low eGFR, dialysis was not started. The true GFR was likely higher than the estimated GFR because of his good muscle bulk. The relatively high urea (BUN) was related to his good protein intake.

Table 21.1 Laboratory results from Mr. Shaw

	Concentration	Normal range	Non-SI units
Sodium	145 mmol/L	133–146	145 mEq/L
Potassium	5.2 mmol/L	3.5–5.3	5.2 mEq/L
Urea	34.7 mmol/L	2.5–7.8	BUN 97 mg/dL
Creatinine	850 μmol/L	64–111	9.6 mg/dL
eGFR	5.0 mL/min/1.73 m²		
Bicarbonate	22.5 mmol/L	22.0–29.0	22.5 mEq/L
Albumin	39 g/L	35–50	3.9 g/dL
Calcium (corrected for serum albumin)	2.51 mmol/L	2.20–2.60	10.0 mEq/L
Phosphate	1.40 mmol/L	0.80–1.50	4.3 mEq/L
Haemoglobin	111 g/L	135–180	11.1 g/dL

Care of the Whole Person

It would be wrong not to emphasise the importance of psychosocial factors in the progression and treatment of kidney failure. Observational studies have shown a strong association between the amount of social support a person has and their risk of developing kidney failure [40] and of having a poorer quality of life and dying when on dialysis [41].

Anxiety and depression are common amongst people with kidney disease. Being depressed is one of the strongest markers for mortality in people on dialysis [42].

Replacing kidney function is only one aspect of the care needed by people with kidney failure. Support in the form of exercise programs [43] and psychological therapies [44] are an important part of the package of care (Fig. 21.10). Involving patients in their own care is, for some patients, an effective way of improving the experience of dialysis [45].

Death: Not the End of the Story

Patients receiving long term kidney care often develop strong relationships with their clinical team. Indeed, this is one of the many reasons why a clinical career in nephrology is so rewarding. These relationships do not cease at the time of death. The death of a dialysis patient can have a profound effect on the staff as well as on other patients in the dialysis unit, and the bereavement needs of the patient's family should not be overlooked [47].

Staff from the dialysis unit may attend the patient's funeral, to represent the clinical team and pay their respects. Our nephrology department holds an annual memorial service, led by medical and nursing staff and supported by a hospital chaplain and an imam, to which the relatives of all patients who have died in the previous year are invited. It is very much appreciated by those who attend.

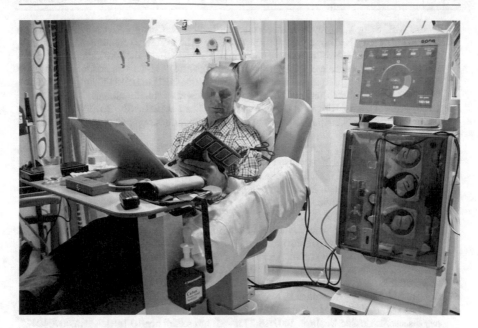

Fig. 21.10 Dialysis is one part of holistic care for patients with kidney failure. Time spent having dialysis can be put to good use with activities such as exercise or, as here, art [46]

References

1. Harper SJ, Bates DO. Endothelial permeability in uremia. Kidney Int. 2003;63:S41–4. https://doi.org/10.1046/j.1523-1755.63.s84.15.x. http://www.nature.com/ki/journal/v63/n84s/abs/4493766a.html.
2. Iseki K, Ikemiya Y, Iseki C, Takishita S. Proteinuria and the risk of developing end-stage renal disease. Kidney Int. 2003;63:1468–74. http://www.nature.com/ki/journal/v63/n4/full/4493578a.html.
3. Hallan SI, Matsushita K, Sang Y, Mahmoodi BK, Black C, Ishani A, Kleefstra N, Naimark D, Roderick P, Tonelli M, Wetzels JFM, Astor BC, Gansevoort RT, Levin A, Wen C-P, Coresh J, for the CKD Prognosis Consortium. Age and the association of kidney measures with mortality and end-stage renal disease. JAMA. 2012;308(22):2349–60. https://doi.org/10.1001/jama.2012.16817. http://jama.jamanetwork.com/article.aspx?articleid=1387683.
4. Garg AX, Meirambayeva A, Huang A, Kim J, Prasad GVR, Knoll G, et al. Cardiovascular disease in kidney donors: matched cohort study. BMJ. 2012;344:e1203. http://www.bmj.com/content/344/bmj.e1203.
5. Moody WE, Ferro CJ, Edwards NC, Chue CD, Lin ELS, Taylor RJ, Cockwell P, Steeds RP, Townend JN, on behalf of the CRIB-Donor Study Investigators. Cardiovascular effects of unilateral nephrectomy in living kidney donors. Hypertension. 2016;67:368–77. https://doi.org/10.1161/HYPERTENSIONAHA.115.06608.
6. Garg AX, Nevis IF, McArthur E, Sontrop JM, Koval JJ, Lam NN, Hildebrand AM, Reese PP, Storsley L, Gill JS, Segev DL, Habbous S, Bugeja A, Knoll GA, Dipchand C, Monroy-Cuadros M, Lentine KL, for the DONOR Network. Gestational hypertension and preeclampsia in living kidney donors. NEJM. 2014; https://doi.org/10.1056/NEJMoa1408932. http://www.nejm.org/doi/full/10.1056/NEJMoa1408932.

7. Grams ME, Sang Y, Levey AS, Matsushita K, Ballew S, Chang AR, Chow EK, Kasiske BL, Kovesdy CP, Nadkarni GN, Shalev V, Segev DL, Coresh J, Lentine KL, Garg AX, Chronic Kidney Disease Prognosis Consortium. Kidney-failure risk projection for the living kidney-donor candidate. N Engl J Med. 2016;374(5):411–21. https://doi.org/10.1056/NEJMoa1510491. https://www.nejm.org/doi/10.1056/NEJMoa1510491?url_ver=Z39.88-2003&rfr_id=ori:rid:crossref.org&rfr_dat=cr_pub%3dwww.ncbi.nlm.nih.gov.

8. Fu H, Liu Y. Loss of Klotho in CKD breaks one's heart. JASN ASN. 2015020200. https://doi.org/10.1681/ASN.2015020200. http://jasn.asnjournals.org/content/early/2015/03/23/ASN.2015020200.

9. Beckett NS, Peters R, Fletcher AE, Staessen JA, Liu L, Dumitrascu D, Stoyanovsky V, Antikainen RL, Nikitin Y, Anderson C, Belhani A, Forette F, Rajkumar C, Thijs L, Banya W, Bulpitt CJ, HYVET Study Group. Treatment of hypertension in patients 80 years of age or older. N Engl J Med. 2008;358:1887–98. http://www.nejm.org/doi/full/10.1056/NEJMoa0801369#t=article.

10. De Nicola L, Minutolo R, Chiodini P, Borrelli S, Zoccali C, Postorino M, Iodice C, Nappi F, Fuiano G, Gallo C, Conte G, for the Italian Society of Nephrology Study Group 'TArget Blood pressure LEvels (TABLE) in CKD. The effect of increasing age on the prognosis of non-dialysis patients with chronic kidney disease receiving stable nephrology care. Kidney Int. 2012;82:482–8. https://doi.org/10.1038/ki.2012.174. http://www.nature.com/ki/journal/v82/n4/full/ki2012174a.html.

11. O'Hare AM, Choi AI, Bertenthal D, Bacchetti P, Garg AX, Kaufman JS, Walter LC, Mehta KM, Steinman MA, Allon M, McClellan WM, Landefeld CS. Age affects outcomes in chronic kidney disease. J Am Soc Nephrol. 2007;18:2758–65. https://doi.org/10.1681/ASN.2007040422. http://jasn.asnjournals.org/content/18/10/2758.long.

12. Hsu JY, Roy JA, Xie D, Yang W, Shou H, Anderson AH, Landis JR, Jepson C, Wolf M, Isakova T, Rahman M, Feldman HI; Chronic Renal Insufficiency Cohort (CRIC) Study Investigators. Statistical methods for cohort studies of CKD: Survival analysis in the setting of competing risks. Clin J Am Soc Nephrol 2017;12(7):1181–1189. https://doi.org/10.2215/CJN.10301016. Epub 2017 Feb 27. https://cjasn.asnjournals.org/content/12/7/1181.long.

13. Bikbov B, Perico N, Remuzzi G, on behalf of the GBD Genitourinary Diseases Expert Group. Disparities in chronic kidney disease prevalence among males and females in 195 countries: analysis of the global burden of disease 2016 study. Nephron. 2018;139:313–8. PMID: 29791905. https://www.karger.com/Article/FullText/489897.

14. Tomlinson LA, Clase CM. Sex and the incidence and prevalence of kidney disease. CJASN 2019:CJN.11030919. https://doi.org/10.2215/CJN.11030919. https://cjasn.asnjournals.org/content/early/2019/10/23/CJN.11030919?papetoc.

15. Antlanger M, Noordzij M, van de Luijtgaarden M, Carrero JJ, Palsson R, Finne P, Hemmelder MH, Aresté-Fosalba N, Varberg Reisæter A, Cases A, Traynor JP, Kramar R, Massy Z, Jager KJ, Hecking M and on behalf of the ERA-EDTA Registry. Sex differences in kidney replacement therapy initiation and maintenance. CJASN 2019:CJN.04400419; https://doi.org/10.2215/CJN.04400419. https://cjasn.asnjournals.org/content/early/2019/10/23/CJN.04400419.full.

16. Tangri N, Stevens LA, Griffith J, Tighiouart H, Djurdjev O, Naimark D, Levin A, Levey AS. A predictive model for progression of chronic kidney disease to kidney failure. JAMA. 2011;305:1553–9. https://jamanetwork.com/journals/jama/fullarticle/897102.

17. Sawhney S, Beaulieu M, Black C, Djurdjev O, Espino-Hernandez G, Marks A, McLernon DJ, Sheriff Z, Levin A. Predicting kidney failure risk after acute kidney injury among people receiving nephrology clinic care. Nephrol Dial Transplant. 2018; https://doi.org/10.1093/ndt/gfy294. https://academic.oup.com/ndt/advance-article/doi/10.1093/ndt/gfy294/5133052.

18. Ravani P, Fiocco M, Liu P, Quinn RR, Hemmelgarn B, James M, Lam N, Manns B, Oliver MJ, Strippoli GFM, Tonelli M. Influence of mortality on estimating the risk of kidney failure in people with stage 4 chronic kidney disease. JASN 2019:ASN.2019060640. https://doi.org/10.1681/ASN.2019060640. https://jasn.asnjournals.org/content/early/2019/09/19/ASN.2019060640.full

19. Bansal N, Katz R, De Boer IH, Peralta CA, Fried LF, Siscovick DS, Rifkin DE, Hirsch C, Cummings SR, Harris TB, Kritchevsky SB, Sarnak MJ, Shlipak MG, Joachim H. Development and validation of a model to predict 5-year risk of death without ESRD among older adults with CKD. CJASN CJN.04650514. https://doi.org/10.2215/CJN.04650514. http://cjasn.asn-journals.org/content/early/2015/02/18/CJN.04650514.abstract.

20. Couchoud CG, Beuscart JB, Aldigier JC, Brunet PJ, Moranne OP, REIN Registry. Development of a risk stratification algorithm to improve patient-centered care and decision making for incident elderly patients with end-stage renal disease. Kidney Int. 2015;88(5):1178–86. https://doi.org/10.1038/ki.2015.245. Epub 2015 Sep 2. https://www.kidney-international.org/article/S0085-2538(15)61002-X/fulltext.

21. Kovesdy CP, Coresh J, Ballew SH, Woodward M, Levin A, Naimark DM, Nally J, Rothenbacher D, Stengel B, Iseki K, Matsushita K, Levey AS, CKD Prognosis Consortium. Past decline versus current eGFR and subsequent ESRD risk. J Am Soc Nephrol. 2016;27(8):2447–55. https://doi.org/10.1681/ASN.2015060687. Epub 2015 Dec 11. https://jasn.asnjournals.org/content/27/8/2447.long.

22. Naimark DM, Grams ME, Matsushita K, Black C, Drion I, Fox CS, Inker LA, Ishani A, Jee SH, Kitamura A, Lea JP, Nally J, Peralta CA, Rothenbacher D, Ryu S, Tonelli M, Yatsuya H, Coresh J, Gansevoort RT, Warnock DG, Woodward M, de Jong PE, CKD Prognosis Consortium. Past decline versus current eGFR and subsequent mortality risk. J Am Soc Nephrol. 2016;27(8):2456–66. https://doi.org/10.1681/ASN.2015060688. Epub 2015 Dec 11. https://jasn.asnjournals.org/content/27/8/2456.long.

23. Inker LA, Heerspink HJL, Tighiouart H, Levey AS, Coresh J, Gansevoort RT, Simon AL, Ying J, Beck GJ, Wanner C, Floege J, Li PK, Perkovic V, Vonesh EF, Greene T. GFR slope as a surrogate end point for kidney disease progression in clinical trials: a meta-analysis of treatment effects of randomized controlled trials. J Am Soc Nephrol. 2019. pii: ASN.2019010007. https://doi.org/10.1681/ASN.2019010007. https://jasn.asnjournals.org/content/early/2019/07/09/ASN.2019010007.long.

24. Carrero JJ, Grams ME, Sang Y, Ärnlöv J, Gasparini A, Matsushita K, Qureshi AR, Evans M, Barany P, Lindholm B, Ballew SH, Levey AS, Gansevoort RT, Elinder CG, Coresh J. Albuminuria changes are associated with subsequent risk of end-stage renal disease and mortality. Kidney Int. 2017;91(1):244–51. https://doi.org/10.1016/j.kint.2016.09.037. https://www.ncbi.nlm.nih.gov/pmc/articles/PMC5523054.

25. Brankovic M, Kardys I, Hoorn EJ, Baart S, Boersma E, Rizopoulos D. Personalized dynamic risk assessment in nephrology is a next step in prognostic research. Kidney Int. 2018;94(1):214–7. https://doi.org/10.1016/j.kint.2018.04.007. Epub 2018 May 24. https://www.kidney-international.org/article/S0085-2538(18)30284-9/fulltext.

26. Tangri N, Inker LA, Hiebert B, Wong J, Naimark D, Kent D, Levey AS. A dynamic predictive model for progression of CKD. Am J Kidney Dis. 2017;69(4):514–20. https://doi.org/10.1053/j.ajkd.2016.07.030. Epub 2016 Sep 29. https://www.ajkd.org/article/S0272-6386(16)30417-6/fulltext.

27. Potok OA, Nguyen HA, Abdelmalek JA, Beben T, Woodell TB, Rifkin DE. Patients, 'nephrologists,' and predicted estimations of ESKD Risk Compared with 2-Year Incidence of ESKD. Clin J Am Soc Nephrol. 2019. pii: CJN.07970718. https://doi.org/10.2215/CJN.07970718. https://cjasn.asnjournals.org/content/14/2/206.long.

28. Javier AD, Figueroa R, Siew ED, Salat H, Morse J, Stewart TG, Malhotra R, Jhamb M, Schell JO, Cardona CY, Maxwell CA, Ikizler TA, Abdel-Kader K. Reliability and utility of the surprise question in CKD stages 4 to 5. Am J Kidney Dis. 2017;70(1):93–101. https://doi.org/10.1053/j.ajkd.2016.11.025. https://www.ncbi.nlm.nih.gov/pmc/articles/PMC5771496/.

29. Mitch WE, Walser M, Buffington GA, Lemann J Jr. A simple method of estimating progression of chronic renal failure. Lancet. 1976;2(7999):1326–8. https://www.thelancet.com/journals/lancet/article/PIIS0140-6736(76)91974-7/fulltext.

30. Kennedy DM, Chatha K, Rayner HC. Laboratory database population surveillance to improve detection of progressive chronic kidney disease. J Ren Care. 2013;39(Suppl 2):23–9. https://doi.org/10.1111/j.1755-6686.2013.12029.x.   https://onlinelibrary.wiley.com/doi/full/10.1111/j.1755-6686.2013.12029.x.
31. https://www.kidneyresearchuk.org/research/assist-ckd.
32. Brown EA, Farrington K. Geriatric assessment in advanced kidney disease. CJASN 2019:CJN.14771218. https://doi.org/10.2215/CJN.14771218. https://cjasn.asnjournals.org/content/clinjasn/early/2019/05/21/CJN.14771218.full.pdf.
33. Farrington K, Covic A, Aucella F, Clyne N, de Vos L, Findlay A, Fouque D, Grodzicki T, Iyasere O, Jager KJ, Joosten H, Macias JF, Mooney A, Nitsch D, Stryckers M, Taal M, Tattersall J, Van Asselt D, Van den Noortgate N, Nistor I, Van Biesen W, for the ERBP Guideline Development Group. Clinical Practice Guideline on management of older patients with chronic kidney disease stage 3b or higher (eGFR <45 mL/min/1.73 m2). Nephrol Dial Transplant. 2016;31(Suppl 2):ii1–ii66. https://doi.org/10.1093/ndt/gfw356. https://academic.oup.com/ndt/article/32/1/9/2931168.
34. Please, write to me. Writing outpatient letters to patients. Guidance. https://www.aomrc.org.uk/wp-content/uploads/2018/09/Please_write_to_me_Guidance_010918.pdf.
35. Rayner H, Hickey M, Logan I, Mathers N, Rees P, Shah R. Writing outpatient letters to patients. BMJ 2020; 368. https://www.bmj.com/content/368/bmj.m24.
36. Rayner HC, Zepel L, Fuller DS, Morgenstern H, Karaboyas A, Culleton BF, Mapes DL, Lopes AA, Gillespie BW, Hasegawa T, Saran R, Tentori F, Hecking M, Pisoni RL, Robinson BM. Recovery time, quality of life, and mortality in hemodialysis patients: the Dialysis Outcomes and Practice Patterns Study (DOPPS). Am J Kidney Dis. 2014;64(1):86–94. https://doi.org/10.1053/j.ajkd.2014.01.014. Epub 2014 Feb 14. http://www.ajkd.org/article/S0272-6386(14)00031-6/abstract.
37. Okamoto I, Tonkin-Crine S, Rayner H, Murtagh FEM, Farrington K, Caskey F, Tomson C, Loud F, Greenwood R, O'Donoghue DJ, Roderick P. Conservative Care for ESRD in the United Kingdom: a national survey. CJASN CJN.05000514; published ahead of print November 11, 2014. https://doi.org/10.2215/CJN.05000514. http://cjasn.asnjournals.org/content/early/2014/11/10/CJN.05000514.abstract.
38. Cooper BA, Branley P, Bulfone L, Collins JF, Craig JC, Fraenkel MB, Harris A, Johnson DW, Kesselhut J, Li JJ, Luxton G, Pilmore A, Tiller DJ, Harris DC, Pollock CA, for the IDEAL Study. A randomized, controlled trial of early versus late initiation of dialysis. N Engl J Med. 2010;363:609–19. https://doi.org/10.1056/NEJMoa1000552. http://www.nejm.org/doi/full/10.1056/NEJMoa1000552.
39. Winnicki E, Johansen KL, Cabana MD, Warady BA, McCulloch CE, Grimes B, Ku E. Higher eGFR at dialysis initiation is not associated with a survival benefit in children. JASN 2019:ASN.2018111130. https://doi.org/10.1681/ASN.2018111130. https://jasn.asnjournals.org/content/early/2019/07/17/ASN.2018111130.
40. Dunkler D, Kohl M, Heinze G, Teo KK, Rosengren A, Pogue J, Gao P, Gerstein H, Yusuf S, Oberbauer R, Mann JF. Modifiable lifestyle and social factors affect chronic kidney disease in high-risk individuals with type 2 diabetes mellitus. Kidney Int. 2015;87(4):784–91. https://doi.org/10.1038/ki.2014.370. Epub 2014 Dec 10. http://www.nature.com/ki/journal/v87/n4/full/ki2014370a.html.
41. Untas A, Thumma J, Rascle N, Rayner H, Mapes D, Lopes AA, Fukuhara S, Akizawa T, Morgenstern H, Robinson BM, Pisoni RL, Combe C. The associations of social support and other psychosocial factors with mortality and quality of life in the dialysis outcomes and practice patterns study. CJASN. 2011;6(1):142–52. https://doi.org/10.2215/CJN.02340310. http://www.ncbi.nlm.nih.gov/pmc/articles/PMC3022236.
42. Lopes AA, Bragg J, Young E, Goodkin D, Mapes D, Combe C, Piera L, Held P, Gillespie B, Port FK. Depression as a predictor of mortality and hospitalization among hemodialysis patients in the United States and Europe. Kidney Int. 2002;62(1):199–207. http://www.nature.com/ki/journal/v62/n1/full/4493090a.html.

43. Jung T-D, Park S-H. Intradialytic exercise programs for hemodialysis patients. Chonnam Med J. 2011;47(2):61–5. https://doi.org/10.4068/cmj.2011.47.2.61. http://www.ncbi.nlm.nih.gov/pmc/articles/PMC3214879/.
44. Cukor D, Ver Halen N, Asher DR, Coplan JD, Weedon J, Wyka KE, Saggi SJ, Kimmel PL. Psychosocial intervention improves depression, quality of life, and fluid adherence in hemodialysis. JASN. 2014;25:196–206. https://doi.org/10.1681/ASN.2012111134. http://jasn.asnjournals.org/content/25/1/196.abstract.
45. Wilkie M, Barnes T. Shared hemodialysis care. Increasing patient involvement in center-based dialysis. CJASN 2019:CJN.02050219. https://doi.org/10.2215/CJN.02050219. https://cjasn.asnjournals.org/content/clinjasn/early/2019/07/25/CJN.02050219.full.pdf.
46. Williams T, Bird K, Martin J, Bishop H, Bieber B, Rayner HC. Art and craft activities during haemodialysis: an untapped potential to improve patients' experience. Br J Renal Med. 2018;23(3):85–7.
47. Hudson P, Remedios C, Zordan R, Thomas K, Clifton D, Crewdson M, Hall C, Trauer T, Bolleter A, Clarke DM, Bauld C. Guidelines for the psychosocial and bereavement support of family caregivers of palliative care patients. J Palliat Med. 2012;15(6):696–702. https://doi.org/10.1089/jpm.2011.0466. https://www.liebertpub.com/doi/full/10.1089/jpm.2011.0466?url_ver=Z39.88-2003&rfr_id=ori%3Arid%3Acrossref.org&rfr_dat=cr_pub%3Dpubmed&.

Kidney Replacement Therapy: Common Problems in Dialysis and Transplant Patients

22

There are three types of kidney replacement therapy—haemodialysis, peritoneal dialysis and a kidney transplant. In this chapter, we explain the clinical aspects of these treatments that may be encountered by a non-specialist doctor, either incidentally when seeing the patient for another problem or in the emergency department.

Haemodialysis

Haemodialysis involves removing blood from the body and passing it though an artificial kidney (Fig. 22.1). The 'dialyser' contains thousands of semi-permeable hollow fibres. Blood flows through the fibres and back to the patient while dialysis fluid flows around the fibres in the opposite direction. Diffusion and ultrafiltration occur across the fibre membrane, removing waste products and excess fluid, and correcting electrolyte abnormalities. Adequate dialysis is usually achieved by having three treatments per week, each 4 h long.

Vascular Access

Having a reliable means of accessing the circulation is a crucial issue in haemodialysis. The ideal method is to insert a large needle into an arteriovenous (AV) fistula or graft. Second best is to insert a catheter into a large vein.

An AV fistula is created by joining an artery to an adjacent vein (Fig. 22.2). Strictly speaking, the fistula is the anastomosis but the word is used to refer to the enlarged vein. If an anastomosis is not feasible, a piece of artificial vessel—a graft—may be inserted between the artery and vein.

The increased pressure in the vein causes it to enlarge and develop thickened walls. Over time and with repeated needling, the fistula vein can become massively enlarged.

© Springer Nature Switzerland AG 2020
H. C. Rayner et al., *Understanding Kidney Diseases*,
https://doi.org/10.1007/978-3-030-43027-6_22

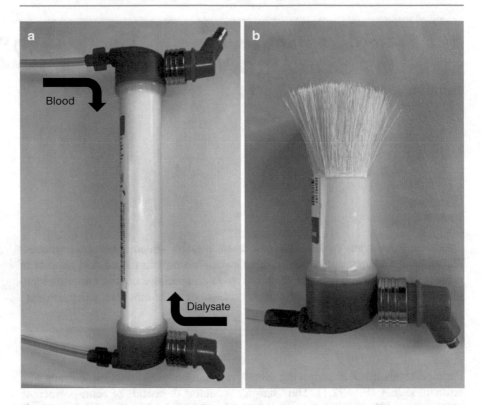

Fig. 22.1 A hollow fibre dialyser. (**a**) Blood flows from the patient into the dialyser through the tube at the top, through the hollow fibres and back to the patient through the tube at the bottom. Dialysate solution flows into the dialyser through the large connector at the bottom and out at the top. (**b**) Dialyser cut open to show the thousands of hollow fibres through which the blood flows. The fibres are bathed in dialysate fluid flowing in the opposite direction

Having an AV fistula formed in good time and ready to use from the start of dialysis provides big benefits for patients, greatly reducing the risk of complications.

The main problems that arise with an AV fistula are [1]:

- Infection—cellulitis or superficial pustules
- Steal syndrome—reduced perfusion of the hand when collateral flow cannot compensate for the blood diverted into the fistula (Fig. 22.3)
- Ischaemic painful polyneuropathy—commoner with an upper arm fistula and in patients with diabetes or vascular disease whose nerves are more easily damaged
- High output cardiac failure—uncommon but may require the fistula to be tied off

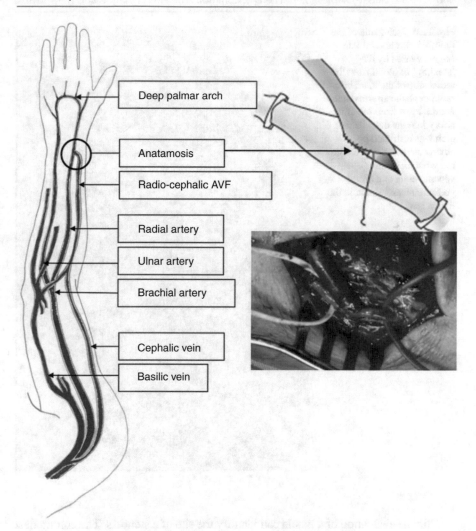

Fig. 22.2 The anatomy of an arteriovenous fistula (AVF). The ideal site for the anastomosis is between the radial artery and the cephalic vein near the wrist, as shown here. Blood returns up the vein rather than continuing into the hand. Perfusion of the hand is normally maintained by flow in the deep palmar arch via a branch from the ulnar artery. Other options for an anastomosis are between the brachial artery and the cephalic vein, and between the brachial artery and the basilic vein

- Clotting—usually due to slow flow caused by a stenosis in the fistula vein; requires urgent specialist attention to salvage the fistula
- Stenosis and aneurysm—often occur together, the aneurysm forming upstream of a stenosis. A rapidly growing aneurysm covered with thin or dusky skin may rupture and requires urgent specialist attention

Fig. 22.3 Ischaemia of the thumb, index and middle fingers caused by the 'stealing' of blood from the radial side of the hand by a radio-cephalic arteriovenous fistula. Flow from the ulnar artery into the deep palmar arch was restricted by atherosclerotic disease. The red wristband warns against venepuncture and blood pressure measurement in the fistula arm

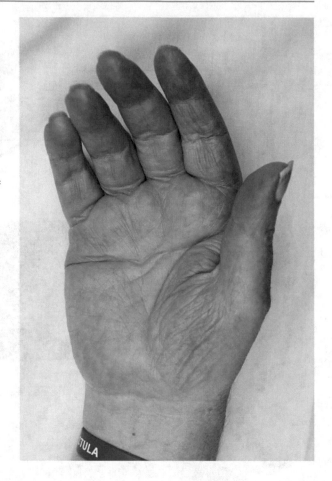

Clinical evaluation of a fistula can identify the site of a stenosis. The commonest site is near the anastomosis because the surgical wound stimulates fibrosis in the vein. The stenosis reduces the flow into the fistula, weakening the thrill that can be felt and the bruit that can be heard with a stethoscope.

Stenosis in a vein downstream of the fistula increases the pressure in the fistula. Normal fistula pressure is about 35 mmHg; if there is a stenosis, the pressure may be over 100 mmHg. This can be detected by elevating the arm. When the arm is above the head, blood should drain out of the fistula into the right atrium with little resistance to flow, and the fistula should collapse (Fig. 22.4). If there is a central stenosis, the fistula does not collapse and feels hard and pulsatile.

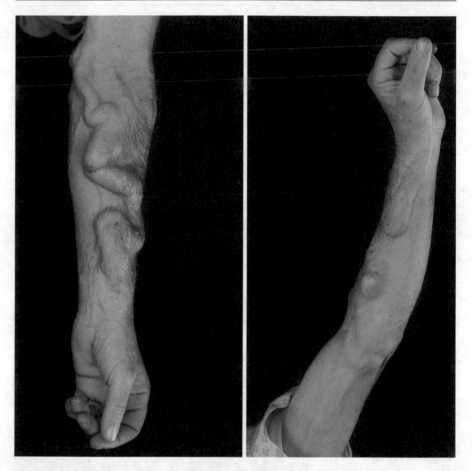

Fig. 22.4 This large radiocephalic fistula is shown with the arm dependent (*left*) and then elevated (*right*). On elevation, the fistula collapses completely except for two distended sections where the vessel wall has been weakened by repeated needling. These were soft, indicating that there was no stenosis obstructing flow. See a video of this examination at vimeo.com/123945414

During dialysis, blood is pumped through the artificial kidney at speeds of about 300 mL/min. If there is a stenosis in a vein downstream of the fistula, some of the blood pumped back into the fistula cannot flow up the arm. Instead some recirculates back round the dialysis circuit (Patient 22.1). The patient appears to be dialysing normally but potassium, urea and other toxins are not cleared [2]. The patient may present later as an emergency with a dangerously high serum potassium concentration. Urgent radiological imaging and intervention are needed to dilate the vein, prevent the fistula clotting and restore effective clearance on dialysis.

Patient 22.1 Recirculation Due to Arteriovenous Fistula Stenosis

The dialysis nurses were increasingly concerned about Mr. Trellis' fistula. The blood flow rate during dialysis was normal but the post-dialysis urea and potassium were 28 and 5.2 mmol/L (BUN = 78 mg/dL, K$^+$ = 5.2 mEq/L) compared to the usual 15 and 3.5 (42 mg/dL, 3.5 mEq/L) respectively. The monitor of recirculation built into the dialysis machine suggested that the percentage of blood recirculating had increased. An urgent fistulagram was performed (Fig. 22.5).

The stenosis restricts the return of blood up the arm towards the heart. During dialysis, a proportion of the blood flowing from the venous needle flows back to the arterial needle and recirculates around the dialyser (Fig. 22.6).

After the angioplasty (Fig. 22.7), flow up the arm was no longer restricted (Fig. 22.8).

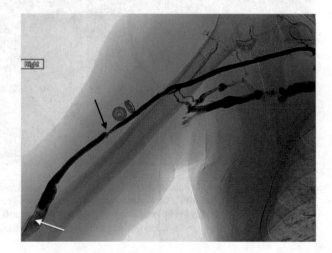

Fig. 22.5 A fistulagram study of the vein draining blood downstream from an arteriovenous fistula. The catheter can be seen in the fistula (*arrow*). There is a tight stenosis in the cephalic vein (*arrow*) related to a venous valve. The round objects next to the vein are fasteners on the patient's gown

Complications of a Haemodialysis Catheter

The main complications of a haemodialysis catheter are infection, clotting, and venous stenosis. Infection tends to track down the catheter from the exit site to form a biofilm around the catheter. This can lead to septicaemia, endocarditis and more distant seeding of infection such as osteomyelitis. Because of the serious consequences of infection, a dialysis catheter should not be used for any purpose other than dialysis.

Fig. 22.6 Recirculation in the dialyser circuit. Blood is removed from the fistula vein via the arterial needle, pumped through the dialyser by the dialysis machine and returned to the fistula via the venous needle. The high resistance to flow up the arm forces some of the returned blood back towards the arterial needle. It then flows round the dialyser circuit again

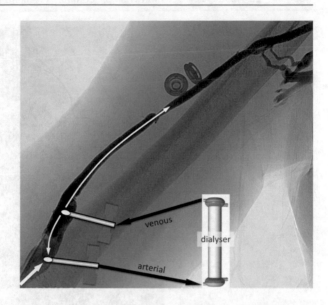

Fig. 22.7 Angioplasty balloon inflated at the site of the stenosis

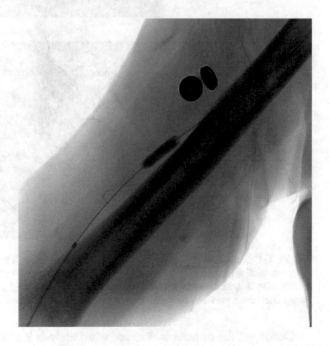

Fig. 22.8 Angiogram following angioplasty showing unobstructed flow up the arm through the cephalic vein

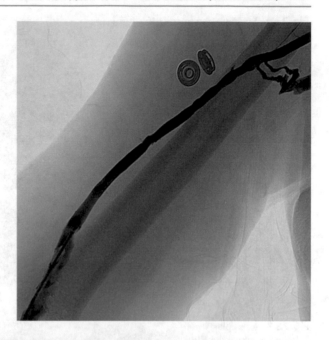

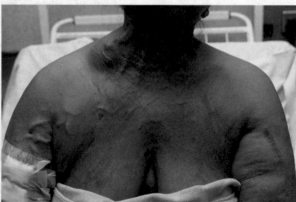

Fig. 22.9 Dilated veins across the right upper chest and neck of a lady due to an occlusion of the right brachial vein in the axilla caused by a previous dialysis catheter. Venous blood flow is increased by an arteriovenous fistula in the right upper arm, covered with dressings. There are scars on her chest from previous catheters, and on her left arm from fistula surgery

Clotting of the catheter is detected when dialysis is attempted. Clotting and stenosis of the surrounding central vein due to trauma can obstruct the flow of blood in one or both lumens of the catheter.

If a catheter is in place for many months, stenosis and eventual occlusion of a central vein may occur. If an arteriovenous fistula is then created on the same side, the increase in venous pressure causes dilatation of veins over the upper chest and neck (Fig. 22.9).

The Effects of Haemodialysis Treatment

Each haemodialysis treatment session is a physical and mental stress on the patient. Blood flow to the heart [3], brain [4] and kidneys [5] can be reduced, causing ischaemia and 'stunning'. This can cause a fall in blood pressure, impaired cognitive function [6] and loss of residual kidney function. Repeated episodes of stunning, combined with the accelerated cardiovascular disease that accompanies end-stage kidney disease, lead to long-term organ damage.

It is useful to ask patients how long it takes them to recover from a dialysis treatment. This can be prolonged, over 12 h in many patients, and is associated with worse quality of life and mortality [7]. It is also strongly correlated with the severity of itching, and both recovery time and itching tend to get worse over years of maintenance dialysis. This linkage suggests that both symptoms are mediated by damage to the central nervous system by uraemia and hemodialysis treatment. Functional MRI scans of haemodialysis patients with severe itching show changes in the density of grey matter in many regions of the brain [8].

The time may come for a patient when the burden and effects of the dialysis treatment are worse than the benefit. In particular, patients with dementia can be made more confused and unwell during and after the dialysis session. A decision may have to be made, in collaboration with the patient and their loved ones, to withdraw dialysis and provide supportive care. This can provide a period of lucid time for the family to share before the end of the patient's life.

Fluid Balance in a Haemodialysis Patient

Regulation of fluid balance is impaired in patients with end-stage kidney failure. Many dialysis patients, especially those who have been on dialysis for less than 3 years, still have some kidney function and pass urine. This residual kidney function significantly improves prognosis and, when assessing a patient, it is useful to ask how much urine they pass [9].

However, the volume of urine is often less than is needed to maintain fluid balance. The excess fluid is removed during each haemodialysis treatment by ultrafiltration, driven by a hydrostatic pressure gradient across the dialyser membrane.

It can be hard to judge accurately a patient's fluid balance from a clinical examination. Blood pressure is not a reliable guide to fluid overload; it may be high due to increased intravascular volume or low due to reduced left ventricular function. Peripheral oedema may not be obvious, especially in younger patients. Techniques such as bioimpedance spectroscopy and lung ultrasound can be used to gain a more reliable estimate of fluid balance. There is some evidence that these techniques are of added benefit compared with careful clinical assessment [10] but the results of clinical trials are awaited [11].

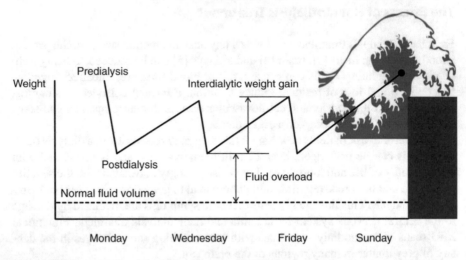

Fig. 22.10 The analogy of the tide and waves of fluid balance, crashing into the quayside

Measurement of changes in weight plays a key role in prescribing haemodialysis treatment. If the volumes of urine and insensible losses together are less than the fluid in food and drink, the patient's body weight will increase between the end of one dialysis treatment and the start of the next. This is called the interdialytic weight gain, which is removed during the next dialysis. The rise and fall in weight across the week are like waves on the sea (Fig. 22.10).

Underneath the waves is the weight that the patient would have without kidney failure—the normal fluid volume. This weight rises and falls over a longer timescale due to gains and losses of lean tissue. The difference between the post-dialysis weight and the normal fluid volume is the fluid overload.

Each dialysis patient has a prescribed target weight that should be reached by the end of each dialysis treatment. If the target weight is lower than the patient's normal fluid volume weight the blood pressure may drop during dialysis—commonly called 'crashing'.

Conversely, if the target weight is above the normal fluid volume weight there will be residual fluid overload. This is like a high tide underneath the waves. As the wave rises before the next treatment on top of the high tide, fluid may flood into the lungs (Fig. 22.11). This is more likely to happen at the weekend when there is a gap of 2 days rather than one between dialysis treatments [12]. Persistent fluid overload is associated with increased mortality [13] and patients who are treated in dialysis units that assess fluid balance regularly have lower mortality [14].

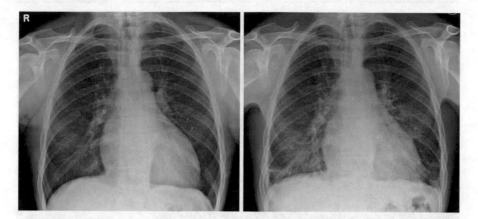

Fig. 22.11 Chest X-rays from a haemodialysis patient taken (*left*) when well and (*right*) when severely short of breath on arrival at the dialysis unit on a Monday. The right X-ray shows features of fluid overload with pulmonary vascular congestion, Kerley B lines and bilateral pleural effusions blunting the costophrenic angles. The heart is enlarged on both X-rays

Peritoneal Dialysis

In peritoneal dialysis (PD), waste products are excreted by diffusion and convective flow across the peritoneal membrane into dialysis fluid in the peritoneal cavity. Fluid is drawn into the peritoneal cavity by an osmotic gradient created by glucose or other osmotic agent in the dialysis fluid.

To achieve adequate dialysis, fluid needs to be exchanged every few hours, every day. Fluid is drained in and out either manually (continuous ambulatory peritoneal dialysis, CAPD) or by a machine overnight (automated peritoneal dialysis, APD).

The catheter lying in the peritoneal cavity should allow dialysis fluid to flow freely in and out. If flow is slow or blocked, a plain abdominal X-ray is taken to check its position (Fig. 22.12).

The commonest complication of PD is infection. It can affect the skin where the catheter emerges from abdomen—the 'exit site' (Fig. 22.13), the tunnel through the abdominal wall, or the peritoneal fluid. If the infection does not respond to antibiotics or the tunnel becomes infected, the PD catheter will have to be removed and a new catheter inserted when the infection has been cleared.

PD peritonitis presents with abdominal pain and cloudy dialysis fluid but seldom leads to septicaemia [15]. Samples of PD fluid should be taken and antibiotic treatment started immediately to cover Gram-positive and Gram-negative organisms, including *Pseudomonas* species, whilst the results of a culture are awaited. Antibiotics are preferably given via the peritoneal fluid, usually for 2–3 weeks.

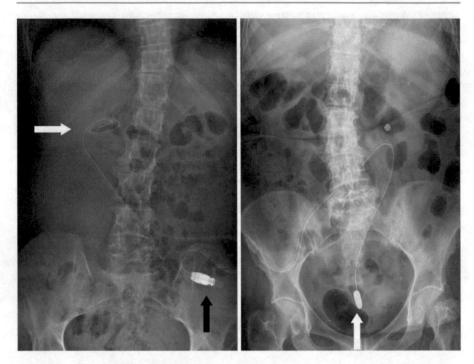

Fig. 22.12 Plain abdominal X-rays of two patients having peritoneal dialysis. The catheter on the left is malpositioned. Draining fluid in was slow and caused discomfort; fluid would not drain out. The curled end (*white arrow*) lies in the right upper quadrant under the liver. The radio-opaque tube connector (*black arrow*) is outside the body. The catheter on the right is correctly located. The radio-opaque weighted end of the catheter (*white arrow*) helps to keep it in the pelvic cavity

Prophylaxis with oral nystatin helps to prevent secondary fungal peritonitis, which is very hard to clear [16].

If peritonitis does not respond or comes back after antibiotics have been stopped, the catheter will have to be removed and the patient treated with haemodialysis. A new PD catheter can sometimes be inserted later but often the change to haemodialysis is permanent.

Kidney Transplant

The most complete replacement of kidney function is achieved with a kidney transplant. Best results are obtained using kidneys donated by a live donor who is related to the recipient. Kidneys are otherwise obtained from deceased donors, either brain-dead or after the heart has stopped beating.

A detailed explanation of the transplant procedure and subsequent patient management are outside the scope of this book. We have limited this section to problems that may present to a non-specialist clinician.

Fig. 22.13 Peritoneal catheter exit sites. (**a**) a healthy exit site—the skin around the catheter is dry and not inflamed. The dried exudate ('crusting') below the catheter does not indicate infection. The catheter is clean. (**b**) an unhealthy exit site— swollen granulation tissue is secreting purulent exudate and blood. There is dried material adherent to the catheter. A culture grew *Staphylococcus aureus*

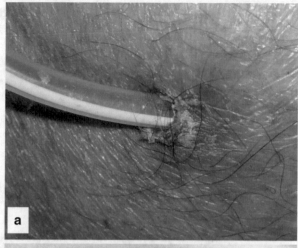

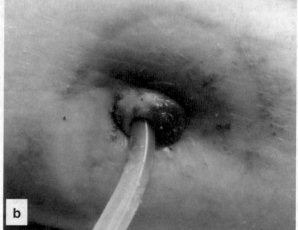

Causes of a Decline in Transplant Function

The most likely cause of a decline in transplant kidney function changes with time after transplantation.

Acute kidney injury in the first week is usually due to:

- Hypovolaemia or acute tubular necrosis
- Hyperacute rejection
- Surgical problems with the blood supply or ureter

Declining function during the first 3 months is usually due to:

- Hypovolaemia
- Acute rejection—antibody or T cell-mediated
- Calcineurin inhibitor toxicity
- Interstitial nephritis
- Ureteric obstruction
- Recurrent focal segmental glomerulosclerosis (FSGS)
- Bacterial pyelonephritis
- BK virus infection

After 3 months, the following additional causes become increasingly common.

- Chronic rejection
- Chronic allograft nephropathy—interstitial fibrosis and tubular atrophy
- Non-adherence to immunosuppression
- Recurrent or de-novo glomerulonephritis
- Transplant artery stenosis

Immunosuppressive drugs prevent a decline in transplant function due to rejection but increase the risk of two other complications: infection and malignancy.

Infection

The most likely type of infection also changes with time after transplantation [17]:

- Within the first month, infections are usually due to environmental pathogens, such as catheter or wound infections and *Clostridium difficile* diarrhoea.
- Between 1 and 6 months, the type of infection depends upon the immunosuppressive treatment and whether the patient is taking prophylactic antimicrobial drugs. Cotrimoxazole is usually given to prevent *Pneumocystis jiroveci* pneumonia (PJP), formerly known as *Pneumocystis carinii* pneumonia (PCP). Antivirals such as valganciclovir may be given to prevent infection by herpes viruses such as cytomegalovirus (CMV).
- After the first 6 months, infections are more often due to conventional organisms such as community-acquired pneumonia and urinary tract infection. Late viral infections may appear, e.g. colitis or retinitis due to CMV, and herpes encephalitis (Patient 22.2). Opportunistic infections are commoner in patients who have had more intensive immunosuppression or particular environmental exposures, such as to fungi.

Patient 22.2 Epstein-Barr Viral Encephalitis

Mr. Blackman had a kidney transplant in 2000. Ciclosporin and pred-nisolone were used for immunosuppression. The kidney did not function very well, eGFR was at best 25 mL/min/1.73 m². After 6 years, ciclo-sporin was substituted by mycophenolate mofetil to avoid calcineurin nephrotoxicity.

Ten years after the transplant, he presented with a month's history of pro-gressive difficulty swallowing solids and liquids, and hoarseness of his voice. He had lost 7 kg in weight.

He had been anticoagulated with warfarin for atrial fibrillation but during courses of antibiotics the INR was hard to control so warfarin had been stopped.

An MRI scan was reported as showing changes consistent with infarcts in the left cerebral hemisphere and the left side of the medulla (Fig. 22.14).

He was treated with aspirin and dipyridamole with a plan to restart warfarin, and required feeding via a nasogastric tube. Over the next 3 months his condition did not improve; his legs became weaker and his gait more unsteady. He was increasingly confused and so was readmitted to hospital.

A repeat MRI scan showed much more extensive white matter changes in the posterior fossa and cerebral hemispheres, consistent with encephalitis (Fig. 22.15).

His cerebrospinal fluid (CSF) contained 7 red blood cells per mm³ and 139 white blood cells, of which 138 were lymphocytes. Epstein-Barr virus DNA (EBV, also called human herpesvirus 4 HHV-4) was detected in large amounts in the CSF (23,000 copies/mL). There was no EBV DNA in the blood but IgG against EBV was present, indicating previous infection.

He was treated with 4 weeks of intravenous ganciclovir and then oral val-ganciclovir. Mycophenolate mofetil was stopped. Antiviral drugs were con-tinued until EBV DNA was not detectable in the CSF. An MRI scan after 6 months showed marked improvement in the white matter changes (Fig. 22.16).

After a prolonged period of nasogastric feeding and intensive physiother-apy he made an excellent recovery.

After years of immunosuppression, warts caused by human papillomavirus can be very troublesome (Fig. 22.17). They are most common in patients treated with azathioprine [18] and may improve with reduction in the dose.

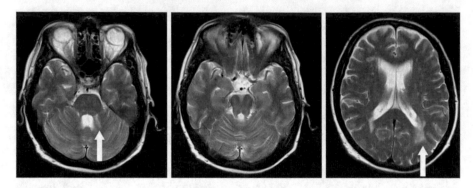

Fig. 22.14 MRI scan showing changes in the left side of the medulla and the left cerebral hemisphere (*arrows*)

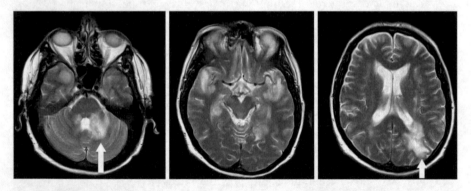

Fig. 22.15 MRI scan showing extensive white matter changes in the posterior fossa and cerebral hemispheres, consistent with encephalitis

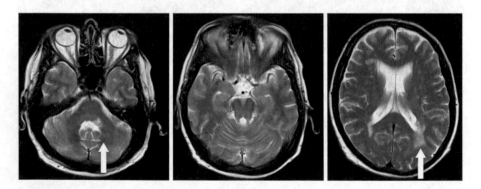

Fig. 22.16 MRI scan after 6 months showing improvement in the white matter changes

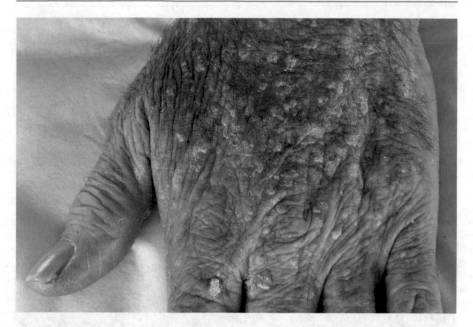

Fig. 22.17 Extensive warts on the hand of a kidney transplant patient who had taken prednisolone and azathioprine as immunosuppression for over 20 years

Malignancy

Long-term treatment with calcineurin inhibitors (tacrolimus and ciclosporin) may allow B cells infected with Epstein-Barr virus to proliferate, causing post-transplant lymphoproliferative disease (PTLD). Polyclonal PTLD may present with symptoms caused by a mass of lymph nodes, such as bowel obstruction. The nodes may regress if the immunosuppressants are stopped or reduced in dose [19]. Sometimes a clone of cells proliferates to become a monoclonal malignant lymphoma (Patient 22.3).

Patient 22.3 Post-transplant Lymphoproliferative Disease
Mr. Park's kidney transplant had functioned perfectly for 19 years, thanks to immunosuppression with prednisolone and ciclosporin. He developed symptoms of nausea and vomiting 1–2 h after meals and lost four kilograms in weight. A CT scan showed a stricture at the duodenal/jejunal flexure with thickening of the bowel wall (Fig. 22.18).

A biopsy of the thickened bowel showed high-grade diffuse large B cell lymphoma (non-germinal centre type). Further scans and a bone marrow trephine showed no sign of spread.

Ciclosporin was stopped and he was treated with R-CHOP chemotherapy—Rituximab, Cyclophosphamide, doxorubicin (Hydroxydaunomycin), vincristine (Oncovin®) and Prednisolone. His tumour regressed completely without perforation of the bowel wall, a complication that can result from tumour lysis.

A low dose of ciclosporin was restarted and prednisolone continued, but his transplant kidney function declined (Fig. 22.19).

A biopsy of the transplant kidney confirmed chronic rejection. He eventually restarted haemodialysis.

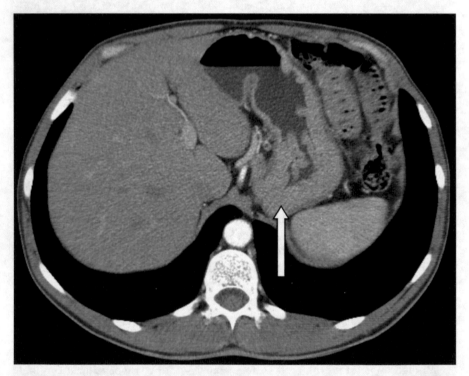

Fig. 22.18 Contrast CT scan showing thickening of the small bowel wall at the junction of the duodenum and jejunum (*arrow*) causing an obstruction to flow and fluid level in the dilated duodenum

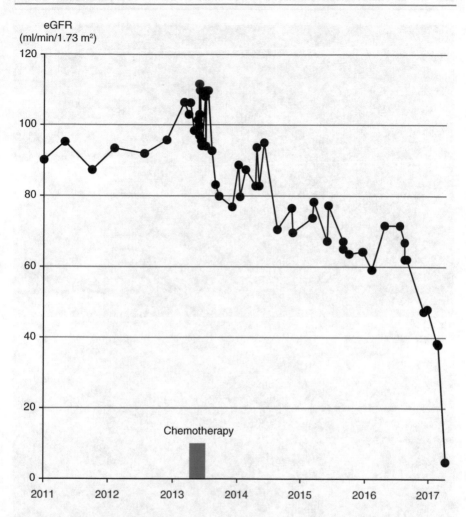

Fig. 22.19 Changes in kidney function after treatment for post-transplant lymphoprolifera-tive disease

Long-term immunosuppression increases the risk of all forms of cancer. The commonest site is the skin, usually a basal cell or squamous cell carcinoma (Fig. 22.20). Death from malignancy, such as lymphoma, lung or kidney cancer, is more common than in the general population [20].

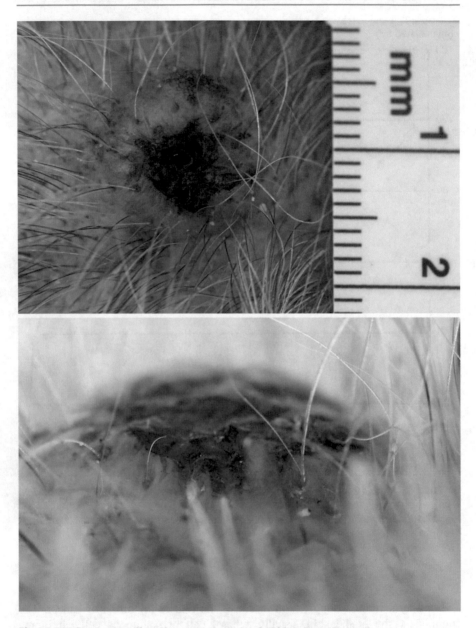

Fig. 22.20 Squamous cell carcinoma on the scalp of a kidney transplant patient

References

1. Siddiky A, Sarwar K, Ahmad N, Gilbert J. Management of arteriovenous fistulas. BMJ. 2014;349:g6262. https://doi.org/10.1136/bmj.g6262. http://www.bmj.com/content/349/bmj.g6262.
2. Zeraati A, Beladi Mousavi SS, Beladi MM. A review article: access recirculation among end stage renal disease patients undergoing maintenance hemodialysis. Nephrourol Mon. 2013;5(2):728–32. https://doi.org/10.5812/numonthly.6689. http://www.ncbi.nlm.nih.gov/pmc/articles/PMC3703129/.
3. Buchanan C, Mohammed A, Cox E, Köhler K, Canaud B, Taal MW, Selby NM, Francis S, McIntyre CW. Intradialytic cardiac magnetic resonance imaging to assess cardiovascular responses in a short-term trial of hemodiafiltration and hemodialysis. J Am Soc Nephrol. 2017;28(4):1269–77. https://doi.org/10.1681/ASN.2016060686. Epub 2016 Nov 10. https://jasn.asnjournals.org/content/28/4/1269.long.
4. Findlay MD, Dawson J, Dickie DA, Forbes KP, McGlynn D, Quinn T, Mark PB. Investigating the relationship between cerebral blood flow and cognitive function in hemodialysis patients. J Am Soc Nephrol. 2019;30(1):147–58. https://doi.org/10.1681/ASN.2018050462. Epub 2018 Dec 7. https://jasn.asnjournals.org/content/30/1/147.long.
5. Marants R, Qirjazi E, Grant CJ, Lee T-Y, McIntyre DW. Renal perfusion during hemodialysis: intradialytic blood flow decline and effects of dialysate cooling. JASN 2019:ASN.2018121194; https://doi.org/10.1681/ASN.2018121194. https://jasn.asnjournals.org/content/early/2019/05/02/ASN.2018121194.
6. Dasgupta I, Patel M, Mohammed N, Baharani J, Subramanian T, Thomas GN, Tadros G. Cognitive function declines significantly during haemodialysis in a majority of patients: a call for further research. Blood Purif. 2018;45(4):347–55. https://doi.org/10.1159/000485961. Epub 2018 Feb 16. https://www.karger.com/Article/Abstract/485961.
7. Rayner HC, Zepel L, Fuller DS, Morgenstern H, Karaboyas A, Culleton BF, et al. Recovery time, quality of life, and mortality in hemodialysis patients: the Dialysis Outcomes and Practice Patterns Study (DOPPS). Am J Kidney Dis. 2014;64(1):86–94. https://www.ncbi.nlm.nih.gov/pmc/articles/PMC4069238/.
8. Papoiu AD, Emerson NM, Patel TS, Kraft RA, Valdes-Rodriguez R, Nattkemper LA, Coghill RC, Yosipovitch G. Voxel-based morphometry and arterial spin labeling fMRI reveal neuropathic and neuroplastic features of brain processing of itch in end-stage renal disease. J Neurophysiol. 2014;112(7):1729–38. https://doi.org/10.1152/jn.00827.2013. Epub 2014 Jun 18. https://www.physiology.org/doi/pdf/10.1152/jn.00827.2013.
9. Hecking M, McCullough KP, Port FK, Bieber B, Morgenstern H, Yamamoto H, Suri RS, Jadoul M, Gesualdo L, Perl J, Robinson BM. Self-reported urine volume in hemodialysis patients: predictors and mortality outcomes in the International Dialysis Outcomes and Practice Patterns Study (DOPPS). Am J Kidney Dis. https://www.ajkd.org/article/S0272-6386(19)30614-6/fulltext.
10. Charalampos L, Sarafidis PA, Ekart R, Papadopoulos C, Sachpekidis V, Alexandrou ME, Papadopoulou D, Efstratiadis G, Papagianni A, London G, Zoccali C. The effect of dry-weight reduction guided by lung ultrasound on ambulatory blood pressure in hemodialysis patients: a randomized controlled trial. Kidney Int. 95(6):1505–13. https://www.kidney-international.org/article/S0085-2538(19)30270-4/pdf.
11. Tabinor M, Davies SJ. The use of bioimpedance spectroscopy to guide fluid management in patients receiving dialysis. Curr Opin Nephrol Hypertens. 2018;27(6):406–12. https://doi.org/10.1097/MNH.0000000000000445. https://insights.ovid.com/pubmed?pmid=30063488.
12. Fotheringham J, Sajjad A, Stel VS, McCullough K, Karaboyas A, Wilkie M, Bieber B, Robinson BM, Massy ZA, Jager KJ. The association between longer haemodialysis treatment times and hospitalization and mortality after the two-day break in individuals receiving three times a week haemodialysis. Nephrol Dial Transplant. 2019:1–8. https://doi.org/10.1093/ndt/gfz007. https://academic.oup.com/ndt/advance-article/doi/10.1093/ndt/gfz007/5366963.

13. Hecking M, Moissl U, Genser B, Rayner H, Dasgupta I, Stuard S, Stopper A, Chazot C, Maddux FW, Canaud B, Port FK, Zoccali C, Wabel P. Greater fluid overload and lower inter-dialytic weight gain are independently associated with mortality in a large international hemo-dialysis population. Nephrol Dial Transplant. 2018;33(10):1832–42. https://doi.org/10.1093/ndt/gfy083. https://www.ncbi.nlm.nih.gov/pmc/articles/PMC6168737/.
14. Dasgupta I, Thomas GN, Clarke J, Sitch A, Martin J, Bieber B, Hecking M, Karaboyas A, Pisoni R, Port F, Robinson B, Rayner H. Associations between hemodialysis facility prac-tices to manage fluid volume and intradialytic hypotension and patient outcomes. Clin J Am Soc Nephrol. 2019;14(3):385–93. https://doi.org/10.2215/CJN.08240718. Epub 2019 Feb 5. https://cjasn.asnjournals.org/content/14/3/385.long.
15. Szeto CC, Li PK. Peritoneal dialysis–associated peritonitis. CJASN CJN.14631218; https://doi.org/10.2215/CJN.14631218.   https://cjasn.asnjournals.org/content/early/2019/05/07/CJN.14631218.
16. Li PK, Szeto CC, Piraino B, de Arteaga J, Fan S, Figueiredo AE, Fish DN, Goffin E, Kim YL, Salzer W, Struijk DG, Teitelbaum I, Johnson DW. ISPD peritonitis recommendations: 2016 update on prevention and treatment. Perit Dial Int. 2016;36:481–508. http://www.pdi-connect.com/content/36/5/481?ijkey=6c137235a9cf97844ffb262d4ec0183ac6dac41e&keytype2=tf_ipsecsha.
17. Karuthu S, Blumberg EA. Common infections in kidney transplant recipients. CJASN 2012;7(12):2058–70. Published ahead of print September 13, 2012. https://doi.org/10.2215/CJN.04410512. http://cjasn.asnjournals.org/content/7/12/2058.full.
18. Dicle O, Parmaksizoglu B, Gurkan A, Tuncer M, Demirbas A, Yilmaz E. Choice of immu-nosuppressants and the risk of warts in renal transplant recipients. Acta Derm Venereol. 2008;88(3):294–5. https://doi.org/10.2340/00015555-0411. http://www.medicaljournals.se/acta/content/?doi=10.2340/00015555-0411&html=1.
19. Starzl TE, Nalesnik MA, Porter KA, Ho M, Iwatsuki S, Griffith BP, Rosenthal JT, Hakala TR, Shaw BW Jr, Hardesty RL, Atchison RW, Jaffe R, Bahnson HT. Reversibility of lympho-mas and lymphoproliferative lesions developing under cyclosporin-steroid therapy. Lancet. 1984;323(8377):583–7. http://www.ncbi.nlm.nih.gov/pmc/articles/PMC2987704/.
20. Farrugia D, Mahboob S, Cheshire J, Begaj I, Khosla S, Ray D, Sharif A. Malignancy-related mortality following kidney transplantation is common. Kidney Int. 2014;85(6):1395–403. https://doi.org/10.1038/ki.2013.458. http://www.nature.com/ki/journal/v85/n6/full/ki2013458a.html.

Frequently Asked Questions

The following are questions about the kidneys and kidney diseases that are frequently asked by patients.

Answering them is a test of both your knowledge and your ability to explain medical matters in a way that patients can understand. You may find this is not as easy as it sounds!

Beware of making your answers vague and long-winded. They should be factually accurate, but not full of medical jargon.

Check how easy they are to read by running a readability test such as the Flesch Reading Ease score [1]. The score is derived from the lengths of words and sentences.

- A score of 30–50 = text requires college level education to be understood easily;
- 60–70 = easily understood by 13- to 15-year-old students;
- 70–80 = easily understood by 12-year-old students;
- 80–90 = conversational English for consumers.
- Most documents should have a score above 60.

Measuring Kidney Function

Q. I feel well but my kidney function has dropped from 55 to 50. Should I be worried?

A. No. At this level of kidney function, results vary a lot from test to test because of random effects. Look at all your results together on a graph to see if the new result is very different from your other ones.

Flesch Reading Ease score = 73.7

Symptoms

Q. I have CKD and my eGFR is 20. I have terrible itching. I have been told to start using phosphate binders with my meals. Is this correct?

© Springer Nature Switzerland AG 2020
H. C. Rayner et al., *Understanding Kidney Diseases*,
https://doi.org/10.1007/978-3-030-43027-6

A. It used to be thought that kidney itch, also called uraemic pruritus, was caused by high phosphate levels. More recent studies show this is not the case. Phosphate binders will not help your itching.

Flesch Reading Ease score = 78.9

Pregnancy

Q. I want to have a baby but have been told my kidney function is reduced. How can I work out how big are the risks to me and to the baby of getting pregnant?

A. The risks depend on the following things: your blood pressure, the protein in your urine and your kidney function. Other factors to consider are your age and whether this would be your first pregnancy. In general, the more factors that are present and the more advanced they are, the greater is the risk to your kidney function and that the pregnancy will have problems.

Flesch Reading Ease score = 66.4

Polycystic Kidney Disease

Q. I have polycystic kidney disease but my parents are not affected—is this possible?

A. Yes—one in ten people with the disease are the first in their family to have the abnormal gene.

Flesch Reading Ease score = 76.5

Q. I have PKD. When should my children have a scan to see if they have the disease?

A. Wait until they are about 21 years old. If there are no cysts at that age they almost certainly do not have the disease. An ultrasound scan may be done sooner if they have tummy pain or blood in the urine.

Flesch Reading Ease score = 83.8

Q. I have pain and bleeding from my polycystic kidneys. Can anything be done?

A. Treatment with Tolvaptan can reduce the pain. Operations to remove cysts are rarely helpful. In very severe cases one or both the kidney can be removed.

Flesch Reading Ease score = 66.1

Q. I want to have a transplant. Do my polycystic kidneys need to be removed?

A. Not usually. Sometimes there is no room in the tummy for a transplant unless they one is removed.

Flesch Reading Ease score = 76.9

Q. I have had a kidney transplant. Can the disease affect my new kidney?

A. No—your transplant kidney does not have the abnormal gene so will not be affected.

Flesch Reading Ease score = 74.2

Drugs

Q. My kidney function has dropped to 20%. Should I stop taking my ACE inhibitor tablets?

A. Probably not, unless you have a high blood potassium level. Most patients with kidney disease should keep taking these tablets. They do not damage the kidneys but can sometimes affect kidney function.

Flesch Reading Ease score = 64.9

Q. I have diabetes and my kidney function is slowly going down. Should I stop taking metformin?

A. Metformin does not damage the kidneys. Keep taking it until your kidney function is less than 30. Even then, it can sometimes be continued.

Flesch Reading Ease score = 63

High Blood Pressure

Q. Does checking your own blood pressure make you anxious and the blood pressure worse?

A. No—the opposite is the case. Once you are used to doing it, your own blood pressure readings are the most useful. Adjusting your treatment according to your home readings gives the most benefit.

Flesch Reading Ease score = 76.5

Fluid Intake

Q. I have kidney disease and swollen ankles. Should I drink less fluid?

A. Swelling, also called oedema, is caused by having too much salt in your body. Drinking less water will not help. Reducing your salt intake makes more sense.

Flesch Reading Ease score = 79.5

Q. I have kidney disease. Should I drink more water?

A. Most types of kidney disease are not helped by drinking large amounts of water. Exceptions are those diseases where the kidneys are damaged by substances that block the flow of urine. Examples are multiple myeloma and kidney stones.

Flesch Reading Ease score = 65.6

Potassium

Q. I have CKD and my eGFR is 20. Should I have a low potassium diet?

A. This is rarely needed. In fact, a diet high in fruit and vegetables that contain lots of potassium are good for your kidneys and general health.

Flesch Reading Ease score = 74

Protein

Q. I work out at the gym and am trying to bulk up my muscles. Will protein or creatine drinks harm my kidneys?

A. If your blood pressure, kidney function and urine protein tests are all normal, these drinks will not harm your kidneys. If these are not normal, a high protein diet is not a good idea.

Flesch Reading Ease score = 80.3

Anaemia

Q. I have chronic kidney disease, my haemoglobin is 105 g/L. I feel fine and can do all the activities I want. Should I have Epo treatment?

A. No. There is no long-term benefit from increasing your haemoglobin to normal and it may increase the risk of having a stroke.

Flesch Reading Ease score = 70.1

Bone Disease

Q. I have CKD and my eGFR is 20 but I feel well. Should my vitamin D levels be measured?

A. There is no need to check vitamin D levels routinely. A simple bone profile is enough. This is calcium, phosphate, alkaline phosphatase and sometimes parathyroid hormone (PTH).

Flesch Reading Ease score = 55.3

Kidney Stones

Q. I have been told I have got calcium oxalate kidney stones. Should I reduce the calcium in my diet?

A. This seems logical but is the wrong thing to do. In people who have had stones, those on a low-calcium diet are twice as likely to form another stone than those on normal diets. A low calcium diet increases uptake of oxalate in the gut. The oxalate binds to calcium in the urine to form more stones.

It is better to reduce refined carbohydrates, animal protein, fat and salt, and to increase water, fruit, vegetables, nuts and wholegrains.

Flesch Reading Ease score = 68.4

Kidney Replacement Therapy

Q. Which is better—haemodialysis, peritoneal dialysis or managing with medicines alone?

A. The choice is yours. If you are independent and want to keep away from hospital, peritoneal dialysis may suit you. If you live alone and find it hard to care for yourself, assisted peritoneal dialysis or haemodialysis may be a better choice. If you are over 80 or have a lot of medical problems, not having dialysis may be the best option. The decision can be difficult. Don't rush it.

Flesch Reading Ease score = 60.1

Q. What is the best type of kidney transplant?

A. The best kidney transplant is one donated by a living person, such as a friend or relative. The donor is tested thoroughly before the kidney is removed to make sure it is perfectly healthy. Kidneys from donors who have died can also be good, though.

Flesch Reading Ease score = 68.0

Q. When will I need to have a kidney transplant?

A. It is best to do the transplant operation before you start dialysis. You may be made active on the waiting list when your kidney function drops below 15. This can often be predicted by plotting the kidney function (eGFR) graph.

Flesch Reading Ease score = 65.0

Q. When will I need to start dialysis?

A. The best time to start dialysis is when the benefits of the treatment are greater than its bother and inconvenience. There is no set level of eGFR when it is best to start and there is no benefit in starting early. The decision should be based mainly upon how you feel.

Flesch Reading Ease score = 72.1

Reference

1. Kincaid JP, Fishburne RP Jr, Rogers RL, Chissom BS. Derivation of new readability formulas (automated readability index, fog count and Flesch reading ease formula) for navy enlisted personnel. Institute for Simulation and Training. Paper 56. 1975. http://stars.library.ucf.edu/istlibrary/56.

Multiple Choice Questions

Chapter 1

1. At what rate does the GFR typically decline in males after the age of 45 years?
   - (a) 0.1 mL/min/1.73 m² per year
   - (b) 0.3 mL/min/1.73 m² per year
   - (c) 0.6 mL/min/1.73 m² per year
   - (d) 1.2 mL/min/1.73 m² per year
   - (e) 2.0 mL/min/1.73 m² per year
2. Which of the following does not form part of the glomerular filtration barrier?
   - (a) Endothelial cell fenestration
   - (b) Sub-endothelial space
   - (c) Glomerular basement membrane
   - (d) Podocyte foot process slit diaphragm
   - (e) Sub-podocyte space
3. Which of the following cell types does not perform a phagocytic function?
   - (a) Glomerular endothelial cell
   - (b) Mesangial cell
   - (c) Macrophage
   - (d) Podocyte
   - (e) Proximal tubular epithelial cell
4. Which of the following statements about angiotensin II is false?
   - (a) It causes vasoconstriction of the efferent arteriole
   - (b) It increases the amount of albumin filtered by the glomeruli
   - (c) It is increased in renal acidosis
   - (d) It increases aldosterone production
   - (e) It is reduced in people with diabetes

© Springer Nature Switzerland AG 2020
H. C. Rayner et al., *Understanding Kidney Diseases*,
https://doi.org/10.1007/978-3-030-43027-6

Chapter 2

5. Which of the following does not affect the serum creatinine concentration in chronic kidney disease?
   (a) Glomerular filtration rate
   (b) Tubular secretory function
   (c) Fluid overload
   (d) Skeletal muscle mass
   (e) Ethnic origin
6. Which of the following is not required to estimate GFR using the MDRD or CKD-EPI equations?
   (a) Age
   (b) Sex
   (c) Race
   (d) Creatinine
   (e) Body weight
7. In which of the following circumstances is the urea-to-creatinine ratio most likely to increase?
   (a) A malnourished patient with small muscle mass
   (b) A bodybuilder taking protein supplements
   (c) High blood pressure treated with vasodilator drugs
   (d) When the rate of flow of filtrate along the nephron is slowed
   (e) Trimethoprim therapy

Chapter 3

8. Which of the following indicates that a series of data points is not stable?
   (a) The mean is decreasing slowly over time
   (b) The control limits lie outside the data points
   (c) Three consecutive points are below the mean
   (d) Three consecutive points are in a decline
   (e) The mean is greater than the median

Chapter 4

9. An adult female with previously normal kidney function is admitted to hospital in cardiogenic shock. She passes an average of 300 mL of urine per 24 h. How long after the cardiac arrest will the serum creatinine concentration reach a new equilibrium, assuming her GFR does not improve and she receives no dialysis treatment?
   (a) 6 h
   (b) 12 h
   (c) 24 h

    (d) 6 days

    (e) 10 days

10. An adult male who normally has a serum creatinine of 120 μmol/L (1.4 mg/dL) presents to hospital with a serum creatinine of 320 μmol/L (3.6 mg/dL). According to the Kidney Disease Improving Global Outcomes (KDIGO) criteria, what stage of acute kidney injury has been reached?

    (a) Stage 1

    (b) Stage 2

    (c) Stage 3

    (d) Stage 4

    (e) Stage 5

11. Which if the following statements about acute kidney injury (AKI) is correct?

    (a) Continuous haemodiafiltration leads to better survival than acute peritoneal dialysis

    (b) Starting dialysis immediately after stage 3 AKI has been diagnosed leads to better survival than waiting until the blood urea is greater than 40 mmol/L (112 mg/dL) or the pH <7.15

    (c) Pre-renal AKI is only likely to occur if the systolic blood pressure falls below 110 mmHg

    (d) Patients who develop AKI often have multiple factors affecting their kidney function

    (e) If the eGFR fully recovers to its previous level after an episode of AKI, the risk of future chronic kidney disease is not increased

Chapter 5

12. Which of the following statements is correct?

    (a) The serum prostate specific antigen test is specific for prostate cancer antigen

    (b) Someone with diabetes insipidus may pass 20 L of urine per day

    (c) Urinary frequency is another term for polyuria

    (d) Stress incontinence occurs when women are stressed

    (e) A child with a congenital dermal sinus should be investigated for a developmental spinal abnormality

13. At a routine checkup, a 42-year-old male with diabetes is found to have an eGFR of 32 mL/min/1.73 m². When repeated 3 months later it is 35 mL/min/1.73 m². His albumin: creatinine ratio (ACR) is 35 mg/mmol (310 mg/g). Macroalbuminuria is defined as ACR >30 mg/mmol (>300 mg/g). What stage of CKD does he have?

    (a) Stage G4A2

    (b) Stage G2A1

    (c) Stage G4A3

    (d) Stage G3A3

    (e) Stage G3A2

14. Which of the following is not a typical symptom of kidney failure?
    (a) Insomnia
    (b) Hallucinations
    (c) Itching
    (d) Restless legs
    (e) Nausea

Chapter 6

15. In a patient with diabetic nephropathy and proteinuria, which of the following is not associated with the rate of decline in GFR?
    (a) Glycated haemoglobin (HbA1c) concentration
    (b) Mean arterial pressure
    (c) Serum bicarbonate
    (d) Serum total CO_2
    (e) Urinary angiotensinogen
16. Which of the following is an indication for renal artery angioplasty?
    (a) Systolic blood pressure >240 mmHg
    (b) Flash pulmonary oedema
    (c) eGFR <30 mL/min/1.73 m2
    (d) Decline in eGFR of >10 mL/min/1.73 m2per year
    (e) Blood pressure requiring >3 different antihypertensives
17. Which of the following is not a typical feature of cholesterol crystal embolisation?
    (a) Elevated CRP
    (b) Eosinophilia
    (c) Peripheral vascular atherosclerosis
    (d) Positive ANA
    (e) Decline in eGFR over weeks

Chapter 7

18. Which of the following is not associated with an increased risk of pre-eclampsia?
    (a) Fourth pregnancy
    (b) New paternity
    (c) Multiple pregnancy
    (d) Obesity
    (e) Chronic kidney disease
19. Which of the following is not associated with chronic kidney disease?
    (a) Polyhydramnios
    (b) Intrauterine growth retardation
    (c) Premature delivery

(d) Down's syndrome
(e) Spontaneous abortion

Chapter 8

20. Which of the following is not a feature of Alport syndrome?
    (a) Deafness
    (b) Visual impairment
    (c) Proteinuria
    (d) Microscopic haematuria
    (e) Kidney failure
21. Polycystic kidney disease is thought to be due primarily to a genetic abnormality of:
    (a) Sodium transport
    (b) Cell division
    (c) Tubular membrane structure
    (d) Epithelial permeability
    (e) Cilial function
22. Which of the following is not an inherited disease affecting nephron function?
    (a) Von Hippel Lindau syndrome
    (b) Gitelman syndrome
    (c) Liddle syndrome
    (d) Bartter syndrome
    (e) Dent disease
23. Furosemide acts on which part of the nephron?
    (a) Proximal tubule
    (b) Descending limb of the loop of Henle
    (c) Ascending limb of the loop of Henle
    (d) Distal tubule
    (e) Collecting duct

Chapter 9

24. Which of the following causes a fall in serum potassium concentration (hypokalaemia)?
    (a) Losartan
    (b) Spironolactone
    (c) Acute kidney injury with oliguria
    (d) Furosemide
    (e) Amiloride
25. An 80-year-old lady was prescribed ramipril 10 mg daily. Which of the following suggests this drug was adversely affecting her kidney function?
    (a) High urea-to-creatinine ratio

    (b) eGFR <15 mL/min/1.73 m^2

    (c) Systolic blood pressure <110 mmHg

    (d) An irritating dry cough

    (e) Bilateral loin pain

26. Which of the following drugs is a common cause of interstitial nephritis?

    (a) Metformin

    (b) Ranitidine

    (c) Lithium

    (d) Omeprazole

    (e) Ondansetron

27. Which of the following is not nephrotoxic?

    (a) Gentamicin

    (b) Cadmium

    (c) Metformin

    (d) Lithium

    (e) Orellanine

Chapter 10

28. Which of the following is not associated with impaired growth in children?

    (a) Congenital nephrotic syndrome

    (b) Vesico-ureteric reflux

    (c) Autosomal recessive polycystic kidney disease

    (d) Steroid therapy

    (e) Social deprivation

29. Which of the following statements about obesity is false?

    (a) It is associated with proteinuria

    (b) Weight loss reduces the risk of kidney disease in people with diabetes

    (c) In increases the risk of complications after transplant surgery

    (d) It increases the risk of mortality in dialysis patients

    (e) It is associated with hypertension

Chapter 11

30. Which of the following statements about hypertension is false?

    (a) Antihypertensive medication is better taken before bed

    (b) Nocturnal hypertension is more common in CKD

    (c) The arm with the lower pressure should be used to monitor blood pressure

    (d) Patient self-management improves control of blood pressure

    (e) High blood pressure increases the risk of end-stage kidney disease

Chapter 12

31. In IgA nephropathy, which of the following does not indicate an increased risk of kidney failure?
    (a) Proteinuria
    (b) High blood pressure
    (c) Reduced glomerular filtration rate
    (d) Interstitial fibrosis on kidney biopsy
    (e) Macroscopic haematuria
32. Which of the following statements about myoglobin is false?
    (a) It is freely filtered by glomeruli
    (b) It is glomerulotoxic
    (c) It is reabsorbed by the proximal tubule
    (d) It colours urine dark red
    (e) It is detected by the urine dipstick test for blood
33. Which of the following is not a feature of the nephrotic syndrome?
    (a) Proteinuria greater than 5 g per day
    (b) Hypercholesterolaemia
    (c) Microscopic haematuria
    (d) Peripheral oedema
    (e) Hypoalbuminaemia
34. Whom of the following should be treated with antibiotics?
    (a) A man with a urinary catheter and a positive urine culture
    (b) A woman with diabetes and a positive urine culture from a mid-stream urine specimen
    (c) A man with a culture of 104 CFU/mL from a mid-stream urine specimen
    (d) A woman with frequency, dysuria, fever and a negative urine culture
    (e) A man with a positive dipstick test for nitrites and leucocytes

Chapter 13

35. Which of the following statements is correct?
    (a) Raised jugular venous pressure is a reliable marker of fluid overload
    (b) High blood pressure indicates increased total body sodium
    (c) Increased total body sodium usually causes high blood pressure
    (d) Lymphoedema is incompressible
    (e) Sleeping in a chair worsens leg oedema
36. Which of the following statements about the loop diuretic furosemide is true?
    (a) It is mainly used to treat hypertension
    (b) Intestinal oedema reduces its absorption in oedematous patients
    (c) It takes 1–2 h to have a diuretic effect

(d) It enters the tubule by glomerular filtration

(e) It causes a diuresis in an all–or-nothing manner

37. Which of the following statements about a vasculitic rash is false?

(a) It is found on the legs in Henoch-Schönlein purpura

(b) It blanches when compressed

(c) It may cause necrotic ulcers

(d) IgA is deposited in the skin in Henoch-Schönlein purpura

(e) Blood and protein in the urine means urgent referral is required

Chapter 14

38. Which of the following statements about erythropoietin production in an adult is true?

(a) It is divided between the liver and the kidneys

(b) It is inhibited by NSAIDs

(c) It is stimulated by muscle hypoxia

(d) It is located in the interstitial cells of the kidney medulla

(e) It is down-regulated in chronic kidney disease

Chapter 15

39. Which of the following statements regarding acid base disorder is false?

(a) In metabolic acidosis, a normal anion gap indicates excessive loss of bicarbonate may be the cause

(b) In metabolic acidosis, a high anion gap indicates an excess of acid may be the cause

(c) In type 4 renal tubular acidosis, the serum potassium concentration is usually increased

(d) Excess alcohol can cause ketoacidosis

(e) In metabolic alkalosis, the serum chloride concentration is usually increased

40. Which of the following does not cause metabolic acidosis?

(a) Tranexamic acid

(b) Aspirin overdose

(c) Paracetamol (acetaminophen) overdose

(d) Paracetamol (acetaminophen) at regular dose

(e) Methanol

41. Which of the following statements about treatment of renal acidosis is false?

(a) Fruit and vegetable diet is effective

(b) Sodium bicarbonate lowers angiotensin production in the kidney

(c) Sodium bicarbonate reduces the rate of decline in GFR

(d) Sodium bicarbonate increases muscle mass

(e) Sodium bicarbonate causes heart failure

Chapter 16

42. Which of the following statements about parathyroid hormone synthesis is true?
    (a) It is stimulated by hypocalcaemia
    (b) It is stimulated by activated vitamin D_3
    (c) It is inhibited by hyperphosphataemia
    (d) It is stimulated by FGF-23
    (e) It is autonomous in secondary hyperparathyroidism
43. Which of the following statements about hypercalcaemia is false?
    (a) It reduces GFR due to vasoconstriction
    (b) It impairs urinary concentration
    (c) It can be caused by loop diuretics
    (d) It is associated with raised alkaline phosphatase with metastatic carcinoma
    (e) It is associated with normal alkaline phosphatase in multiple myeloma

Chapter 17

44. Which of the following statements about myeloma is false?
    (a) Free light chains are filtered by glomeruli
    (b) Free light chains form casts with uromodulin
    (c) Bence Jones proteinuria is not detected by urine protein dipsticks
    (d) Kidney function can recover with chemotherapy treatment
    (e) A significantly raised concentration of serum free light chains is diagnostic
45. Which of the following statements about amyloid is false?
    (a) It develops in the skeleton of some patients in the first 5 years of dialysis
    (b) When deposited in the kidney, it causes proteinuria
    (c) It is shown by Congo red staining on histology
    (d) It is composed of proteins arranged in a beta-pleated sheet
    (e) Chronic inflammation causes AA type amyloid
46. Which of the following antibodies is found in post-streptococcal glomerulo-nephritis?
    (a) Anti-streptolysin B
    (b) Anti-DNAse B
    (c) Anti-hyaluronic acid
    (d) Anti-staphylokinase
    (e) Anti-adenine dinucleotidase
47. Which of the following statements about ANCA-associated vasculitis is true?
    (a) C-ANCA is associated with microscopic polyangiitis
    (b) MPO-ANCA is usually C-ANCA
    (c) PR3-ANCA is usually C-ANCA
    (d) A rising titre of MPO-ANCA indicates a need to increase immuno-suppression
    (e) ANCA-associated vasculitis is usually cured by a prolonged course of cyclophosphamide

Chapter 18

48. Which of the following is the modality of choice for detecting kidney stones?
    (a) Ultrasound
    (b) Doppler ultrasound
    (c) CT scanning
    (d) Isotope renography
    (e) MRI scanning
49. Which of the following statements about contrast-induced nephropathy is true?
    (a) It can be ameliorated by sodium chloride infusion before the procedure
    (b) It often requires temporary dialysis
    (c) It is commoner in women
    (d) It is less likely with hyper-osmolar contrast medium
    (e) It is rare if the eGFR is <30 mL/min/1.73 m^2

Chapter 19

50. Which of the following statements about kidney biopsy is true?
    (a) It is usually required to confirm a diagnosis of diabetic nephropathy
    (b) It causes bleeding in a minority of patients
    (c) It is essential to diagnose anti-glomerular basement membrane disease
    (d) It requires a general anaesthetic
    (e) It should only be performed if it will change patient management

Chapter 20

51. Which of the following is not associated with an increased risk of kidney stone formation?
    (a) Previous antibiotic usage
    (b) Gastric bypass surgery
    (c) Female sex compared with male
    (d) Inflammatory bowel disease
    (e) Gout
52. Which if the following is incorrect advice for someone with a calcium oxalate kidney stone?
    (a) Eat a low calcium diet
    (b) Drink more than two litres of mainly clear fluid per day
    (c) Eat more fruit and vegetables
    (d) Eat less animal protein
    (e) Reduce your salt intake

Chapter 21

53. In someone aged 35 years with an eGFR of 65 mL/min/1.73 m², by how much does an albumin:creatinine ratio of 42 mg/mmol increase the risk of mortality compared to no albuminuria?
    - (a) 1.5 times
    - (b) 2 times
    - (c) 4 times
    - (d) 9 times
    - (e) 12 times
54. Clinic letters are best written directly to the patient. Which of the following statements is false? You should aim to:
    - (a) Keep paragraphs short, explaining one topic3 in each
    - (b) Keep sentences short and avoid long technical words
    - (c) Achieve a Flesch Reading Ease Score of less than 50
    - (d) Use the active rather than passive voice
    - (e) Provide a list of diagnoses and problems
55. When should a patient be transferred to the multidisciplinary team to prepare them for dialysis?
    - (a) When the eGFR goes below 20 mL/min/1.73 m²
    - (b) When the patient develops symptoms of uraemia
    - (c) When the eGFR goes below 10 mL/min/1.73 m²
    - (d) When the rate of decline in eGFR is greater than 10 mL/min/1.73 m² per year
    - (e) When dialysis is likely to be needed within the next 12 months
56. Which of the following statements about kidney replacement therapy is true?
    - (a) It is unethical not to treat someone with dialysis with an eGFR less than 5 mL/min/1.73 m²
    - (b) Mortality is less with a kidney transplant than dialysis
    - (c) Mortality is less with peritoneal dialysis than haemodialysis
    - (d) The minimum frequency of haemodialysis is three times per week
    - (e) Peritoneal dialysis is done 5 days per week

Chapter 22

57. Which of the following statements about haemodialysis treatment is true?
    - (a) Urine volume is usually insignificant after maintenance dialysis has been started
    - (b) Fluid overload can be monitored by measuring systolic blood pressure
    - (c) Recurrent intradialytic hypotension can cause permanent organ damage
    - (d) Having some fluid overload is protective and reduces mortality
    - (e) The risk of pulmonary oedema is highest on a Friday night

58. Which of the following statements about an arterio-venous fistula is true?
    (a) It is contraindicated if the left ventricular ejection fraction is less than 40 %
    (b) The blood flow is good if it remains full of blood when the arm is elevated
    (c) The thrill should only be felt in systole
    (d) The dialysis needle is inserted as near to the anastomosis as possible
    (e) The risk of infection is lower than with a dialysis catheter
59. Which of the following statements about a peritoneal dialysis catheter is true?
    (a) Fluid should take under 20 min to drain out
    (b) The tip should be located in the centre of the abdomen
    (c) Fluid should be slightly cloudy on draining out
    (d) Dried exudate ('crusting') at the exit site should be treated with antibiotics
    (e) It should be replaced once a year to reduce the risk of infection
60. Which of the following statements about a kidney transplant patient is false?
    (a) Infections after 12 months are usually due to conventional organisms
    (b) Post-transplant lymphoproliferative disease is due to T cell proliferation
    (c) Cotrimoxazole is used to prevent *Pneumocystis jiroveci* pneumonia (PJP)
    (d) The commonest site of malignancy is the skin
    (e) Post-transplant lymphoproliferative disease may regress if immunosuppressive drugs are stopped

Answers

Question	Answer
1	d
2	b
3	a
4	e
5	c
6	e
7	d
8	a
9	d
10	b
11	d
12	b
13	d
14	b
15	a
16	b
17	d
18	a
19	d
20	b
21	e
22	a
23	c
24	d
25	a
26	d
27	c
28	b
29	d
30	c

© Springer Nature Switzerland AG 2020
H. C. Rayner et al., *Understanding Kidney Diseases*,
https://doi.org/10.1007/978-3-030-43027-6

Question	Answer
31	e
32	b
33	c
34	d
35	e
36	e
37	b
38	d
39	e
40	a
41	e
42	a
43	c
44	e
45	a
46	b
47	c
48	c
49	a
50	e
51	c
52	a
53	c
54	c
55	e
56	b
57	c
58	e
59	a
60	b

Case Reports

ACE inhibitor effect	6.2, 9.1, 11.2, 12.6
Acute kidney injury	3.3, 4.1, 9.1–9.4, 16.1
Anaemia	14.1
Anticoagulant-related nephropathy	9.4
Cervical carcinoma	12.7
Cholesterol crystal embolisation	6.3
Chronic kidney disease	2.1–2.4, 3.1–3.5, 5.2, 10.2
Crescentic glomerulonephritis	17.3, 17.4, 19.1
Diabetic nephropathy	6.1, 6.2, 19.1
eGFR graph interpretation	3.1–3.5, 21.1, 21.2
End-stage kidney disease	21.1–21.3
Epstein-Barr viral encephalitis	22.2
Growth retardation	10.1–10.4
Haematuria	12.1–12.5
Haemodialysis	22.1
Haemolytic uraemic syndrome	14.2, 14.3
Hypercalcaemia	16.5, 16.6, 17.1
Hyperparathyroidism	16.2–16.4
Hypertension	11.1–11.3
Hypocalcaemia	16.1, 16.2
IgA nephropathy	12.2–12.4
Interstitial nephritis	19.2
Intravenous fluids	3.4
Lactic acidosis	4.1
Lithium	9.5
Magnesium	16.1

© Springer Nature Switzerland AG 2020
H. C. Rayner et al., *Understanding Kidney Diseases*,
https://doi.org/10.1007/978-3-030-43027-6

Malignancy	16.5
Metabolic acidosis	4.1, 15.1, 15.2
Multiple myeloma	17.1
Nephrotic syndrome	10.1, 11.2, 17.2
Normal kidneys with low eGFR	2.3
NSAID	9.2, 9.3
Obstructive uropathy	12.7, 18.1
Parathyroidectomy	16.4
Post-transplant lymphoproliferative disease	22.3
Pregnancy	7.1
Pruritus	5.1
Puberty	10.4
Renal bone disease	16.2–16.4
Renal tubular acidosis	15.1, 15.2
Retroperitoneal fibrosis	18.1
Rhabdomyolysis	12.5
Sarcoidosis	16.6
Sepsis	4.1
Systemic lupus erythematosis	17.2
Thin glomerular basement membrane disease	12.1
Transplant kidney	2.4, 10.2, 10.3, 22.2, 22.3
Trimethoprim	2.4
Urinary infection	12.7
Uromodulin kidney disease	8.1
Vasculitis	17.3, 17.4
Vesico-ureteric reflux	8.2

Index

© Springer Nature Switzerland AG 2020
H. C. Rayner et al., *Understanding Kidney Diseases*,
https://doi.org/10.1007/978-3-030-43027-6

Printed in the United States
by Baker & Taylor Publisher Services